Lecture Notes in Computer Science　　13769

Founding Editors

Gerhard Goos
Juris Hartmanis

The series Lecture Notes in Computer Science (LNCS), including its subseries Lecture Notes in Artificial Intelligence (LNAI) and Lecture Notes in Bioinformatics (LNBI), has established itself as a medium for the publication of new developments in computer science and information technology research, teaching, and education.

LNCS enjoys close cooperation with the computer science R & D community, the series counts many renowned academics among its volume editors and paper authors, and collaborates with prestigious societies. Its mission is to serve this international community by providing an invaluable service, mainly focused on the publication of conference and workshop proceedings and postproceedings. LNCS commenced publication in 1973.

Spyridon Bakas · Alessandro Crimi ·
Ujjwal Baid · Sylwia Malec · Monika Pytlarz ·
Bhakti Baheti · Maximilian Zenk ·
Reuben Dorent
Editors

Brainlesion:
Glioma, Multiple Sclerosis, Stroke and Traumatic Brain Injuries

8th International Workshop, BrainLes 2022
Held in Conjunction with MICCAI 2022
Singapore, September 18, 2022
Revised Selected Papers, Part I

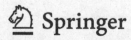

Editors

Spyridon Bakas (iD)
University of Pennsylvania
Philadelphia, PA, USA

Ujjwal Baid (iD)
University of Pennsylvania
Philadelphia, PA, USA

Monika Pytlarz (iD)
Sano, Center for Computational Personalised
Medicine
Kraków, Poland

Maximilian Zenk (iD)
German Cancer Research Center
Heidelberg, Germany

Alessandro Crimi (iD)
Sano, Center for Computational Personalised
Medicine
Kraków, Poland

Sylwia Malec (iD)
Sano, Center for Computational Personalised
Medicine
Kraków, Poland

Bhakti Baheti (iD)
University of Pennsylvania
Philadelphia, PA, USA

Reuben Dorent (iD)
Harvard Medical School
Boston, MA, USA

ISSN 0302-9743   ISSN 1611-3349 (electronic)
Lecture Notes in Computer Science
ISBN 978-3-031-33841-0   ISBN 978-3-031-33842-7 (eBook)
https://doi.org/10.1007/978-3-031-33842-7

This Springer imprint is published by the registered company Springer Nature Switzerland AG
The registered company address is: Gewerbestrasse 11, 6330 Cham, Switzerland

Preface

This volume contains articles from the Brain Lesion workshop (BrainLes), as well as the Brain Tumor Segmentation (BraTS) Challenge, the Brain Tumor Sequence Registration (BraTS-Reg) Challenge, the Cross-Modality Domain Adaptation (CrossMoDA) Challenge, and the Federated Tumor Segmentation (FeTS) Challenge. All these events were held in conjunction with the Medical Image Computing and Computer Assisted Intervention (MICCAI) conference on the 18th–22nd of September 2022 in Singapore.

The submissions for each conference were reviewed through a rigorous double-blind peer-review process. The review process involved the evaluation of the submitted papers by at least three independent reviewers, ensuring high quality and reliability of the accepted papers. The average number of papers reviewed by each reviewer was two, which helped to maintain the consistency and fairness of the review process.

The presented manuscripts describe the research of computational scientists and clinical researchers working on brain lesions, and specifically glioma, multiple sclerosis, cerebral stroke, traumatic brain injuries, vestibular schwannoma, and white matter hyperintensities of presumed vascular origin. This compilation does not claim to provide a comprehensive understanding from all points of view; however, the authors present their latest advances in segmentation, registration, federated learning, disease prognosis, and other applications to the clinical context.

The volume is divided into five chapters: The first chapter comprises the accepted paper submissions to the BrainLes workshop, and the second through the fifth chapters contain a selection of papers regarding methods presented at the BraTS, BraTS-Reg, CrossMoDA, and FeTS challenges, respectively.

The aim of the **first chapter**, focusing on the accepted **BrainLes workshop submissions**, is to provide an overview of new advances of medical image analysis in all the aforementioned brain pathologies. It brings together researchers from the medical image analysis domain, neurologists, and radiologists working on at least one of these diseases. The aim is to consider neuroimaging biomarkers used for one disease applied to the other diseases. This session did not have a specific dataset to be used. BrainLes workshop received 15 submissions, out of which 10 papers were accepted.

The **second chapter** focuses on a selection of papers from the **BraTS 2022** challenge participants. BraTS 2022 had a two-fold intention: a) to report a snapshot of the state-of-the-art developments in the continuous evaluation schema of the RSNA-ASNR-MICCAI BraTS challenge, which made publicly available the largest ever manually annotated dataset of baseline pre-operative brain glioma scans from 20 international institutions, and b) to quantify the generalizability performance of these algorithms on out-of-sample independent multi-institutional sources covering underrepresented Sub-Saharan African adult patient populations of brain diffuse glioma and from a pediatric population of diffuse intrinsic pontine glioma (DIPG) patients. All challenge data were routine clinically acquired, multi-institutional, skull-stripped multi-parametric magnetic resonance imaging (mpMRI) scans of brain tumor patients (provided in NIfTI file format). Total number of manuscript sent to review in BraTS were 16, from which 9 were accepted.

The **third chapter** contains a selection of papers from the **BraTS-Reg 2022** challenge participants. BraTS-Reg 2022 intended to establish a benchmark environment for deformable registration algorithms, focusing on estimating correspondences between baseline pre-operative and follow-up scans of the same patient diagnosed with a brain glioma. The challenge data comprise de-identified multi-institutional mpMRI scans, curated for each scan's size and resolution, according to a canonical anatomical template (similarly to BraTS). The unique difficulty here comes from the induced tumor mass effect that harshly shifts brain tissue in unknown directions. Extensive landmarks points annotations within the scans were provided by the clinical experts of the organizing committee. Among 13 papers submitted in BraTS-Reg challenge, 9 were accepted.

The **fourth chapter** contains a selection of papers from the **CrossMoDA 2022** challenge participants. CrossMoDA 2022 was the continuation of the first large and multi-class benchmark for unsupervised cross-modality domain adaptation for medical image segmentation. Compared to the previous CrossMoDA instance, which used single-institution data and featured a single segmentation task, the 2022 edition extended the segmentation task by including multi-institutional data and introduced a new classification task. The segmentation task aims to segment two key brain structures involved in the follow-up and treatment planning of vestibular schwannoma (VS): the VS tumour and the cochleas. The goal of the classification challenge is to automatically classify T2 images with VS according to the Koos grade. The training dataset provides annotated T1 scans (N=210) and unpaired non-annotated T2 scans (N=210). CrossMoDA received 8 submissions, from which 7 were accepted.

The **fifth chapter** contains a selection of papers from the **FeTS 2022** challenge participants. This was the continuation of the first computational challenge focussing on federated learning, and ample multi-institutional routine clinically acquired pre-operative baseline multi-parametric MRI scans of radiographically appearing glioblastoma (from the RSNA-ASNR-MICCAI BraTS challenge) were provided to the participants, along with splits on the basis of the site of acquisition. The goal of the challenge was two-fold: i) identify the best way to aggregate the knowledge coming from segmentation models trained on the individual institutions, and ii) find the best algorithm that produces robust and accurate brain tumor segmentations across different medical institutions, MRI scanners, image acquisition parameters, and populations. Interestingly, the second task was performed by actually circulating the containerized algorithms across different institutions, leveraging the collaborators of the largest to-date real-world federation (https://www.fets.ai) and in partnership with the largest open community effort for ML, namely MLCommons. FeTS challenge received a total of 13 submissions, out of which 11 papers were accepted.

We heartily hope that this volume will promote further exciting computational research on brain-related pathologies.

The BrainLes organizers,

Ujjwal Baid
Spyridon Bakas
Alessandro Crimi
Sylwia Malec
Monika Pytlarz

The original version of this book was revised: The frontmatter and cover is revised with subtitle "8th International Workshop, BrainLes 2022, Held in Conjunction with MICCAI 2022, Singapore, September 18, 2022, Revised Selected Papers, Part I" and backmatter is revised with combined author names of part 1 and part 2.

Organization

Main BrainLes Organizing Committee

Ujjwal Baid   University of Pennsylvania, USA
Spyridon Bakas   University of Pennsylvania, USA
Alessandro Crimi   Sano Science, Poland
Sylwia Malec   Sano Science, Poland
Monika Pytlarz   Sano Science, Poland

BrainLes Program Committee

Maruf Adewole   University of Lagos, Nigeria
Bhakti Baheti   University of Pennsylvania, USA
Ujjwal Baid   University of Pennsylvania, USA
Florian Kofler   Technical University of Munich, Germany
Hugo Kuijf   University Medical School of Utrecht,
                             The Netherlands
Andreas Mang   University of Houston, USA
Zahra Riahi Samani   University of Pennsylvania, USA
Maciej Szymkowski   Sano Science, Poland
Siddhesh Thakur   University of Pennsylvania, USA
Benedikt Wiestler   Technical University of Munich, Germany

Challenges Organizing Committee

Brain Tumor Segmentation (BraTS) Challenge

Ujjwal Baid   University of Pennsylvania, USA
Spyridon Bakas (Lead Organizer) University of Pennsylvania, USA
Evan Calabrese*   University of California San Francisco, USA
Christopher Carr*   Radiological Society of North America (RSNA),
                                   USA
Errol Colak*   Unity Health Toronto, Canada
Keyvan Farahani   National Institutes of Health (NIH), USA
Adam E. Flanders*   Thomas Jefferson University Hospital, USA
Anahita Fathi Kazerooni   University of Pennsylvania, USA

Felipe C Kitamura*	Diagnósticos da América SA (Dasa) and Universidade Federal de São Paulo, Brazil
Marius George Linguraru	Children's National Hospital, USA
Bjoern Menze	University of Zurich, Switzerland
Luciano Prevedello*	Ohio State University, USA
Jeffrey Rudie*	University of California San Francisco, USA
Russell Taki Shinohara	University of Pennsylvania, USA

* These organizers were involved in the BraTS 2021 Challenge, the data of which were used here, but were not directly involved in the BraTS 2022 Continuous Challenge.

The Brain Tumor Sequence Registration (BraTS-Reg) Challenge

Hamed Akbari	University of Pennsylvania, USA
Bhakti Baheti	University of Pennsylvania, USA
Spyridon Bakas	University of Pennsylvania, USA
Satrajit Chakrabarty	Washington University in St. Louis, USA
Bjoern Menze	University of Zurich, Switzerland
Aristeidis Sotiras	Washington University in St. Louis, USA
Diana Waldmannstetter	University of Zurich, Switzerland

Cross-Modality Domain Adaptation (CrossMoDA) Challenge

Spyridon Bakas	University of Pennsylvania, USA
Stefan Cornelissen	Elisabeth-TweeSteden Hospital, The Netherlands
Reuben Dorent (Lead Organizer)	King's College London, UK
Ben Glocker	Imperial College London, UK
Samuel Joutard	King's College London, UK
Aaron Kujawa	King's College London, UK
Patrick Langenhuizen	Elisabeth-TweeSteden Hospital, The Netherlands
Nicola Rieke	NVIDIA, Germany
Jonathan Shapey	King's College London, UK
Tom Vercauteren	King's College London, UK

Federated Tumor Segmentation (FeTS) Challenge

Ujjwal Baid	University of Pennsylvania, USA
Spyridon Bakas (Task 1 Lead Organizer)	University of Pennsylvania, USA
Timothy Bergquist	Sage Bionetworks, USA
Yong Chen	University of Pennsylvania, USA
Verena Chung	Sage Bionetworks, USA

James Eddy	Sage Bionetworks, USA
Brandon Edwards	Intel, USA
Ralf Floca	German Cancer Research Center (DKFZ), Germany
Patrick Foley	Intel, USA
Fabian Isensee	DKFZ, Germany
Alexandros Karargyris	IHU Strasbourg, France
Klaus Maier-Hein	DKFZ, Germany
Lena Maier-Hein	DKFZ, Germany
Jason Martin	Intel, USA
Peter Mattson	Google, USA
Bjoern Menze	University of Zurich, Switzerland
Sarthak Pati	University of Pennsylvania, USA
Annika Reinke	DKFZ, Germany
Prashant Shah	Intel, USA
Micah J Sheller	Intel, USA
Russell Taki Shinohara	University of Pennsylvania, USA
Maximilian Zenk (Task 2 Lead Organizer)	DKFZ, Germany
David Zimmerer	DKFZ, Germany

Contents – Part I

BraTS

Contents – Part II

FeTS

BrainLes

Deep Quality Estimation: Creating Surrogate Models for Human Quality Ratings

Florian Kofler[1,2,3,7(✉)], Ivan Ezhov[1,2], Lucas Fidon[4], Izabela Horvath[1,5], Ezequiel de la Rosa[1,8], John LaMaster[1,12], Hongwei Li[1,12], Tom Finck[5,6], Suprosanna Shit[1,2], Johannes Paetzold[1,2,5,6], Spyridon Bakas[9,10,11], Marie Piraud[7], Jan Kirschke[3], Tom Vercauteren[4], Claus Zimmer[3], Benedikt Wiestler[3], and Bjoern Menze[1,12]

[1] Department of Informatics, Technical University Munich, Munich, Germany
florian.kofler@tum.de
[2] TranslaTUM - Central Institute for Translational Cancer Research, Technical University of Munich, Munich, Germany
[3] Department of Diagnostic and Interventional Neuroradiology, School of Medicine, Klinikum rechts der Isar, Technical University of Munich, Munich, Germany
[4] School of Biomedical Engineering and Imaging Sciences, King's College London, London, UK
[5] Insitute for Tissue Engineering and Regenerative Medicine, Helmholtz Institute Munich (iTERM), Munich, Germany
[6] Imperial College London, South Kensington, London, UK
[7] Helmholtz AI, Helmholtz Zentrum München, Munich, Germany
[8] icometrix, Leuven, Belgium
[9] Center for Biomedical Image Computing and Analytics (CBICA), University of Pennsylvania, Philadelphia, PA, USA
[10] Department of Radiology, Perelman School of Medicine, University of Pennsylvania, Philadelphia, PA, USA
[11] Department of Pathology and Laboratory Medicine, Perelman School of Medicine, University of Pennsylvania, Philadelphia, PA, USA
[12] Department of Quantitative Biomedicine, University of Zurich, Zürich, Switzerland

Abstract. Human ratings are abstract representations of segmentation quality. To approximate human quality ratings on scarce expert data, we train surrogate quality estimation models. We evaluate on a complex multi-class segmentation problem, specifically glioma segmentation, following the BraTS annotation protocol. The training data features quality ratings from 15 expert neuroradiologists on a scale ranging from 1 to 6 stars for various computer-generated and manual 3D annotations. Even though the networks operate on 2D images and with scarce training data, we can approximate segmentation quality within a margin of error comparable to human intra-rater reliability. Segmentation quality prediction has broad applications. While an understanding of segmentation quality is imperative for successful clinical translation of automatic segmentation

---

B. Wiestler and B. Menze—Contributed equally as senior authors.

© The Author(s), under exclusive license to Springer Nature Switzerland AG 2023
S. Bakas et al. (Eds.): BrainLes 2022, LNCS 13769, pp. 3–13, 2023.
https://doi.org/10.1007/978-3-031-33842-7_1

quality algorithms, it can play an essential role in training new segmentation models. Due to the split-second inference times, it can be directly applied within a loss function or as a fully-automatic dataset curation mechanism in a federated learning setting.

Keywords: automatic quality control · quality estimation · segmentation quality metrics · glioma · BraTS

1   Introduction

Large and long-standing community challenges, such as BraTS [2], have created a multitude of fully-automatic segmentation algorithms over the years. To fully exploit the potential of these task-specific algorithms, be it for clinical or scientific purposes, it is essential to understand the quality of their predictions and account for segmentation failures.[1]

As individual segmentation quality metrics are only able to cover isolated aspects of segmentation quality, most segmentation challenges evaluate on a combination of metrics [15]. Human expert quality ratings have become a prominent tool to complement conventional analysis, among others [14,17,20] for segmentation outputs [13]. In contrast, to narrowly defined quality metrics, these more holistic measures capture various quality aspects. However, they are prohibitively expensive regarding data acquisition times and financials to be deployed regularly.

Related Work: Therefore, previous research tried to approximate segmentation performance by other means. Reverse classification accuracy (RCA) has been proposed to evaluate segmentation accuracy for applications of multi-organ segmentation in magnetic resonance imaging (MRI) [21] and cardiac MRI segmentation [19]. The authors used the maximum predicted segmentation quality metric estimated by a multi-atlas-based registration method as a proxy to estimate the true quality metric. However, the application of RCA is so far limited to organ segmentation. Further, the analysis is restricted to established segmentation quality metrics such as DSC and Hausdorff distance. It is unclear how it would generalize to expert scoring and to lesion segmentation.

A method to estimate the Dice score of an ensemble of convolutional neural networks (CNNs) for segmentation has also been proposed [7]. They propose to train a linear classifier regression model to predict the Dice score for every CNN in the ensemble. Here, the Dice scores for every pair of segmentation predictions of the models in the ensemble serve as input for the regressor. Further, Audelan et al. proposed an unsupervised learning method for predicting DSC using Bayesian learning [1].

---

[1] Models often output uncertainty levels to account for this. However, we believe the judgment of external entities is more trustworthy for quality assurance purposes. Remarkably, while this separation of concerns is a well-established practice in other fields, it remains largely ignored in machine learning. For instance, imagine a world where aircraft pilots could self-certify their ability to fly.

The above methods are coupled with segmentation algorithms for the estimation of segmentation quality metrics. Unlike this, Fournel et al. predict the segmentation quality metric directly from the input image and segmentation map using a CNN [5]. Similarly, it is possible to predict an ensemble's segmentation performance from discord between individual segmentation maps, even when ignoring the image data [12].

The BraTS challenge [16] features the multi-class segmentation problem of glioma segmentation. Distinguishing between *enhancing tumor*, *necrosis*, and *edema* is a complex subtask scattered over multiple imaging modalities. It is evaluated using Sørensen-Dice coefficient (DSC) and Hausdorff distance (HD) for the *whole tumor*, *tumor core* and *enhancing tumor* channels. Previous research revealed that BraTS tumor segmentation algorithms typically perform well when monitoring established segmentation quality ratings such as DSC, HD, and others. However, when they fail, they fail spectacularly [2,4,11,12,16]. These findings reflecting multiple established segmentation quality metrics are supported by surveys with expert neuroradiologists [13]. Here, the multi-faceted concept of segmentation quality was condensed to a single expert quality rating. To this end, BraTS glioma segmentation is a good candidate for studying how a holistic rating can complement or replace them.

Contribution: In contrast to the above-mentioned methods, which predict narrowly defined quality metrics such as DSC or HD, we focus on the approximation of more holistic expert neuroradiologists' ratings. We build surrogate regression models for these abstract human quality ratings to estimate the segmentation quality of MICCAI BraTS segmentation algorithms. A sophisticated augmentation pipeline compensates for the scarce 2D training data available. Despite these obstacles, our model manages to create robust estimates for 3D segmentation quality on an internal and external test set. While our models are agnostic to the segmentation method and are even compatible with 2D manual segmentations, split-second inference times enable broad downstream applications in scientific and clinical practice.

2 Methods: Network Training

We train multiple regression networks to approximate the human quality ratings.

Segmentation Quality Rating: We use human quality ratings provided by Kofler et al. [13]. In this study, expert radiologists rated the quality of glioma segmentations in two experiments. In the first experiment, 15 neuroradiologists rated the segmentations' center of mass for 25 exams with four different segmentations from axial, sagittal, and coronal views, resulting in 300 trials. The experiment featured one manual and three computer-generated segmentations. In the second experiment, three neuroradiologists rated another 50 exams with one manual and five computer-generated segmentations only on axial views, again resulting in 300 trials. The rating scale ranges from 1 star for very bad to 6 stars for very good segmentations.

Network Input and Output: To predict the above-mentioned quality rating, the network receives the four MR modalities, namely T1, T1c, T2, and FLAIR. The tumor segmentations are either supplied in a single label channel encoding the different tumor tissues or with three label channels following BraTS annotation concepts, as illustrated by Fig. 1. We try this style of encoding the tumor segmentations as this approach has been proven successful for training BraTS segmentation algorithms [2].

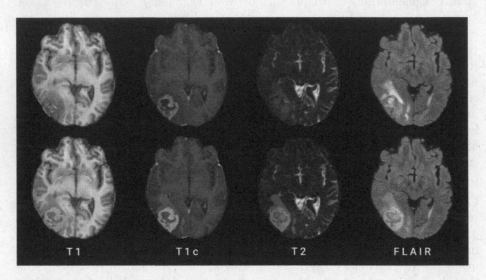

Fig. 1. Example inputs for the CNN training - axial center of mass slices of a glioma exam. Besides the illustrated T1, T1c, T2, and FLAIR MR sequences, the tumor segmentations are supplied to the network. The different tumor tissue types are visualized in colors: Red: *necrosis*; Yellow: *enhancing tumor*; Green: *edema*. For BraTS label encoding, the *enhancing tumor* is encoded in a binary label channel, while a second *tumor core* channel is formed by combining *enhancing tumor* and *necrosis* and a third *whole tumor* channel is calculated by combining all three tumor tissue labels. (Color figure online)

Training Constants: The dataset is randomly split into 80% (60) of the 75 exams for training and 20% (15) for testing. Batch size is kept constant at *80* and learning rate at *1e-3*. To compensate for the scarce training data, we employ a heavy augmentation pipeline featuring Gaussian noise, flips, and random affine plus elastic transformations. Additionally, we use *batchgenerators* [9] to augment with contrast, brightness, gamma, low resolution, and rician noise. Further, we simulate MR artifacts with *TorchIO* [18], specifically motion, ghosting, spikes, and bias fields. We employ a Mean Square Error (MSE) loss for all training runs to especially penalize far-off predictions. The human quality ratings serve as reference annotations for the loss computations. Due to the scarcity of training data, we do not conduct model selection and use the last checkpoint after *500* epochs of training across all training runs.

Training Variations: Between training runs we experiment with three optimizers, namely Ranger21 [22], AdamW, and SGD with a momentum of 0.95. We use DenseNet121 and DenseNet201 [8] to investigate whether the performance profits from more trainable parameters. Moreover, we try a channel-wise min/max, and a *nn-Unet* [9] inspired percentile-based normalization using the 0.5 and 99.5 percentiles for minimum and maximum, respectively.

Software: All computations happen with *NVIDIA Driver v470.103.01, CUDA v11.4* with *PyTorch 1.9.0*. The networks are implemented via *MONAI* [3] *0.6.0*. Segmentation metrics are computed with *pymia 0.3.1* [10] and regression metrics via *scikit-learn 0.24.2*.

Hardware: All computations take place on a small workstation with an *8-core Intel(R) Xeon(R) W-2123 CPU @ 3.60GHz* with *256GB RAM* and a *NVIDIA Quadro P5000* GPU.

Computation Times: A training run takes approximately two hours. The above machine infers four 3D exams per second, including mass computation. Without the extraction of 2D slices, the inference performance increases to 25 per second. Note that the implementation is not fully-optimized for computation time, as the split-second inference times are in no way impeding our purposes.

Memory Consumption: With the *batch size* of 80 we use most of the 16gb CUDA memory of the *NVIDIA Quadro P5000* GPU.

3 Evaluation Experiments

We conduct two experiments to evaluate the performance of our models. In the first experiment we identify and evaluate our best performing model. In the second experiment we validate its generalization capabilities on an external test set. In both experiments, we generate network predictions for the axial, coronal, and sagittal views and compute a mean rating for each exam.

3.1 Internal Evaluation Experiment

To investigate which of the six hyperparameter combinations works best by evaluating on an internal test set.

Dataset: We use the previously held-back 20% of the training data for evaluation, as described in Sect. 2.

Procedure: We run inference on the test set for each model. Following, we evaluate using established regression metrics, namely mean absolute error (MAE), root mean square error (RMSE). We further compute Pearson r (r) to measure the linear correlation between network predictions and ground truth labels.

Results: Table 1 illustrates the performance differences between training runs. We observe that the simple DenseNet121 trained with percentile-based normalization, Ranger21 optimizer, and BraTS label encoding approximates the human rating best.

Figure 2 visualizes the model's predictions compared to the averaged human star ratings.

Table 1. Training results for different training parameters. We report mean absolute error (MAE), root mean square error (RMSE), and Pearson r (r). The selected model is highlighted in pink.

architecture	optimizer	normalization	labels	MAE	RMSE	r
DenseNet121	SGD	percentile	tissue	0.65	0.88	0.64
DenseNet121	AdamW	percentile	tissue	0.59	**0.80**	0.62
DenseNet121	Ranger21	percentile	tissue	0.60	0.83	0.58
DenseNet201	Ranger21	percentile	tissue	0.59	**0.80**	0.63
DenseNet121	Ranger21	min.max	BraTS	0.57	0.82	0.61
DenseNet121	Ranger21	percentile	BraTS	**0.51**	**0.80**	**0.66**

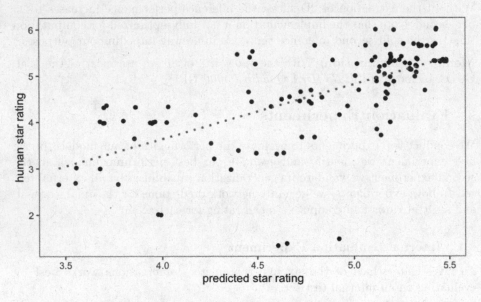

Fig. 2. Scatter plot: Network predicted vs. average human star rating. Even though we have only scarce training data, the model can approximate the human segmentation quality rating quite well. The dotted cyan line symbolizes a linear model fitted through the data. We observe a Pearson r of 0.66.

According to the scatter plot, illustrated in Fig. 2, the model performs more accurately for better segmentations. This is also reflected by a Bland-Altman plot, see Fig. 3. It is important to note that the variance in human quality assessment also increases for lower quality segmentations, see Fig. 4.

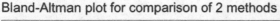

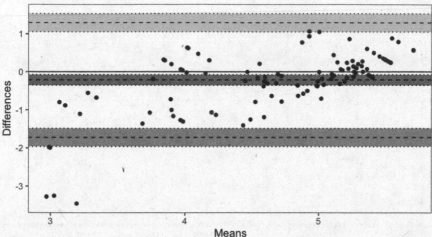

Fig. 3. Bland-Altman plot: Network predictions vs. human star rating. The model reveals higher prediction accuracy for better-quality segmentations. This is not surprising given that human raters also display higher agreement for such cases and that these are better represented in the training data, compare Fig. 4.

3.2   External Evaluation Experiment

To better understand our model's generalizability, we further evaluate an external dataset.

Data Set: The dataset features manual annotations for 68 exams generated by two expert radiologists in consensus voting. It includes 15 high-grade glioma (GBM) and 13 low-grade glioma (LGG) from *University Hospital rechts der Isar*. Furthermore, 25 GBM and 15 LGG from the publicly available Rembrandt dataset [6] are added to the analysis. We obtain five segmentations from BraTS algorithms and four fusions from BraTS Toolkit [11]. This way, we have a total of 612 segmentations to evaluate.

Procedure: We select the best model obtained from the first experiment. We feed 2D views of the 3D augmentations' center of mass to the network to obtain an axial, sagittal, and coronal quality rating. As there are no human quality ratings for this dataset, we measure segmentation performance using established quality metrics, namely Sørensen-Dice coefficient (DSC) and surface Dice coefficient (SDSC).

Results: We find a strong correlation between the quality ratings predicted by the network and DSC, see Fig. 5. We observe a Pearson r of 0.75 for the axial, 0.76 for the coronal, and 0.77 for the sagittal view, while the averaged rating across views has a 0.79 correlation. This is supported by a high correlation between the mean rating and SDSC (Pearson r: 0.85), suggesting that the model generalizes well to the external data set.

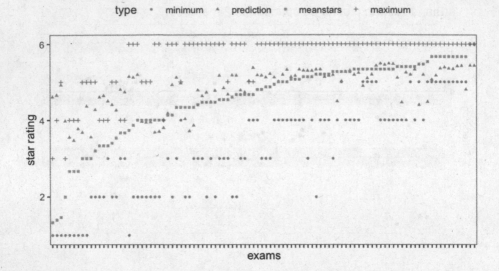

Fig. 4. Network predictions vs. minimum, mean, and maximum human rating. For lower quality segmentations, human raters disagree more. In most cases, the network's predictions are in the range or close to the human ratings. As already visible in Fig. 3, the network tends to overestimate the quality of bad segmentations. However, they are still assigned systematically lower scores. In practice, this difference is sufficient to distinguish between good and bad segmentations by employing a simple thresholding operation.

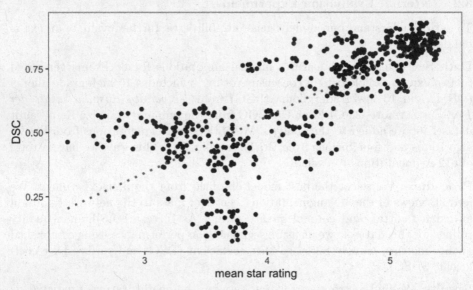

Fig. 5. Scatter plot: Predicted star rating averaged across views vs. DSC for 612 segmentations. Even though we observe moderate heteroscedasticity, a linear model is able to describe the data well, as illustrated by the dotted pink line. We observe a Pearson r of 0.79 between the variables, meaning our model can predict the segmentation quality as measured by DSC quite well. Again we observe more accurate predictions for better segmentations. (Color figure online)

4   Discussion

We demonstrate that a simple *DenseNet121* is able to serve as a surrogate model for the abstract human segmentation quality rating under a scarce training data regime. Notably, the mean absolute error deviation is lower than the difference Kofler et al. [13] reported for individual human raters from the mean human rating. Apparently, the 3D segmentation quality is sufficiently encoded in the 2D center of mass slices. Our experiments show that the choice of hyperparameters is not critical as all networks reach solid performance.

Expert radiologists are among the highest-paid doctors and are notoriously hard to come by. Given that the inference of the approximated quality rating only takes split seconds, there are broad potential applications for *deep quality estimation (DQE)* networks:

One obvious application for *DQE* is quality monitoring during inference. Even though fully-automatic glioma segmentation algorithms, on average, tend to outperform human annotators [13], they sometimes fail spectacularly. For successful clinical translation of such algorithms, detection and mitigation of failure cases is imperative.

Another potential use case for *DQE* is dat aset curation. Data set curation is an important aspect of model training, as broken ground truth labels can destroy model performance. As we demonstrate in the evaluation experiments, *DQE* can differentiate between trustworthy and broken ground truth cases in a fully-automatic fashion. This property becomes especially valuable in a federated learning setting, where researchers have no access to the ground truth labels. *DQE* allows training models only on trustworthy exams by applying a simple thresholding operation on the estimated quality score.

Limitations: It is unclear how well our approach generalizes to other (segmentation) tasks and quality metrics. Taking into account that glioma segmentation is a complex multi-class segmentation problem, the scarce training data, the 3D to 2D translation, and the abstract nature of the human-generated quality judgments, we believe there is a slight reason for optimism.

The proposed model performs better for predicting high-quality segmentations. This is perhaps not surprising given that humans agree more on the quality of such cases and that these are better represented in the training data, as visible in Figs. 2, 3 and 4. Nevertheless, in practice, simple thresholding of the predicted star ratings can sufficiently distinguish segmentation qualities. ,

Outlook: As we demonstrated, *DQE* can approximate non-differentiable quality metrics, such as the abstract human segmentation quality rating, with a differentiable CNN. This promises the possibility of training new (segmentation) networks with surrogates of non-differentiable quality metrics by using *DQE* within the loss function.[2] Future research should address these open questions.

---

[2] A big advantage here (compared to, e.g., *GAN* training) is the possibility to train the networks sequentially and thereby stabilize the training process.

Acknowledgement. BM, BW and FK are supported through the SFB 824, subproject B12.

Supported by Deutsche Forschungsgemeinschaft (DFG) through TUM International Graduate School of Science and Engineering (IGSSE), GSC 81.

LF, SS, EDLR and IE are supported by the Translational Brain Imaging Training Network (TRABIT) under the European Union's 'Horizon 2020' research & innovation program (Grant agreement ID: 765148).

IE and SS are funded by DComEX (Grant agreement ID: 956201).

Supported by Anna Valentina Lioba Eleonora Claire Javid Mamasani.

With the support of the Technical University of Munich - Institute for Advanced Study, funded by the German Excellence Initiative.

EDLR is employed by ico**metrix** (Leuven, Belgium).

JP and SS are supported by the Graduate School of Bioengineering, Technical University of Munich.

JK has received Grants from the ERC, DFG, BMBF and is Co-Founder of Bonescreen GmbH.

BM acknowledges support by the Helmut Horten Foundation.

Research reported in this publication was partly supported by the National Institutes of Health (NIH) under award numbers NIH/NCI:U01CA242871 and NIH/NINDS:R01NS042645.

Research reported in this publication was partly supported by AIME GPU cloud services.

References

1. Audelan, B., Delingette, H.: Unsupervised quality control of image segmentation based on bayesian learning. In: Shen, D., et al. (eds.) MICCAI 2019. LNCS, vol. 11765, pp. 21–29. Springer, Cham (2019). https://doi.org/10.1007/978-3-030-32245-8_3
2. Bakas, S., et al.: Identifying the best machine learning algorithms for brain tumor segmentation, progression assessment, and overall survival prediction in the BRATS challenge (2019)
3. The MONAI Consortium: Project MONAI (2020). https://doi.org/10.5281/zenodo.4323059
4. Fidon, L., Shit, S., Ezhov, I., Paetzold, J.C., Ourselin, S., Vercauteren, T.: Generalized Wasserstein dice loss, test-time augmentation, and transformers for the brats 2021 challenge (2021)
5. Fournel, J., et al.: Medical image segmentation automatic quality control: a multidimensional approach. Med. Image Anal. **74**, 102213 (2021)
6. Gusev, Y., Bhuvaneshwar, K., Song, L., Zenklusen, J.C., Fine, H., Madhavan, S.: The rembrandt study, a large collection of genomic data from brain cancer patients. Sci. Data **5**(1), 1–9 (2018)
7. Hann, E., et al.: Deep neural network ensemble for on-the-fly quality control-driven segmentation of cardiac MRI T1 mapping. Med. Image Anal. **71**, 102029 (2021)
8. Huang, G., Liu, Z., Van Der Maaten, L., Weinberger, K.Q.: Densely connected convolutional networks. In: Proceedings of the IEEE Conference on Computer Vision and Pattern Recognition, pp. 4700–4708 (2017)
9. Isensee, F., et al.: batchgenerators - a python framework for data augmentation (2020). https://doi.org/10.5281/zenodo.3632567

10. Jungo, A., et al.: pymia: a python package for data handling and evaluation in deep learning-based medical image analysis. Comput. Methods Programs Biomed. **198**, 105796 (2021)
11. Kofler, F., et al.: Brats toolkit: translating brats brain tumor segmentation algorithms into clinical and scientific practice. Front. Neurosci. 125 (2020)
12. Kofler, F., et al.: Robust, primitive, and unsupervised quality estimation for segmentation ensembles. Front. Neurosci. **15**, 752780 (2021)
13. Kofler, F., et al.: Are we using appropriate segmentation metrics? Identifying correlates of human expert perception for CNN training beyond rolling the dice coefficient (2021)
14. Li, H., et al.: DiamondGAN: unified multi-modal generative adversarial networks for MRI sequences synthesis. In: Shen, D., et al. (eds.) MICCAI 2019. LNCS, vol. 11767, pp. 795–803. Springer, Cham (2019). https://doi.org/10.1007/978-3-030-32251-9_87
15. Maier-Hein, L., et al.: Why rankings of biomedical image analysis competitions should be interpreted with care. Nat. Commun. **9**(1), 1–13 (2018)
16. Menze, B.H., et al.: The multimodal brain tumor image segmentation benchmark (BRATS). IEEE Trans. Med. Imaging **34**(10), 1993–2024 (2014)
17. Möller, M., et al.: Reliable saliency maps for weakly-supervised localization of disease patterns. In: Cardoso, J., et al. (eds.) IMIMIC/MIL3ID/LABELS -2020. LNCS, vol. 12446, pp. 63–72. Springer, Cham (2020). https://doi.org/10.1007/978-3-030-61166-8_7
18. Pérez-García, F., Sparks, R., Ourselin, S.: Torchio: a python library for efficient loading, preprocessing, augmentation and patch-based sampling of medical images in deep learning. Comput. Methods Programs Biomed. **208**, 106236 (2021). https://doi.org/10.1016/j.cmpb.2021.106236
19. Robinson, R., et al.: Automated quality control in image segmentation: application to the UK biobank cardiovascular magnetic resonance imaging study. J. Cardiovasc. Magn. Reson. **21**(1), 1–14 (2019)
20. Thomas, M.F., et al.: Improving automated glioma segmentation in routine clinical use through artificial intelligence-based replacement of missing sequences with synthetic magnetic resonance imaging scans. Invest. Radiol. **57**(3), 187–193 (2022)
21. Valindria, V.V., et al.: Reverse classification accuracy: predicting segmentation performance in the absence of ground truth. IEEE Trans. Med. Imaging **36**(8), 1597–1606 (2017)
22. Wright, L., Demeure, N.: Ranger21: a synergistic deep learning optimizer (2021)

Unsupervised Anomaly Localization with Structural Feature-Autoencoders

Felix Meissen[1,2(✉)], Johannes Paetzold[1,2], Georgios Kaissis[1,2,3], and Daniel Rueckert[1,2,3]

[1] Technical University of Munich (TUM), Munich, Germany
{felix.meissen,g.kaissis,daniel.rueckert}@tum.de
[2] Klinikum Rechts der Isar, Munich, Germany
[3] Imperial College London, London, UK

Abstract. Unsupervised Anomaly Detection has become a popular method to detect pathologies in medical images as it does not require supervision or labels for training. Most commonly, the anomaly detection model generates a "normal" version of an input image, and the pixel-wise l^p-difference of the two is used to localize anomalies. However, large residuals often occur due to imperfect reconstruction of the complex anatomical structures present in most medical images. This method also fails to detect anomalies that are not characterized by large intensity differences to the surrounding tissue. We propose to tackle this problem using a feature-mapping function that transforms the input intensity images into a space with multiple channels where anomalies can be detected along different discriminative feature maps extracted from the original image. We then train an Autoencoder model in this space using structural similarity loss that does not only consider differences in intensity but also in contrast and structure. Our method significantly increases performance on two medical data sets for brain MRI. Code and experiments are available at https://github.com/FeliMe/feature-autoencoder.

Keywords: Semi-Supervised Learning · Anomaly Localization · Anomaly Detection

1 Introduction

For computed aided decision support systems, accurate detection and localization of pathologies is crucial to assist the radiologist in their work and to build trust in the underlying machine learning algorithms. Supervised methods require large amounts of labeled data. However, manual labeling of medical images – especially pixel- or voxel-wise segmentation – is expensive, time-consuming, and can be ambiguous if two raters don't agree on the same contour of a certain pathology. Unsupervised anomaly localization algorithms can detect regions in images that deviate from the normal appearance without ever seeing anomalous samples of any class during training. These algorithms use machine learning models to learn the normative distribution of the data from normal samples

S. Bakas et al. (Eds.): BrainLes 2022, LNCS 13769, pp. 14–24, 2023.
https://doi.org/10.1007/978-3-031-33842-7_2

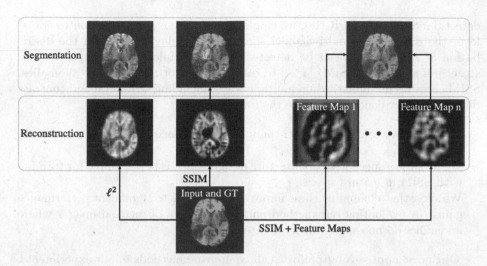

Fig. 1. A sample of a brain MR image showing a tumor (bottom) is reconstructed by a model trained to minimize the L_2-loss (left) SSIM-loss (middle) and to reconstruct feature maps in a multi-channel feature space with SSIM-loss (right). The combination of n anomaly maps gives the most accurate and focused localization.

only. Generative machine learning models, such as Autoencoders (AE) or Generative Adversarial Networks (GAN), have been proven successful for this task. For a new input image, these models usually generate a reconstruction that lies within the distribution of the "normal" data and detect anomalies from pixelwise residual maps between the input- and the reconstructed image. In [16] and [17], Schlegl *et al.* apply this principle by training a GAN on images of retinal OCT scans. They generate the reconstruction during inference by mapping the new sample to the latent space of the GAN. In [13], Pawlowski *et al.* use an Autoencoder to detect anomalies in CT images of the brain. Zimmerer *et al.* [23] train a Variational Autoencoder (VAE) to maximize the likelihood of the normal training data. They experiment with different anomaly scoring functions and found the gradient of the evidence lower bound (ELBO) with respect to the pixels of the input image to improve detection performance. In [3], Baur *et al.* present a thorough comparison of different anomaly localization approaches. However, for detecting tumors and lesions in brain MRI, Saase *et al.* and Meissen *et al.* have independently shown that these methods can be outperformed by simple statistical methods [9,15]. In later work, Meissen *et al.* have identified that small reconstruction inaccuracies at edges and complex anatomical structures yield large residuals that hinder the detection of anomalies that are not characterized by high-contrast intensity regions [10]. They also hypothesize that this problem is more pronounced for single-channel images than for multichannel images because, in the latter one, the anomaly-contributions of different channels to each pixel add up. To alleviate these problems, we apply two changes to the standard Autoencoder framework that were successful in industrial defect detection. Similar to DFR [18], we employ a feature-mapping function to transform the data into a multi-channel space, so that deviations from the distribution of healthy data can be detected along multiple feature maps. We use structural similarity (SSIM) [4, 22] to train our network and localize anomalies. SSIM captures dissimilarities in multiple ways, including structural and contrast differences. Our contributions are the following:

- We combine working in a multi-channel feature space with SSIM for anomaly localization.
- We propose a specialized architecture design which is better suited for training with SSIM in feature spaces.
- We show that combining these improvements leads to significant performance gains, by evaluating our method on two data sets of medical images where anomalies do not appear as hyperintense regions.

Our novel approach outperforms all comparing methods in our experiments. Figure 1 shows the effectiveness of our proposed Structural Feature-Autoencoder on a sample from the Multimodal Brain Tumor Image Segmentation Benchmark (BraTS) data set [1, 2, 11].

2   Methodology

We train a vanilla convolutional Autoencoder to reconstruct feature maps extracted from the input images as shown in Fig. 2.

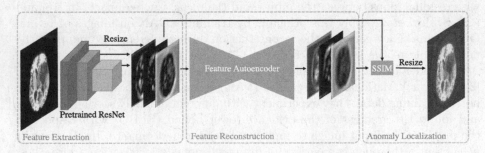

Fig. 2. Pipeline of our proposed method: First, we extract image feature maps with a pre-trained CNN, then we reconstruct these features using an Autoencoder. Finally, we localize anomalies via SSIM between the extracted and the reconstructed feature maps.

2.1   Feature Extraction

We use a pre-trained CNN to transform our initial input image $x \in \mathbb{R}^{c \times h \times w}$ into a multi-channel space with discriminative hierarchical features. The CNN can be seen as a combination of L sequential feature mapping functions, each of them outputting a feature map $\phi_l(\mathbf{x})$ with size $c_l \times h_l \times w_l$. While early layers with small receptive fields capture local facets of the input image, later layers encode more global information. Our extractor combines feature maps from different scales by resizing all maps $\phi_l(\mathbf{x})$ to the spatial size of the largest feature map $\phi_1(\mathbf{x})$ using bilinear interpolation.

2.2 SSIM Loss

The Structural Similarity Index (SSIM) [22] is a metric to measure the perceptual similarity of two images by comparing them on a patch level. For every patch $\mathbf{p}$ in the first image and their corresponding patch $\mathbf{q}$ in the second image, SSIM computes their similarity in terms of luminance $l(\mathbf{p}, \mathbf{q})$, contrast $c(\mathbf{p}, \mathbf{q})$, and structure $s(\mathbf{p}, \mathbf{q})$, and aggregates them into a single score. Similarity in luminance is calculated by comparing the means of the two patches $\mu_{\mathbf{p}}$ and $\mu_{\mathbf{q}}$, contrast by comparing the variances $\sigma_{\mathbf{p}}$ and $\sigma_{\mathbf{q}}$, and for structure, the covariance $\sigma_{\mathbf{pq}}$ is used. Together with two constants C_1 and C_2 for numerical stability, SSIM equates to:

$$\text{SSIM}(\mathbf{p}, \mathbf{q}) = l(\mathbf{p}, \mathbf{q})c(\mathbf{p}, \mathbf{q})s(\mathbf{p}, \mathbf{q}) = \frac{(2\mu_{\mathbf{p}}\mu_{\mathbf{q}} + C_1)(2\sigma_{\mathbf{pq}} + C_2)}{(\mu_{\mathbf{p}}^2 + \mu_{\mathbf{q}}^2 + C_1)(\sigma_{\mathbf{p}}^2 + \sigma_{\mathbf{q}}^2 + C_2)}$$

By computing a score for every pixel-location in the input- and reconstructed image $\mathbf{x}$ and $\hat{\mathbf{x}} \in \mathbb{R}^{c \times h \times w}$, the algorithm outputs an anomaly map $\mathbf{a} \in \mathbb{R}^{h \times w}$, or a scalar loss term when computing the mean SSIM (MSSIM) that evaluates the overall similarity and is differentiable.

$$\text{MSSIM}(\mathbf{x}, \hat{\mathbf{x}}) = \frac{1}{M} \sum_{j=1}^{M} \text{SSIM}(\mathbf{x}_j, \hat{\mathbf{x}}_j)$$

$M = h \times w$. We use MSSIM as a loss function to train our model and the anomaly maps $\mathbf{a}$ to localize anomalies in the image.

3 Experiments

3.1 Datasets

We evaluate our method on two publicly available data sets of brain MRI. First, we use the data of the MOOD Analysis Challenge 2020 [24]. It consists of 800 T2-weighted scans of healthy young adults from which we use 640 for training and split the remaining into 10% validation and 90% test. As part of the preprocessing, we perform histogram equalization on every scan and use a subset of 80 slices around the center of the brain because the majority of lesions are usually accumulated in this region. We then resize all slices to 128×128 pixels and add an artificial sink deformation anomaly from FPI [19] to half of the resulting images in the validation and test sets. Note that the sink deformation anomaly has similar pixel intensities as the surrounding tissue and can therefore not easily be detected via thresholding [10]. Apart from that, the MOOD evaluation data does not contain any anomalies.

The second evaluation is performed on a real world data set. Here, we use the Cambridge Centre for Ageing and Neuroscience (Cam-CAN) dataset [21] for training. It contains scans from 653 healthy women and men between the age of 18 and 87. Both reported genders and all age groups are approximately uniformly distributed. All scans were acquired with a 3T Siemens Magnetom TrioTim syngo MR machine at the Medical Research Council Cognition and Brain Sciences Unit in Cambridge, UK. For evaluation, we use the training set of the 2020 version of the Multimodal Brain Tumor Image Segmentation Benchmark (BraTS) [1,2,11]. Here, scans of 371 patients were acquired with different clinical protocols and various scanners from 19 institutions. The BraTS dataset has manual segmentations from up to four raters. 36 of the BraTS-scans are used for validation, the remainder is used for testing. We only use T1-weighted scans for training and evaluation of the BraTS dataset to assess the detection performance of our method on anomalies that are not necessarily hyperintense. All scans in Cam-CAN and BraTS are registered to the SRI atlas [14] and the scans in Cam-CAN are additionally skull-stripped using ROBEX [7] beforehand. We perform the same pre-processing as for the MOOD data. It is important to note that the distributions of the Cam-CAN training and BraTS evaluation data are likely to be different because of varying scanner types and protocols in the respective acquisition sites. This poses difficulties for Unsupervised Anomaly Detection models since they are designed to detect out-of-distribution samples and even slight distributions shifts might be picked up by the them.

3.2   Implementation

As feature-mapping function, we choose a ResNet18 [6] pre-trained on ImageNet [5]. If not specified otherwise, we use the feature maps of the first three layers (layer0, layer1, and layer2) with a spatial resolution of 32×32, 32×32, and 16×16 respectively. The Feature-Autoencoder is a fully convolutional Autoencoder with four layers in the encoder and the decoder. All encoder layers consist of a 5×5 convolution with stride 2, same padding, and without bias, followed by a batch normalization layer, leaky ReLU activations with a negative slope of 0.01, and dropout with a probability of 0.1. This contrasty DFR which only uses 1×1 convolutions and no spatial down- and upsampling. The encoder is wrapped up by a convolution with a 5×5 kernel and stride 1. The numbers of channels for the encoder layers are 100, 150, 200, and 300. The decoder mirrors the encoder in the number of channels and has four layers with strided transpose convolutions for upsampling, followed by batch normalization, leaky ReLU activations, and dropout as in the encoder. The decoder additionally has a final 1 by 1 convolution which outputs the reconstructed feature maps. We implement our model in PyTorch [12] and train it using the Adam optimizer [8] with a learning rate of 0.0002, and a batch size of 64 for 10.000 steps.

3.3 Baselines

We compare our method against several baselines for semi- and self-supervised anomaly localization: We choose the VAE proposed by Zimmerer *et al.* [23] as a method that uses likelihood-measures to detect anomalies. We use the best-performing methods from their paper ("combi" for localization and the KL-term for detection). For image reconstruction-based variants, we compare against a Vanilla AE with L_2-loss (AE MSE) and one with SSIM-loss (AE SSIM) [4]. We select the same architectures as for the VAE but exchange the variational bottleneck. Results are also compared against those of f-AnoGAN [17]. We further compare against DFR [18] and DFR trained with SSIM-loss to quantify the influence of our architectural contribution. Next, we use the recently proposed self-supervised methods Foreign Patch Interpolation (FPI) [19] and Poisson Image Interpolation (PII) [20] that train a segmentation model on synthetic anomalies. Lastly, we evaluate the statistical baseline method (BM) from Saase *et al.* [15] that previously outperformed several reconstruction-based methods. For all baselines that require training, we choose Adam with a learning rate of 0.0002 as an optimizer, set the batch size to 64, and train for 10.000 steps. Only DFR uses the original batch size of 4 from the paper, because of its large memory footprint.

3.4 Evaluation Metrics

For evaluating anomaly localization performance of the models, we resort to standard metrics used in the literature. First, we use the pixel-wise average precision (Pixel-AP) which is equivalent to the area under the precision-recall curve and is threshold-independent. We also report the Sørensen-Dice coefficient at a false positive rate of 5% (Dice @ 5% FPR). Sample-wise performance is measured via the area under the receiver operating characteristics curve (Image-AUROC). We considered every slice that contains at least one anomalous pixel as abnormal. All metrics are computed over the whole test data set.

4 Results

We repeat the training- and evaluation procedure for each method with $N = 5$ different random seeds. The results for the MOOD and BraTS data sets are shown in Table 1 and Fig. 3 respectively. On MOOD, only the self-supervised methods FPI outperform our proposed model. However, it is crucial to note that at FPI was designed to achieve good performance on this anomaly type. For the real-world data set, our model outperforms all competing methods from Sect. 3.3 both in the pixel- and in the sample-wise setting. We perform a two-sided, heteroscedastic t-test with $p \leq 0.05$ to show that the results are statistically significant. We also added the performance a random uniform classifier would get (Random Classifier) for comparison.

Table 1. Performance of all compared models and a random classifier, including standard deviations over $N = 5$ runs with different random seeds, on the MOOD data set with sink deformation anomalies.

	Pixel-AP	Dice @ 5% FPR	Image-AUROC
Random	0.019 ± 0.000	0.028 ± 0.000	0.500 ± 0.000
VAE [23]	0.051 ± 0.000	0.092 ± 0.001	0.482 ± 0.003
AE MSE	0.048 ± 0.001	0.088 ± 0.001	0.572 ± 0.006
AE SSIM [4]	0.090 ± 0.010	0.155 ± 0.022	0.624 ± 0.004
f-AnoGAN [17]	0.052 ± 0.001	0.071 ± 0.001	0.580 ± 0.007
FPI [19]	$\mathbf{0.474 \pm 0.048}$	0.320 ± 0.017	$\mathbf{0.879 \pm 0.046}$
PII [20]	0.338 ± 0.146	0.268 ± 0.064	0.808 ± 0.078
DFR [18]	0.080 ± 0.001	0.138 ± 0.003	0.560 ± 0.004
DFR SSIM	0.080 ± 0.002	0.140 ± 0.003	0.556 ± 0.004
BM [15]	0.048 ± 0.000	0.090 ± 0.000	0.544 ± 0.000
Ours	0.431 ± 0.007	$\mathbf{0.336 \pm 0.004}$	0.775 ± 0.007

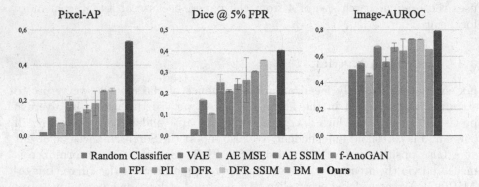

Fig. 3. Performance of all compared models and a random classifier, including error bars that indicate one standard deviation over $N = 5$ runs with different random seeds, on the BraTS data set. Our method performs significantly better than all compared methods (t-test; $p \leq 0.05$).

4.1 Ablation - Feature Extractor Layers

We perform an ablation study to evaluate the influence of the feature-mapping function on the performance of our method. We use feature maps from different layers of the pre-trained ResNet (Indicated by "layer x, y, z"). The results are shown in Fig. 4.

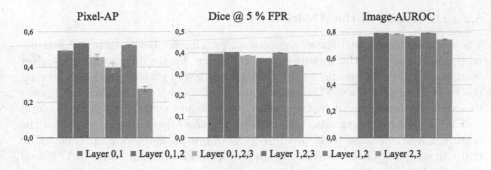

Fig. 4. Ablation study using different layers of the feature-mapping function. The error bars indicate one standard deviation.

5   Discussion

The above experiments provide evidence that our contributions significantly improve anomaly detection and localization performance on anomalies that are mainly characterized by textural differences. Although the anomalies are not hyperintense and despite the domain shift between training and evaluation data, our model achieves strong performance on both data sets.

5.1   Discussion of the Main Experiments

The results of our method and DFR have low variance compared to others, which demonstrates that anomaly localization in a multi-channel feature space is more robust than in image space. The two self-supervised methods perform well in detecting the artificial sink anomalies. This is not surprising as they have been designed and optimized for this exact type of artifical anomaly. Importantly, however, they fail in detecting real-world anomalies, which indicates that the self-supervision task does not generalize beyond synthetic anomalies. They also consistently exhibit the largest variance in the pixel- and the sample-wise task. Their performance, therefore, is more random and less reliable than our method. Noticeably, DFR with SSIM-loss performs worse than our method and only slightly better than vanilla DFR (Fig. 3). This is a result of the architecture choices of both methods: DFR uses only 1 by 1 convolutions with no spatial interconnections. However, a scoring function like SSIM – that works on patches – benefits from an architecture like ours with a large receptive field provided by spatial convolutions, and down- and upsampling. SSIM captures interdependencies between neighboring pixels and combines differences along three dimensions (luminance, contrast, and structure), while the pixel-wise residual scores pixels isolated and only based on their intensity. Combining this process on multiple channels multiplies the beneficial effect.

5.2 Discussion of the Ablation

The ablation experiment shows a consistent ranking for both pixel- and sample-wise performance of the feature-extractor layers. Earlier layers of the ResNet seem to provide more useful features than later layers with layers 1 and 2 being the most important ones. This makes sense as CNN-based backbones are known to extract a hierarchy of features with lower layers containing more textural and later ones more semantic information. On the other, a larger depth of the feature maps is harder to fit as it requires more parameters and, thus, more training samples. That is why a drop in performance between "layer 0, 1, 2" and "layer 0, 1, 2, 3" can be observed.

5.3 Limitations

While working in multi-channel feature spaces improves robustness and performance of anomaly detection methods for brain MRI, the loss of spatial resolution through the feature mapping function leads to coarse segmentations and can cause models to miss small anomalies as shown in Fig. 5. Another failure case shown here happens at slices far away from the center of the brain. Since the structure there differs significantly from the rest of the brain, large regions get misclassified as anomalous.

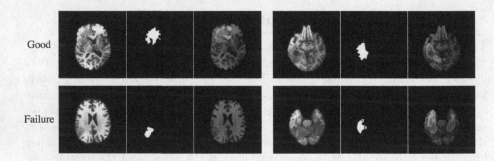

Fig. 5. Two successful samples (first row) and two failure cases (second row). On the left, the model fails to detect a small anomaly. On the right, a slice far away from the center shows false positives. Each with input image, manual segmentation, and anomaly map thresholded at $t = 0.75$ from left to right.

6 Conclusion

This work has shown that using SSIM in a multi-channel discriminative feature space improves localization of non-hyperintense anomalies on brain MRI significantly and sets a new state-of-the-art in this domain. While we are aware that for unsupervised detection of brain tumors other MR sequences, such as fluid-attenuated inversion recovery (FLAIR) images are available, we argue that our method can easily be transferred to other modalities and pathologies, such as CT, where this isn't the case. We deem anomaly detection from feature spaces a promising research direction and will further explore methods to increase the spatial resolution of these approaches. We will also apply our findings to different modalities and pathologies and study their behavior.

References

1. Bakas, S., et al.: Advancing the cancer genome atlas glioma MRI collections with expert segmentation labels and radiomic features. Sci. Data **4**, 2052–4463 (2017). https://doi.org/10.1038/sdata.2017.117
2. Bakas, S., et al.: Identifying the best machine learning algorithms for brain tumor segmentation, progression assessment, and overall survival prediction in the brats challenge (2019)
3. Baur, C., Denner, S., Wiestler, B., Navab, N., Albarqouni, S.: Autoencoders for unsupervised anomaly segmentation in brain MR images: a comparative study. Med. Image Anal. **69**, 101952 (2021). https://doi.org/10.1016/j.media.2020.101952
4. Bergmann, P., Löwe, S., Fauser, M., Sattlegger, D., Steger, C.: Improving unsupervised defect segmentation by applying structural similarity to autoencoders. In: Proceedings of the 14th International Joint Conference on Computer Vision, Imaging and Computer Graphics Theory and Applications (2019). https://doi.org/10.5220/0007364503720380
5. Deng, J., Socher, R., Fei-Fei, L., Dong, W., Li, K., Li, L.: Imagenet: a large-scale hierarchical image database. In: 2009 IEEE Conference on Computer Vision and Pattern Recognition (CVPR), pp. 248–255 (2009). https://doi.org/10.1109/CVPR.2009.5206848
6. He, K., Zhang, X., Ren, S., Sun, J.: Deep residual learning for image recognition. In: Proceedings of the IEEE Conference on Computer Vision and Pattern Recognition, pp. 770–778 (2016)
7. Iglesias, J.E., Liu, C.Y., Thompson, P.M., Tu, Z.: Robust brain extraction across datasets and comparison with publicly available methods. IEEE Trans. Med. Imaging **30**, 1617–1634 (2011). https://doi.org/10.1109/TMI.2011.2138152
8. Kingma, D.P., Ba, J.: Adam: a method for stochastic optimization (2017)
9. Meissen, F., Kaissis, G., Rueckert, D.: Challenging current semi-supervised anomaly segmentation methods for brain MRI. In: Crimi, A., Bakas, S. (eds.) Brainlesion: Glioma, Multiple Sclerosis, Stroke and Traumatic Brain Injuries, pp. 63–74. Springer, Cham (2022). https://doi.org/10.1007/978-3-031-08999-2_5
10. Meissen, F., Wiestler, B., Kaissis, G., Rueckert, D.: On the pitfalls of using the residual as anomaly score. In: Medical Imaging with Deep Learning (2022). https://openreview.net/forum?id=ZsoHLeupa1D
11. Menze, B.H., et al.: The multimodal brain tumor image segmentation benchmark (BRATS). IEEE Trans. Med. Imaging **34**(10), 1003 2024 (2015). https://doi.org/10.1109/TMI.2014.2377694
12. Paszke, A., et al.: Pytorch: an imperative style, high-performance deep learning library. In: Wallach, H., Larochelle, H., Beygelzimer, A., d' Alché-Buc, F., Fox, E., Garnett, R. (eds.) Advances in Neural Information Processing Systems, vol. 32, pp. 8024–8035. Curran Associates, Inc. (2019)
13. Pawlowski, N., et al.: Unsupervised lesion detection in brain CT using Bayesian convolutional autoencoders. In: MIDL 2018 Conference Book. MIDL (2018)

14. Rohlfing, T., Zahr, N.M., Sullivan, E.V., Pfefferbaum, A.: The SRI24 multichannel atlas of normal adult human brain structure. Hum. Brain Mapp. **31**, 798–819 (2010). https://doi.org/10.1002/hbm.20906
15. Saase, V., Wenz, H., Ganslandt, T., Groden, C., Maros, M.E.: Simple statistical methods for unsupervised brain anomaly detection on MRI are competitive to deep learning methods (2020)
16. Schlegl, T., Seeböck, P., Waldstein, S., Schmidt-Erfurth, U., Langs, G.: Unsupervised anomaly detection with generative adversarial networks to guide marker discovery. In: International Conference on Information Processing in Medical Imaging, pp. 146–157 (2017)
17. Schlegl, T., Seeböck, P., Waldstein, S.M., Langs, G., Schmidt-Erfurth, U.: f-AnoGAN: fast unsupervised anomaly detection with generative adversarial networks. Med. Image Anal. **54**, 30–44 (2019). https://doi.org/10.1016/j.media.2019.01.010
18. Shi, Y., Yang, J., Qi, Z.: Unsupervised anomaly segmentation via deep feature reconstruction. Neurocomputing (2020). https://doi.org/10.1016/j.neucom.2020.11.018
19. Tan, J., Hou, B., Batten, J., Qiu, H., Kainz, B.: Detecting outliers with foreign patch interpolation. arXiv preprint arXiv:2011.04197 (2020)
20. Tan, J., Hou, B., Day, T., Simpson, J., Rueckert, D., Kainz, B.: Detecting outliers with poisson image interpolation. In: de Bruijne, M., et al. (eds.) MICCAI 2021. LNCS, vol. 12905, pp. 581–591. Springer, Cham (2021). https://doi.org/10.1007/978-3-030-87240-3_56
21. Taylor, J.R., et al.: The Cambridge centre for ageing and neuroscience (cam-CAN) data repository: structural and functional MRI, MEG, and cognitive data from a cross-sectional adult lifespan sample. NeuroImage **144**, 262–269 (2017). https://doi.org/10.1016/j.neuroimage.2015.09.018. Data Sharing Part II
22. Wang, Z., Bovik, A.C., Sheikh, H.R., Simoncelli, E.P.: Image quality assessment: from error visibility to structural similarity. IEEE Trans. Image Process. **13**(4), 600–612 (2004)
23. Zimmerer, D., Isensee, F., Petersen, J., Kohl, S., Maier-Hein, K.: Unsupervised anomaly localization using variational auto-encoders. In: Shen, D., et al. (eds.) MICCAI 2019. LNCS, vol. 11767, pp. 289–297. Springer, Cham (2019). https://doi.org/10.1007/978-3-030-32251-9_32
24. Zimmerer, D., et al.: Medical out-of-distribution analysis challenge (2020). https://doi.org/10.5281/zenodo.3784230

Transformer Based Models for Unsupervised Anomaly Segmentation in Brain MR Images

Ahmed Ghorbel[1]([envelope]) [ID], Ahmed Aldahdooh[1] [ID], Shadi Albarqouni[2,3,4] [ID], and Wassim Hamidouche[1] [ID]

[1] Univ. Rennes, INSA Rennes, CNRS, IETR - UMR 6164,
20 Av. des Buttes de Coesmes, 35700 Rennes, France
{ahmed.ghorbel,ahmed.aldahdooh,wassim.hamidouche}@insa-rennes.fr
[2] University Hospital Bonn, Venusberg-Campus 1, 53127 Bonn, Germany
shadi.albarqouni@ukbonn.de
[3] Helmholtz Munich, Ingolstädter Landstraße 1, 85764 Neuherberg, Germany
[4] Technical University of Munich, Boltzmannstr. 3, 85748 Garching, Germany

Abstract. The quality of patient care associated with diagnostic radiology is proportionate to a physician's workload. Segmentation is a fundamental limiting precursor to both diagnostic and therapeutic procedures. Advances in machine learning (ML) aim to increase diagnostic efficiency by replacing a single application with generalized algorithms. The goal of unsupervised anomaly detection (UAD) is to identify potential anomalous regions unseen during training, where convolutional neural network (CNN) based autoencoders (AEs), and variational autoencoders (VAEs) are considered a de facto approach for reconstruction based-anomaly segmentation. The restricted receptive field in CNNs limits the CNN to model the global context. Hence, if the anomalous regions cover large parts of the image, the CNN-based AEs are not capable of bringing a semantic understanding of the image. Meanwhile, vision transformers (ViTs) have emerged as a competitive alternative to CNNs. It relies on the self-attention mechanism that can relate image patches to each other. We investigate in this paper Transformer's capabilities in building AEs for the reconstruction-based UAD task to reconstruct a coherent and more realistic image. We focus on anomaly segmentation for brain magnetic resonance imaging (MRI) and present five Transformer-based models while enabling segmentation performance comparable to or superior to state-of-the-art (SOTA) models. The source code is made publicly available on GitHub.

Keywords: Unsupervised Learning · Anomaly Segmentation · Deep-Learning · Transformers · Neuroimaging

1 Introduction

In recent years, significant progress has been achieved in developing deep learning approaches for tackling various tasks. Anomaly segmentation is one of the most

S. Bakas et al. (Eds.): BrainLes 2022, LNCS 13769, pp. 25–44, 2023.
https://doi.org/10.1007/978-3-031-33842-7_3

challenging tasks in computer vision applications. It seeks to act like experienced physicians to identify and delineate various anomalies on medical images, such as tumors on brain magnetic resonance (MR) scans. Therefore, it is crucial to constantly improve the accuracy of medical image segmentation by developing novel deep learning (DL) techniques. Since the advent of DL, fully convolutional neural network (FCNN) and in particular U-shaped autoencoder architectures [23,24] have achieved SOTA results in various medical semantic segmentation tasks. Additionally, in computer vision, using Transformers as a backbone encoder is beneficial due to their great capability of modeling long-range dependencies and capturing global context [22].

Detecting and diagnosing diseases, monitoring illness development, and treatment planning are all common uses for neuroimaging. Manually identifying and segmenting diseases in the brain MRI is time-consuming and arduous. The medical image analysis community has offered a wide range of strategies to aid in detecting and delineating brain lesions emerging from multiple sclerosis (MS) lesions or tumors. Many supervised DL techniques have attained outstanding levels of performance like supervised k-nearest neighbors (KNN) and automatic knowledge-guided (KG) for glioma patients and supervised CNN-based methods for multiple sclerosis lesion segmentation described throughout this survey [34]. Nevertheless, these techniques, which are primarily based on supervised DL, have certain drawbacks: 1) A relevant pathology is estimated to be missed in 5–10% of scans [26]. 2) Training supervised models requires large and diverse annotated datasets, which are scarce and expensive to acquire. 3) The resulting models are limited to detecting lesions similar to those seen in the training data.

Furthermore, these methods have a limited generalization since training data rarely covers the whole range of clinical manifestations [27]. To overcome these challenges, recent works [7,9] investigated modeling the distribution of healthy brains to detect pathologies as a deviation from the norm. The challenge of brain anomalies identification and delineation is formulated here as an UAD task based on SOTA deep representation learning, which requires only a set of healthy data. Anomalies are detected and delimited first by computing the pixel-wise L_1-distance between an input image and its reconstruction, and then post-processing the resulting residual image to get a binary segmentation, as illustrated in Fig. 3 and Fig. 2 of Appendix A.

Due to the inherent locality of convolution processes, CNN-based techniques have difficulties modeling explicit long-range relationships, despite their outstanding representational capability. Therefore, these architectures generally yield weak performance, especially for target structures that show significant inter-patient variation in texture, shape, and size. On the other hand, Transformers exempt convolution operators entirely and rely solely on attention mechanisms to capture the interactions between inputs, regardless of their relative position to one another, like pixel recurrent neural networks (PixelRNNs) [37]. Unlike prior CNN-based methods known for creating blurry reconstructions, Transformers are not only effective in modeling global contexts but also show greater transferability for downstream tasks under large-scale pre-training. In this work, we propose a method for unsupervised anomaly segmentation using Transformers, where we learn the distribution of healthy brain MR data. We create and evaluate different Transformer-based models and compare their performance results on real anomalous datasets with recent SOTA unsupervised models [7].

Although Transformers need a large-scale dataset for training, we train our models and SOTA models from scratch on the healthy OASIS-3 [31] dataset, and we don't use extra data for pre-trained models. Two challenging datasets MSLUB [33] and BraTS-20 [32] are tested for detecting two different pathologies. To summarize, our contributions are mainly focusing on building Transformer-based models to answer the following questions:

- Is the basic Transformer architecture capable of modeling the distribution of healthy data? Due to the Transformer's ability to model the global context of the image, we found that it can reconstruct anomalous inputs with the same intensity levels. Thus it fails in modeling the healthy data distribution for the anomaly segmentation task.
- Are the joint Transformer and CNN architectures capable of modeling the distribution of healthy data? Due to the ability to model global and local features in the common architecture, we found that having Dense Convolutional AE between the encoder and the decoder of the Transformer yields superior performance compared to CNN-based AEs in BraTS dataset and comparable performance in MSLUB dataset.
- Is the hierarchical Transformer architecture able to model the latent space of the healthy data? Owing to the ability to capture short/long-range spatial correlations by down/up-sampling and combining the self-attention provided by Transformer layers, respectively, we can say yes, and it yields superior performance in BraTS dataset compared to other CNN and Transformer based architectures.

2 Related Works

CNN-Based UAD Networks: Since the introduction of AEs [6] and their generative siblings [8, 25] for the UAD task, many recent CNN-based UAD networks were proposed [35, 36]. Regardless of their accomplishment, these networks have a weakness in learning long-range spatial dependencies, which can significantly impact segmentation performance for difficult tasks.

Combining CNNs with Self-attention Mechanisms: Various studies have attempted to integrate self-attention mechanisms into CNNs by modeling global interactions of all pixels based on the feature maps. For instance, [17] designed a non-local operator, which can be plugged into multiple intermediate convolution layers. Furthermore, [18] proposed additive attention gate modules built upon the AE u-shaped architecture and integrated into the skip-connections. [4] combined the latent discrete representation from the VQ-VAE model with an auto-regressive Transformer to obtain the likelihood of each latent variable value.

Vision Transformers: For several computer vision tasks, ViTs have rapidly acquired traction. By large-scale pretraining and fine-tuning of a basic Transformer architecture, [22] achieved SOTA on ImageNet classification by directly applying Transformers with global self-attention to full-size images. In object detection, end-to-end Transformer-based models have shown prominence on several benchmarks [15,16]. A few efforts [11,12] have explored the possibility of using Transformers for image segmentation tasks. Furthermore, for medical image segmentation, [10] proposed an axial fusion of Transformer with U-shaped network (U-Net). Recently, [13,14] proposed hierarchical vision Transformers with varying resolutions and spatial embeddings. For instance, instead of applying self-attention globally, [20] used it just in local neighborhoods for each query pixel. [21] proposed Sparse Transformers, which employ scalable approximations to global self-attention.

3   Methodology

We followed the recommended deep generative representation learning methodology, which is mentioned in [6] and illustrated in Fig. 2 (Appendix A), to model the distribution of the healthy brain. This methodology should allow the model to fully reconstruct healthy brain anatomy while failing to reconstruct anomalous lesions in diseased brain MR images. Anomalies are found and delimited by computing the pixel-wise $\mathcal{L}_1$-distance between an input image $\mathbf{x}$ and its reconstruction $\hat{\mathbf{x}} = h_\phi(g_\theta(\mathbf{x}))$, where g_θ and h_ϕ are, respectively, parametric functions of encoder-decoder networks of parameters θ and ϕ

$$\mathcal{L}_{Rec}^{\phi,\theta}(\mathbf{x}, \hat{\mathbf{x}}) = \mathcal{L}_1(\mathbf{x}, \hat{\mathbf{x}}). \tag{1}$$

Then, we post-process the resulting residual image to get a binary segmentation. This method uses healthy data to create a probability density estimate of the input data specified by the uniformity of the landscape. Pathological traits are subsequently registered as deviations from normality, eliminating the need for labels or anomalous cases in training.

3.1   Anomaly Segmentation

First, we train our model to reconstruct healthy preprocessed input samples. This trained model is used to predict samples from anomalous preprocessed data. Then, we compute the residual or pixel-wise discrepancy between the input and the reconstruction. Figure 3 (Appendix A) illustrates this process. Assume that we are working on one channel ($C = 1$), $\mathbf{x} \in \mathcal{R}^{H \times W}$ is the input sample, $\hat{\mathbf{x}} \in \mathcal{R}^{H \times W}$ is the reconstruction (prediction), $\mathbf{r} \in \mathcal{R}^{H \times W}$ is the residual, $\mathbf{l} \in \{0,1\}^{H \times W}$ is the label relative to the ground truth segmentation of $\mathbf{x}$ and $\mathbf{b_{mask}} \in \{0,1\}^{H \times W}$ is the brain mask of the corresponding input $\mathbf{x}$. We calculate the residual $\mathbf{r}$ which is a pixel-wise multiplication of $\mathbf{b_{mask}}$ with the difference between $\mathbf{x}$ and $\hat{\mathbf{x}}$.

$$\mathbf{r} = \mathbf{b_{mask}} \odot (\mathbf{x} - \hat{\mathbf{x}}). \tag{2}$$

3.2   Proposed Architectures

Basic Transformer AE is the first considered architecture, whose overview is depicted in Fig. 4 (Appendix B). This architecture is the simplest one intended to understand the behavior of Transformers alone and see the real effect of the self-attention mechanism and the added value of the global feature extractions on the reconstructions. Introduced in [19], this (B_TAE) receives as input a 1D sequence of token embeddings. To handle 2D images, we reshape the image $\mathbf{x} \in \mathcal{R}^{H \times W \times C}$ into a sequence of flattened 2D patches $\mathbf{x_p} \in \mathcal{R}^{N \times P^2 \times C}$, as proposed in the original ViT [22], where (H, W) is the resolution of the original image, C is the number of channels, (P, P) is the resolution of each image patch, and $N = \frac{H \times W}{P^2}$ is the resulting number of patches, which also serves as the effective input sequence length for the Transformer. The Transformer uses constant latent vector size K through all of its layers, so we flatten the patches and map to K dimensions with a linear projection. We refer to the output of this projection as the patch embeddings. Finally, we have another linear projection layer to project back embeddings into the initial dimension and a patch expanding layer to reconstruct the image with the same size (H, W, C) as the input.

Convolution Inside Transformer AE: Based on the results of B_TAE, we found that the potential anomalous regions are recovered on the reconstructed images with the same intensity levels even after training on the healthy dataset due to the type of features extracted by Transformers (only global features). From these results and inspired by the work in [30], we decided to use the complementary of Transformers and CNNs to improve the reconstruction capability of our B_TAE, and then, going deeper inside the Transformer bottleneck to combine local and global features by adding a mn AE. Different from the methods mentioned in [14,28], where they modeled hybrid CNN-Transformer architectures, we propose a Transformer AE network with CNN AE inside the bottleneck for the anomaly segmentation task. Two types of Convolutional AEs were considered (see Appendix B): spatial convolutional transformer autoencoder (SC_TAE) with a spatial bottleneck (Fig. 5) and dense convolutional transformer autoencoder (DC_TAE) with a dense bottleneck (Fig. 6). These two convolutional autoencoders were implemented using a unified CNN architecture. This unified architecture was also used for the benchmark models and thus

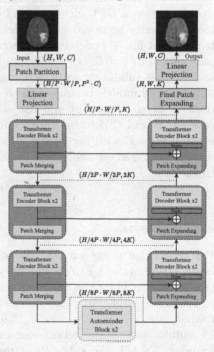

Fig. 1. Hierarchical Transformer Autoencoder with Skip connections (H_TAE_S).

having an accurate comparison as previously done in the comparative study in [7].

Hierarchical Transformer AE: Inspired by Swin-Unet [29], we presented a Hierarchical Transformer as AE (Fig. 1) and (Fig. 7 in Appendix B), with and without skip connections respectively, for gradually learning hierarchical features while reducing the computation complexity of standard Transformers for the medical image segmentation task. Down/Up-sampling will replace the local features retrieved by CNNs, and when combined with the self-attention provided by Transformer layers, we get a fully Transformer architecture that is highly promising for the medical anomaly segmentation challenges. For additional information see the Appendices D and F.

4   Experiments

4.1   Implementation Details

We implemented all models in TensorFlow, and the experimental study was carried out on a GPU cluster including two RTX 8000 devices (see Appendix J for complexity analysis). All models were trained on the same OASIS-3 [31] training-set for 50 epochs with batch-size 12, using the ADAM optimizer, with parameters $\beta_1 = 0.9$, $\beta_2 = 0.999$ and $lr = 10^{-5}$, and mae as loss function. We use the best validation score as a stopping criterion to save the best model. The output of all models is subject to the same post-processing: assuming that only positive pixels were kept and the others were set to zero, we post-process the residual $\mathbf{r}$ (Eq. (2)) to obtain the binary mask $\mathbf{m}$ (Eq. (3)) by applying a 2D median filter $\mathbf{F}$ with kernel $k = 5$, and then applying squashing operator $\mathbf{S}$ to squash the 1% lower intensities. Finally, we evaluate our segmentation according to the label l.

$$\mathbf{m} = \mathbf{S}_{1\%}\left(\mathbf{F}_{k=5}\left(\max(\mathbf{r}, 0)\right)\right) \tag{3}$$

4.2   Datasets

We based our study on the human brain MR scans with FLAIR modality (see Appendix C for the modality use justification), different planes, NIfTI format, and (H, W, C) = (256, 256, 1) sample size. More details can be found in Table 1. We apply the same

Table 1. Considered datasets.

Dataset	Patients/Cohort	Train/Val/Test
OASIS-3	574/Healthy	16896/1280/4805
BraTS-20	31/GB	-/-/4805
MSLUB	18/MS	-/-/3078

preprocessing to all datasets: - the skull has been stripped with ROBEX [3], - the resulting images have been normalized into the range [0,1] and resized using an interlinear interpolation.

4.3   Evaluation Metrics

We use (DSC), with mean and standard deviation, and area under the precision-recall curve (AUPRC) to evaluate segmentation accuracy in our experiments. We report the area under the precision-recall curve (AUPRC) as well. In addition, we use structural similarity image metric (SSIM) to evaluate the reconstruction fidelity on healthy data.

5   Results

5.1   Overall Performance

Table 2 describes the overall performance of our Transformer-based models compared to the SOTA models on each of the BraTS, MSLUB, and healthy unseen OASIS datasets. DC_TAE and H_TAE_S outperform the SOTA models on BraTS dataset, and DC_TAE has comparable performance with the SOTA models on MSLUB. Moreover, the H_TAE_S and SC_TAE have the best reconstruction fidelity performance. Considering the models in [4], we outperform, on BraTS, their Models 1 and 2 but not their Model 3, and on MSLUB, we outperform only the Model 1. It's a relative comparison because we didn't use the same training set. Finally, the qualitative results can be found in (Appendix I) with visual examples of the different reviewed models on BraTS and MSLUB datasets in Fig. 8 and Fig. 9, respectively. For more results about the ablation study and the parameter tuning process, see (Appendix G) and (Appendix H), respectively.

5.2   Quantitative Evaluations

Considering the DSC metric on MSLUB and BraTS test-sets, DC_TAE achieves an overall DSC of 0.337 and outperforms the first and second top-ranked SOTA models by 1.7% and 3.6%, respectively. H_TAE_S achieves an overall DSC of 0.339 and surpasses the first and second top-ranked SOTA models by 1.9% and 3.8%, respectively. Considering the AUPRC metric on MSLUB and BraTS test-sets, DC_TAE achieves an overall AUPRC of 0.313 and achieves better results than the first and second top-ranked SOTA models by 6.4% and 7.4%, respectively. H_TAE_S achieves an overall AUPRC of 0.264 and outperforms the first and second top-ranked SOTA models by 1.5% and 2.5%, respectively. Considering the SSIM on healthy OASIS test-set, H_TAE_S achieves an SSIM score of 0.9958 and surpasses the first and second top-ranked SOTA models by 5.43% and 11.97%, respectively. SC_TAE achieves an SSIM score of 0.9784 and exceeds the first and second top ranked SOTA models by 3.69% and 10.23%, respectively.

5.3   Discussion

CNN-based AEs are known for creating blurry reconstructions. This blurry reconstruction may cause residuals with high values in areas of the image with high frequencies, implying that the model cannot efficiently discriminate between

Table 2. Overall performance on the BraTS and MSLUB and the healthy unseen OASIS dataset. Top-1 and top-2 scores are highlighted in bold/underline and bold, respectively. For each model, we provide an estimate of its theoretically best possible DICE score ($[DSC]$) on each dataset. Models 1, 2 and 3 proposed in [4] correspond to VQ-VAE + Transformer, VQ-VAE + Transformer + Masked Residuals and VQ-VAE + Transformer + Masked Residuals + Different Orderings models, respectively. * Models have not been trained on the same training set as the benchmark and our proposed models.

Approach	BraTS			MSLUB			OASIS
	AUROC ↑	AUPRC ↑	[DSC] $(\mu \pm \sigma)$ ↑	AUROC ↑	AUPRC ↑	[DSC] $(\mu \pm \sigma)$ ↑	SSIM ↑
AE (dense) [7]	0.7648	0.3493	0.4584 ± 0.4017	0.8765	0.1299	0.1687 ± 0.2955	0.8758
AE (spatial) [7]	0.6211	0.0857	0.3646 ± 0.4031	0.7430	0.0347	0.1539 ± 0.2893	0.9415
VAE [7]	0.7733	0.3923	0.4663 ± 0.4041	0.8263	0.0863	**0.1751** ± **0.2985**	0.8761
VQ-VAE [5]	0.6992	0.2549	0.4306 ± 0.3889	**0.8881**	**0.2441**	0.1724 ± 0.2952	0.8724
B_TAE (Ours)	0.6142	0.1221	0.4252 ± 0.4475	0.7272	0.0177	0.1490 ± 0.2747	0.9610
DC_TAE (Ours)	**0.7802**	**0.4250**	**0.5017** ± **0.4056**	**0.8861**	**0.2025**	**0.1728** ± **0.2971**	0.8269
SC_TAE (Ours)	0.6847	0.2561	0.4552 ± 0.4180	0.6669	0.0133	0.1306 ± 0.2682	**0.9784**
H_TAE (Ours)	0.5472	0.0716	0.3593 ± 0.4020	0.5788	0.0374	0.1592 ± 0.2865	0.8987
H_TAE_S (Ours)	**0.7763**	**0.5086**	**0.5296** ± **0.4417**	0.6906	0.0209	0.1489 ± 0.2857	**0.9958**
Model 1* [4]	–	–	0.431	–	–	0.097	–
Model 2* [4]	–	–	**0.476**	–	–	**0.234**	–
Model 3* [4]	–	–	**0.759**	–	–	**0.378**	–

healthy hyper-intensity areas and anomalies. To avoid these areas being mislabelled as anomalous, we conducted our research on three different approaches. We begin at first with the B_TAE architecture and find that modeling only global context yields reconstructions with anomalies. Then, we explored another approach and found that DC_TAE achieves superior performance due to its hybrid architectural design, which not only encodes strong global context by treating, along an attention mechanism, the image features as sequences but also well utilizes the low-level CNN features. The evaluation results indicate that DC_TAE is a stable and powerful network to extract both short and long-range dependencies of MRI scans. Finally, in our H_TAE_S model, we used the spatial information and attention mechanism in a u-shaped architectural design. The extracted context features are fused with multi-scale features from the encoder via skip connections to complement the loss of spatial information caused by down-sampling. By observing the results of anomaly detection scores for the anomalies of different sizes, fully Transformer architecture, i.e., without convolutions, yields less performance than SOTA models for small anomalies. Hence, we can say that local features and small anomalies are correlated. According to BraTS dataset, we can say that better reconstruction fidelity corresponds to the highest segmentation results, but this is not true in MSLUB dataset. To properly study the correlation between SSIM and segmentation metrics, we should do some more experiments on different test sets.

6   Conclusion

In this paper, we have proposed five Transformer-based image reconstruction models for anomaly segmentation. The models are based on three global architectures: basic, convolution inside, and hierarchical Transformer AE. Extensive experiments show that DC_TAE and H_TAE_S achieve better or comparable performance than the SOTA on two representative datasets, especially for small and complex anomalies. However, Transformers are known for modeling pixel dependencies due to their attention mechanism and hence should be able to substitute anomalous pixels with pseudo-healthy ones. However, none of our models succeeded in reconstructing this way. Yet, we can address this weakness as an area of improvement. Finally, we believe our findings will lead to more research into the properties of Transformers for anomaly detection and their application to advanced medical tasks.

A   The Core Concept Behind the Reconstruction-Based Method

The core concept behind the reconstruction method is modeling healthy anatomy with unsupervised deep (generative) representation learning. Therefore, the method leverage a set of healthy MRI scans and learns to project and recover it from a lower dimensional distribution. See Fig. 2 and Fig. 3 for more details.

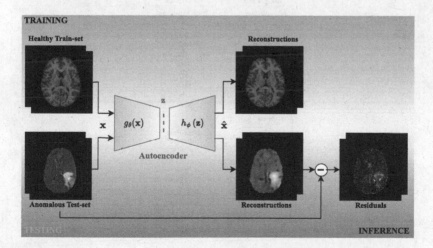

Fig. 2. The concept of AE-based anomaly segmentation: A) model training on healthy samples, B) model testing on anomalous samples, C) and segmentation of anomalies from reconstructions likely to carry an anomaly.

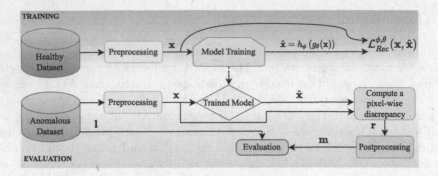

Fig. 3. Unsupervised anomaly segmentation process, where **x**: input, **x̂**: reconstruction, r: residual, l: label, m: mask.

B   Additional Diagrams for the Proposed Transformer Based Architectures

B.1   Basic Transformer Autoencoder Architecture

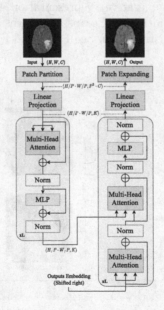

Fig. 4. Basic Transformer Autoencoder (B_TAE).

B.2   Spatial Convolutional Transformer Autoencoder Architecture

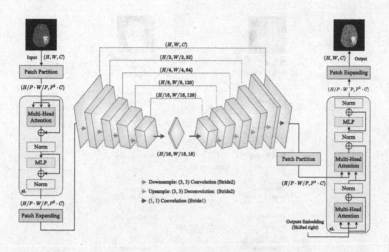

Fig. 5. Spatial Convolutional Transformer Autoencoder (SC_TAE).

B.3   Dense Convolutional Transformer Autoencoder Architecture

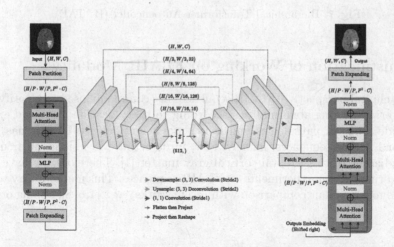

Fig. 6. Dense Convolutional Transformer Autoencoder (DC_TAE).

B.4   Hierarchical Transformer Autoencoder Architecture

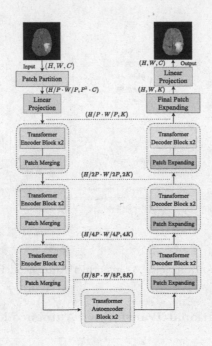

Fig. 7. Hierarchical Transformer Autoencoder (H_TAE).

C   Justification of Working on FLAIR Modality

From a clinical perspective, FLAIR sequences are commonly used to identify and characterize imaging abnormalities according to their location, size, and extent in a wide range of pathologies and lesion manifestations [2]. FLAIR has been superior to other sequences, namely T2w, in detecting MS lesions, particularly those adjacent to the cerebral cortical gray matter [1]. Therefore, we have constrained running our experiments on FLAIR sequences. This methodology would allow us to have a fair comparison with recent works, e.g., [4,6–8], among others.

D   Additional Information on the Hierarchical Transformer Layers

– **Patch Merging:** The patch merging layer decreases the number of tokens by a multiple of $2 \times 2 = 4$ (2 down-sampling of resolution) and increases the feature dimension to half of the input dimension accordingly.
– **Patch Expanding:** The patch expanding layer expands the number of tokens by a multiple of $2 \times 2 = 4$ (2 up-sampling of resolution) and reduces the feature dimension to half of the input dimension accordingly.

E   Contribution of the Transformer Blocks in Each of the Proposed Architectures

Table 3. Role of the Transformer blocks according to each model.

Role	B_TAE	DC_TAE	SC_TAE	H_TAE	H_TAE_S
Encodes strong global context by treating, along an attention mechanism, the image features as sequences	✓	✓	✓	✗	✗
Captures short/long-range spatial correlations by combining the self-attention mechanism with down and up-sampling	✗	✗	✗	✓	✓

F   Architecture Specificities

We compared our five transformer autoencoder (TAE) models with SOTA models as AE(dense), AE(spatial), VAE and variational autoencoder (VQ-VAE) using the same training configurations and a unified CNN architecture [7] for all benchmark models. See Table 4 for additional information about bottleneck size and intermediate dimension.

Table 4. Bottleneck sizes for each of the benchmark and proposed models.

Model	AE (dense)	AE (spatial)	VAE	VQ-VAE	B_TAE	DC_TAE	SC_TAE	H_TAE(_S)
Bottleneck	(512,)	(16, 16, 16)	(512,)	(512,)	(256, 96)	(512,)	(16, 16, 16)	(1024, 768)

G   Ablation Study

Considering that B_TAE is a model deduced from the ablation of the AE(dense) and AE(spatial) respectively inside the D_CTAE and SC_TAE bottlenecks and that the H_TAE is an ablation of the H_TAE_S's skip connections, we can interpret the following Tables 5 and 6 as an ablation study results on the BraTS and MSLUB datasets, respectively. Therefore, we can conclude from these results that the two models DC_TAE and H_TAE_S are globally the best-performing methods on average on the two considered test sets.

Table 5. Ablation study results on the BraTS dataset.

Approach	AUROC ↑	AUPRC ↑	[DSC] $(\mu \pm \sigma)$ ↑
B_TAE	0.6142	0.1221	0.4252 ± 0.4475
DC_TAE	**0.7672**	**0.3498**	**0.4603 ± 0.4022**
SC_TAE	0.6847	0.2561	0.4552 ± 0.4180
H_TAE	0.5472	0.0716	0.3593 ± 0.4020
H_TAE_S	<u>0.7763</u>	<u>0.5086</u>	<u>0.5296 ± 0.4417</u>

Table 6. Ablation study results on the MSLUB dataset.

Approach	AUROC ↑	AUPRC ↑	[DSC] $(\mu \pm \sigma)$ ↑
B_TAE	**0.7272**	0.0177	0.1490 ± 0.2747
DC_TAE	<u>0.8745</u>	<u>0.1609</u>	<u>0.1631 ± 0.2926</u>
SC_TAE	0.6669	0.0133	0.1306 ± 0.2682
H_TAE	0.5788	**0.0374**	**0.1592 ± 0.2865**
H_TAE_S	0.6906	0.0209	0.1489 ± 0.2857

H   Parameters Tuning

We considered, for the parameters tuning process, just for the two DC_TAE and H_TAE_S models according to their performance on the last Tables 5 and 6. You can find the results of the parameters tuning process presented in Table 7 for BraTS test set and Table 8 for MSLUB test set. For the H_TAE_S we were able

Table 7. Parameters tuning results on the BraTS dataset.

Approach	Layers	Patches	Heads	AUROC ↑	AUPRC ↑	[DSC] ($\mu \pm \sigma$) ↑
DC_TAE	8	8	4	0.7755	0.3824	0.4821 ± 0.4058
DC_TAE	8	8	8	**0.8016**	**0.5193**	0.4935 ± 0.4128
DC_TAE	8	16	4	0.7672	0.3498	0.4603 ± 0.4022
DC_TAE	8	16	8	0.7890	0.4673	**0.5060 ± 0.4064**
DC_TAE	12	8	4	0.7773	0.3905	0.4714 ± 0.4052
DC_TAE	12	8	8	**0.8012**	**0.5411**	0.4977 ± 0.4117
DC_TAE	12	16	8	0.7802	0.4250	**0.5017 ± 0.4056**
H_TAE_S	8	4	4	**0.7763**	**0.5086**	**0.5296 ± 0.4417**
H_TAE_S	8	4	8	0.5863	0.1346	0.3444 ± 0.3814

Table 8. Parameters tuning results on the MSLUB dataset.

Approach	Layers	Patches	Heads	AUROC ↑	AUPRC ↑	[DSC] ($\mu \pm \sigma$) ↑
DC_TAE	8	8	4	**0.8909**	0.0975	0.1562 ± 0.2931
DC_TAE	8	8	8	**0.8892**	0.0444	0.1556 ± 0.2920
DC_TAE	8	16	4	0.8745	0.1609	0.1631 ± 0.2926
DC_TAE	8	16	8	0.8765	0.1299	0.1687 ± 0.2955
DC_TAE	12	8	4	0.8776	**0.1812**	**0.1787 ± 0.2958**
DC_TAE	12	8	8	0.8657	0.0329	0.1599 ± 0.2915
DC_TAE	12	16	8	0.8861	**0.2025**	**0.1728 ± 0.2971**
H_TAE_S	8	4	4	**0.6906**	**0.0209**	**0.1489 ± 0.2857**
H_TAE_S	8	4	8	0.5335	0.0046	0.1114 ± 0.2184

to test only two configurations because of the computational cost. Considering the results down below, we can conclude that the best configuration for the H_TAE_S is the one with (8: number of layers, 4: patch size, 4: number of heads) and for DC_TAE is the one with (12: number of layers, 16: patch size, 8: number of heads).

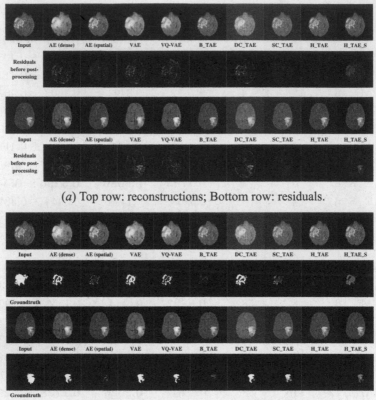

(*a*) Top row: reconstructions; Bottom row: residuals.

(*b*) Top row: reconstructions; Bottom row: masks.

Fig. 8. Visual examples of the different reviewed methods on BraTS dataset.

I   Qualitative Results

Qualitative brain segmentation comparisons are presented in Fig. 8 and Fig. 9. VAE, DC_TAE, and H_TAE_S show improved segmentation performance of the Glioblastoma (GB) on BraTS dataset. Segmenting the lesions in MSLUB dataset seems a little more difficult than detecting the GB on BraTS, given the small size of the lesions. Compared to the basic and spatial Transformer-based models, DC_TAE exhibits higher boundary segmentation accuracy and performs better in capturing the fine-grained details of tumors.

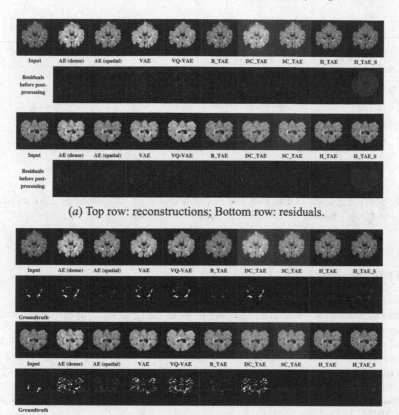

(a) Top row: reconstructions; Bottom row: residuals.

(b) Top row: reconstructions; Bottom row: masks.

Fig. 9. Visual examples of the different reviewed methods on MSLUB dataset.

J   Complexity Analysis

Scatter graphs of the number of parameters (in millions) versus the theoretically best possible DICE-score ([DSC]) for our Transformer-based models and SOTA models according to BraTS (left graph) and MSLUB (right graph) test-sets are displayed on Fig. 10. We are aware of the model complexity that comes with the Transformers. However, we relax this complexity in our investigation, hoping to achieve a significant improvement over the SOTA anomaly detection models. In the future, we would like to incorporate special algorithms into our models to improve performance and reduce computation complexity, as inspired by recent work [13] on innovative Transformer models for the image classification task.

42   A. Ghorbel et al.

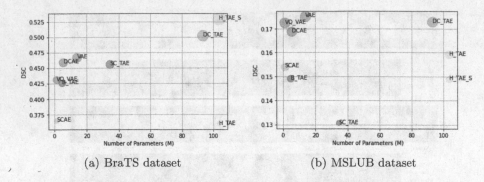

(a) BraTS dataset   (b) MSLUB dataset

Fig. 10. Scatter graphs of the number of parameters M in million vs Dice Similarity Coefficient (DSC) tested on BraTS and MSLUB datasets.

References

1. Bakshi, R., Ariyaratana, S., Benedict, R.H., Jacobs, L.: Fluid-attenuated inversion recovery magnetic resonance imaging detects cortical and juxtacortical multiple sclerosis lesions. Arch. Neurol. **58**(5), 742–748 (2001)
2. Duong, M.T., et al.: Convolutional neural network for automated FLAIR lesion segmentation on clinical brain MR imaging. Am. J. Neuroradiol. **40**(8), 1282–1290 (2019)
3. Iglesias, J.E., Liu, C.Y., Thompson, P.M., Tu, Z.: Robust brain extraction across datasets and comparison with publicly available methods. IEEE Trans. Med. Imaging **30**(9), 1617–1634 (2011)
4. Pinaya, W.H.L., et al.: Unsupervised brain anomaly detection and segmentation with transformers. arXiv preprint arXiv:2102.11650 (2021)
5. Van Den Oord, A., Vinyals, O.: Neural discrete representation learning. In: Advances in Neural Information Processing Systems, vol. 30 (2017)
6. Baur, C., Wiestler, B., Albarqouni, S., Navab, N.: Deep autoencoding models for unsupervised anomaly segmentation in brain MR images. In: Crimi, A., Bakas, S., Kuijf, H., Keyvan, F., Reyes, M., van Walsum, T. (eds.) BrainLes 2018. LNCS, vol. 11383, pp. 161–169. Springer, Cham (2019). https://doi.org/10.1007/978-3-030-11723-8_16
7. Baur, C., Denner, S., Wiestler, B., Navab, N., Albarqouni, S.: Autoencoders for unsupervised anomaly segmentation in brain MR images: a comparative study. Med. Image Anal. **69**, 101952 (2021)
8. Zimmerer, D., Isensee, F., Petersen, J., Kohl, S., Maier-Hein, K.: Unsupervised anomaly localization using variational auto-encoders. In: Shen, D., et al. (eds.) MICCAI 2019. LNCS, vol. 11767, pp. 289–297. Springer, Cham (2019). https://doi.org/10.1007/978-3-030-32251-9_32
9. Baur, C., Wiestler, B., Muehlau, M., Zimmer, C., Navab, N., Albarqouni, S.: Modeling healthy anatomy with artificial intelligence for unsupervised anomaly detection in brain MRI. Radiol. Artif. Intell. **3**(3) (2021)
10. Valanarasu, J.M.J., Oza, P., Hacihaliloglu, I., Patel, V.M.: Medical transformer: gated axial-attention for medical image segmentation. In: de Bruijne, M., et al. (eds.) MICCAI 2021. LNCS, vol. 12901, pp. 36–46. Springer, Cham (2021). https://doi.org/10.1007/978-3-030-87193-2_4

11. Hatamizadeh, A., et al.: UNETR: transformers for 3D medical image segmentation. In: Proceedings of the IEEE/CVF Winter Conference on Applications of Computer Vision, pp. 574–584 (2022)
12. Yan, X., Tang, H., Sun, S., Ma, H., Kong, D., Xie, X.: AFTer-UNet: axial fusion transformer UNet for medical image segmentation. In: Proceedings of the IEEE/CVF Winter Conference on Applications of Computer Vision, pp. 3971–3981 (2022)
13. Liu, Z., et al.: Swin transformer: hierarchical vision transformer using shifted windows. In: Proceedings of the IEEE/CVF International Conference on Computer Vision, pp. 10012–10022 (2021)
14. Wang, W., et al.: Pyramid vision transformer: a versatile backbone for dense prediction without convolutions. In: Proceedings of the IEEE/CVF International Conference on Computer Vision, pp. 568–578 (2021)
15. Carion, N., Massa, F., Synnaeve, G., Usunier, N., Kirillov, A., Zagoruyko, S.: End-to-end object detection with transformers. In: Vedaldi, A., Bischof, H., Brox, T., Frahm, J.-M. (eds.) ECCV 2020. LNCS, vol. 12346, pp. 213–229. Springer, Cham (2020). https://doi.org/10.1007/978-3-030-58452-8_13
16. Dai, X., Chen, Y., Yang, J., Zhang, P., Yuan, L., Zhang, L.: Dynamic DETR: end-to-end object detection with dynamic attention. In: Proceedings of the IEEE/CVF International Conference on Computer Vision, pp. 2988–2997 (2021)
17. Wang, X., Girshick, R., Gupta, A., He, K.: Non-local neural networks. In: Proceedings of the IEEE Conference on Computer Vision and Pattern Recognition, pp. 7794–7803 (2018)
18. Schlemper, J., et al.: Attention gated networks: learning to leverage salient regions in medical images. Med. Image Anal. **53**, 197–207 (2019)
19. Vaswani, A., et al.: Attention is all you need. In: Advances in Neural Information Processing Systems, vol. 30 (2017)
20. Parmar, N., et al.: Image transformer. In: International Conference on Machine Learning, pp. 4055–4064. PMLR (2018)
21. Child, R., Gray, S., Radford, A., Sutskever, I.: Generating long sequences with sparse transformers. arXiv preprint arXiv:1904.10509 (2019)
22. Dosovitskiy, A., et al.: An image is worth 16x16 words: transformers for image recognition at scale. arXiv preprint arXiv:2010.11929 (2020)
23. Isensee, F., Jaeger, P.F., Kohl, S.A., Petersen, J., Maier-Hein, K.H.: nnU-Net: a self-configuring method for deep learning-based biomedical image segmentation. Nat. Methods **18**(2), 203–211 (2021)
24. Siddique, N., Paheding, S., Elkin, C.P., Devabhaktuni, V.: U-net and its variants for medical image segmentation: a review of theory and applications. IEEE Access **9**, 82031–82057 (2021)
25. Chen, X., Konukoglu, E.: Unsupervised detection of lesions in brain MRI using constrained adversarial auto-encoders. arXiv preprint arXiv:1806.04972 (2018)
26. Bruno, M.A., Walker, E.A., Abujudeh, H.H.: Understanding and confronting our mistakes: the epidemiology of error in radiology and strategies for error reduction. Radiographics **35**(6), 1668–1676 (2015)
27. Taboada-Crispi, A., Sahli, H., Hernandez-Pacheco, D., Falcon-Ruiz, A.: Anomaly detection in medical image analysis. In: Handbook of Research on Advanced Techniques in Diagnostic Imaging and Biomedical Applications, pp. 426–446. IGI Global (2009)
28. Zheng, S., et al.: Rethinking semantic segmentation from a sequence-to-sequence perspective with transformers. In: Proceedings of the IEEE/CVF Conference on Computer Vision and Pattern Recognition, pp. 6881–6890 (2021)

29. Cao, H., et al.: Swin-Unet: Unet-like pure transformer for medical image segmentation. arXiv preprint arXiv:2105.05537 (2021)
30. Zhang, Y., Liu, H., Hu, Q.: TransFuse: fusing transformers and CNNs for medical image segmentation. In: de Bruijne, M., et al. (eds.) MICCAI 2021. LNCS, vol. 12901, pp. 14–24. Springer, Cham (2021). https://doi.org/10.1007/978-3-030-87193-2_2
31. LaMontagne, P.J., et al.: OASIS-3: longitudinal neuroimaging, clinical, and cognitive dataset for normal aging and Alzheimer disease. MedRxiv (2019)
32. Menze, B.H., et al.: The multimodal brain tumor image segmentation benchmark (BRATS). IEEE Trans. Med. Imaging **34**(10), 1993–2024 (2014)
33. Lesjak, Ž, et al.: A novel public MR image dataset of multiple sclerosis patients with lesion segmentations based on multi-rater consensus. Neuroinformatics **16**(1), 51–63 (2018)
34. Zhang, H., Oguz, I.: Multiple sclerosis lesion segmentation - a survey of supervised CNN-based methods. In: Crimi, A., Bakas, S. (eds.) BrainLes 2020. LNCS, vol. 12658, pp. 11–29. Springer, Cham (2021). https://doi.org/10.1007/978-3-030-72084-1_2
35. Han, C., et al.: MADGAN: unsupervised medical anomaly detection GAN using multiple adjacent brain MRI slice reconstruction. BMC Bioinform. **22**(2), 1–20 (2021)
36. Tian, Yu., et al.: Constrained contrastive distribution learning for unsupervised anomaly detection and localisation in medical images. In: de Bruijne, M., et al. (eds.) MICCAI 2021. LNCS, vol. 12905, pp. 128–140. Springer, Cham (2021). https://doi.org/10.1007/978-3-030-87240-3_13
37. Van Oord, A., Kalchbrenner, N., Kavukcuoglu, K.: Pixel recurrent neural networks. In: International Conference on Machine Learning, pp. 1747–1756. PMLR (2016)

Weighting Schemes for Federated Learning in Heterogeneous and Imbalanced Segmentation Datasets

Sebastian Otálora[1(✉)], Jonathan Rafael-Patiño[3], Antoine Madrona[3],
Elda Fischi-Gomez[3], Veronica Ravano[2,3,4], Tobias Kober[2,3,4],
Søren Christensen[5], Arsany Hakim[1], Roland Wiest[1], Jonas Richiardi[3],
and Richard McKinley[1]

[1] Support Center for Advanced Neuroimaging (SCAN),
University Institute of Diagnostic and Interventional Neuroradiology,
Inselspital, Bern University Hospital, Bern, Switzerland
juan.otaloramontenegro@insel.ch
[2] Advanced Clinical Imaging Technology, Siemens Healthcare AG,
Lausanne, Switzerland
[3] Department of Radiology, Lausanne University Hospital and University
of Lausanne, Lausanne, Switzerland
[4] LTS5, École Polytechnique Fédérale de Lausanne (EPFL), Lausanne, Switzerland
[5] Stanford Stroke Center, Stanford University School of Medicine, Palo Alto, USA

Abstract. Federated learning allows for training deep learning models
from various sources (e.g., hospitals) without sharing patient information, but only the model weights. Two central problems arise when send-
ing the updated weights to the central node in a federation: the imbalance
of the datasets and data heterogeneity caused by differences in scanners
or acquisition protocols. In this paper, we benchmark the federated average algorithm and adapt two weighting functions to counteract the effect
of data imbalance. The approaches are validated on a segmentation task
with synthetic data from imbalanced centers, and on two multi-centric
datasets with the clinically relevant tasks of stroke infarct core prediction
and brain tumor segmentation. The results show that accounting for the
imbalance in the data sources improves the federated average aggregation in different perfusion CT and structural MRI images in the ISLES
and BraTS19 datasets, respectively.

Keywords: Federated learning · Federated Average · Medical data
imbalance · Medical image segmentation · Deep learning · Perfusion CT

1 Introduction

Deep learning has been shown to be successful in the key computer vision task
of image segmentation [15]. In particular, it excels in applications to medical
image analysis [3]. Robust methods for the automated segmentation of medical images are essential in clinical routine to support the treatment choice and

S. Bakas et al. (Eds.): BrainLes 2022, LNCS 13769, pp. 45–56, 2023.
https://doi.org/10.1007/978-3-031-33842-7_4

ensure a better patient outcome, for example, in thrombectomy eligibility for stroke [6], and for accurate and reproducible measurements of tumor substructures in glioma [1,14]. Despite their undeniable utility, deep learning segmentation models require large training datasets and are sensitive to the shifts in data distribution which can arise from differences in scanner hardware, software, or acquisition protocols between institutions, making it difficult to deploy such tools across multiple institutions. The aggregation of data from all available heterogeneous sources into a single training set is the most commonly used solution to achieve robust models. However, such an approach implies data sharing between different hospitals or institutions, which is typically hindered by privacy, legal, and data security concerns [19], especially when involving international collaborations. Federated learning permits the training of deep learning models from various data sources (e.g., hospitals) without sharing images; only the updated model weights, trained with local data, are shared. Thus the vast amount of centralized data needed to train deep learning models may also be acquired in applications to the medical domain.

Federated Learning (FL) consists of three steps: (1) train an initial model in all the federation clients using their local data. (2) Once the local model is trained for one or few local epochs, each client sends its updated model weights to one of the clients (or single server) that orchestrates the execution of the algorithm [19] and aggregates the model weights, for example, by averaging of the clients' weights. (3) Distribute the aggregated model across the clients and repeat the local training with more rounds. These rounds stop once a convergence criterion is met, see Algorithm 1.

FL can perform similarly to centralized learning using gradient averaging [18]. Nevertheless, in a real-world federation, several constraints such as network availability make the intense communication of gradient averaging infeasible. Federated average is a strong baseline and is used in real-world scenarios [17].

In FL, state-of-the-art approaches often assume many clients, such as smartphones or network sensors, each of which has a small set of local data from which the model should learn [8]. However, this does not describe the situation for a typical medical imaging problem. Here the setup typically consists of a small number of hospitals or centers (fewer than 100). Heterogeneous data due to differences in image count, acquisition protocols, scanners, and patient demographics, among other factors, lead to non-identical client data distributions. In this case, the federated deep learning models must overcome these data disparities to avoid pitfalls such as overfitting to one of the centers or averaging updates from very heterogeneous datasets, preventing the convergence of the global model.

Related Work: In medical imaging, previous FL approaches have tackled the issue of privacy [11] and domain generalisation [12]. In the work of Roth et al. [20], a FL approach was implemented for breast density classification. The authors deliberately did not attempt any data harmonization methods. Their paper shows the effect of different data domains and highlighted the marked differences in intensity distributions due to different mammography systems as well as the need for future research to address the data size heterogeneity in clients.

In HeteroFL [5], the authors proposed an algorithm to update a global model using different local architectures over heterogeneous clients, which may differ in computation power and communication bandwidth in addition to data distribution. Cui et al. [4] proposed a simple yet effective weighting scheme for deep learning model training in the context of datasets with a highly skewed class distribution.

Chang et al. [2] proposed a cyclical weight transfer and showed that it performed comparably to centrally hosted data in the retinal eye fundus imaging Kaggle dataset. Sheller et al. [21] compared the cyclical weight transfer in a dataset where the data is non-iid and obtain better results using the federated average approach, suggesting that more research is needed to understand under which circumstances federated average can overcome the non-iid FL scenario in medical imaging. An extensive survey in FL and the open problems [7] provides a more complete overview of the previous work performed on these lines of research.

In this paper our contributions are the following:

- First benchmark of FL aggregation strategies for stroke infarct core segmentation.
- Study of the efficacy of different weighting schemes with respect to data heterogeneity in FL segmentation algorithms.
- Adaptation of two weighting functions to improve the FedAvg algorithm updates in presence of data-imbalanced and heterogeneous centers.

The source code and data necessary to reproduce our experiments and results can be accessed here: https://github.com/sebastianffx/fedem.

The rest of our paper is organized as follows: in Sect. 2 we provide a description of the federated average algorithm and of the two weighting functions we have devised to address the data size heterogeneity problem. Section 3 gives the details on the datasets used for the experiments and the network architectures. Quantitative and qualitative segmentation results of the experiments are presented in Sect. 4. Finally, we discuss the results and conclude the paper in Sect. 5.

2   Federated Average

The Federated Average (FedAvg) algorithm computes an average of each of the clients' updated model weights and redistributes the updated global model weights to each client, repeating this procedure for several rounds until the global model convergence. McMahan et al. [13] formulated the algorithm, which demonstrated superior robustness in comparison with federated stochastic gradient descent updates to the global model. Pseudo-code of FedAvg with weighting functions is shown in Algorithm 1. FedAvg aggregates the clients' model weights by a weighted average (Line 8 in Algorithm 1), where $n = \sum_{k=1}^{K} n_k$, is the total number of samples in the dataset. This heavily penalizes centers with few data samples and potentially leads to *client-drift* towards those clients where $n_i \gg n_j \forall j \neq i \in [1, ..., K]$. Below, inspired by weighting schemes designed to mitigate class imbalance, we propose two weighting functions that aim to increase the contribution of the clients with less data to the global model update (line 8 in Algorithm 1).

2.1   Federated Average Weighting Functions

Weighted Average: In the formulation of FedAvg [13], the weights are averaged as follows:

$$f(n_k) = \frac{n_k}{n}$$

where n_k is the number of elements in the $k-$th client and n is the total number of samples.

β-**weighting:** In [4], the authors propose to weight the loss of a classifier trained with class-imbalanced data using the concept of the effective number of samples. Instead of weighting the loss with respect to class, here we propose to adapt it to the problem of centre-imbalance. The weight reflects the contribution for each center updates:

$$f(n_k) = \frac{1 - \beta}{1 - \beta^{n_k}}$$

The β hyperparameter ranges between $[0, 1]$, where 0 represents no weight and 1 corresponds to re-weighing by inverse number of samples (inverse class frequency in the original formulation).

Softmax Weighting: We propose the use of a softmax function to transform the vector of number of samples per client to a probability distribution proportional to the exponential of the number of samples per client:

$$f(n_k) = \frac{e^{n_k}}{\sum_{i=1}^{K} e^{n_i}}$$

Normalization Term: The normalization term $\frac{1}{Z}$ (line 8 in Algorithm 1) corresponds to $Z = K$ for FedAvg, i.e., the inverse of the number of clients. For β and the softmax weighting $Z = \sum_{k=1}^{K} f(n_k)$. The weights could diverge when no normalization is applied, becoming too large or extremely small (over-normalization) (Fig. 1).

3   Experimental Setup

Synthetic 3D: We created a synthetic dataset with heterogeneous shapes, composed by overlapping three-dimensional volumes—specifically, spheres and cubes—of varying size and intensity. Each image contained a single type of the two three-dimensional geometries that were randomly placed within a contained

Algorithm 1. Federated Average Training. K centers; W_G global model weights; $\{w\}^k$ are the model weights of the k–th center; η learning rate; f is either the weighted average (FedAvg), β, or softmax weighting functions. Z is the normalization term

1: **Server executes:**
2: Initialize W_G
3: **for** each round $t = 1, 2, \dots$ **do**
4:     Send W_G to each client
5:     **for** each client $k = 1, 2, ..., K$ **do**   ▷ In parallel
6:         $w_{t+1}^k \leftarrow \text{ClientUpdate}(k, W_G)$
7:     **end for**
8:     $W_G \leftarrow \frac{1}{Z} \sum_{k=1}^{K} f(n_k) w_{t+1}^k$
9: **end for**
10: **ClientUpdate**(k, w):
11: **for** each local epoch i from 1 to E **do**   ▷ Runs for each client k
12:     **for** each batch $b \in dataloader_k$ **do**
13:         $w \leftarrow w - \eta \Delta \ell(w; b)$
14:     **end for**
15: **end for**
16: Return w to the server

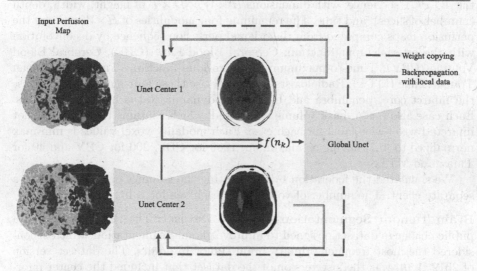

Fig. 1. Federated learning for infarct core prediction: Each of the clients perform a local training epoch with its data. After, the local trained weights (w_k) and the number of local training samples (n_k) of each client are sent to the weighting function $f(n_k)$ to obtain the new global model. For each new round, the clients continue the training with the updated global weights, until convergence.

volume of size $224 \times 224 \times 8$ voxels. Each volume contained an arbitrary number of spheres ranging between three and forty. Additionally, the size of the spheres was randomly chosen between 5 and 10 voxel radius. Similarly, the cubes were randomly placed with a random number between 50 and 80 cubes and a size randomly chosen from a Gamma distribution, $\Gamma(\kappa = 1, \theta = 3)$, where κ and θ are the shape and scale parameters, respectively. The intensities of the spheres and cubes were also randomly chosen between 0.3 and 1. Finally, the images were corrupted using Gaussian noise with $\mu = 0$ and $\sigma = 0.1$. In the case of the federated training, we used a heterogeneous partition of the data by number and shape type.

ISLES2018 Dataset (ISLES): The ISLES dataset was downloaded from the public Ischemic Stroke Lesion Segmentation challenge 2018[1]. The dataset includes data from 4 centers. It consists of 103 acute anterior circulation large artery occlusion stroke patients who underwent diffusion-weighted imaging after the CT perfusion sequence (CTP).

Diffusion-weighted MRI imaging was obtained within three hours of CTP. The stroke lesion was manually segmented on the DWI and was considered as reference standard. A comprehensive description of the dataset and the methods used in the challenge is provided in Hakim et al. [6].

From the training set, 94 cases with their respective annotations were used throughout the experiments. Each perfusion case comprises five input modalities: the 4D PCT sequence, with dimensions $H \times W \times D \times T$ of height, width, depth (number of slices), and time. The remaining four modalities of $H \times W \times D$, are the perfusion maps computed from the original perfusion sequence by deconvolution with the arterial input function: Cerebral Blood Flow (CBF), Cerebral Blood Volume (CBV), Time-to-maximum of the residue function (Tmax), and Mean Transit Time (MTT). Radiologists frequently use these four modalities to assess the infarct core, penumbra and brain hemodynamic status in stroke patients. Each case also has a mask volume associated, which contains the infarcted/not infarcted voxel-wise label for each case. Each modality voxel values is min-max normalized to [0,1] having as maximum: 1200 for CBF, 200 for CBV and 40 for Tmax and MTT.

We simulated the federation by distributing the volumes of each vendor as a separate client. The number of volumes for each vendor is in Table 1.

Brain Tumour Segmentation (BraTS) Dataset: The BraTS dataset is a public challenge dataset designed to improve glioma segmentation, which is considered the most frequent primary brain tumor in adults. The dataset version of 2019 [1,14] was the last version of the dataset that included the center information, and is the one used in our experiments. The BraTS dataset was also used recently [17] in a real-world federation, showing how FL can enable deep learning models to gain knowledge from extensive and diverse data that would otherwise not be available. The number of volumes for each vendor is in Table 2.

Segmentation Network: The deep learning architecture selected for the synthetic and ISLES experiments is the widely-used U-net architecture, with residual unit blocks [10], as implemented in the open-source MONAI (version 0.8)

---

[1] http://www.isles-challenge.org/.

framework[2]. The network has two spatial input dimensions (2D- slice-wise segmentation). Each input corresponds to a perfusion map, i.e.: CBF, Tmax, MTT, or CBV; or a synthetically generated volume, with either randomly generated circular or rectangular patches. The number of network channels is 16, 32, 64, 128, with a (2,2) stride and 3×3 kernel size. The number of residual units is 2. Data augmentation was used by including random rotations of 90°, with a probability of 0.5. A random spatial crop of 224×224 was also included. For BraTS the segmentation network is a 3D-SegResNet [16] with the default parameters as implemented in MONAI. For the three networks, segmentation labels corresponding to tumour annotation for BraTS, infarct lesion segmentation for the ISLES, and the mask for synthetically generated 3D shapes were passed.

Network Training: All networks were trained using the Adam optimizer with a batch size of three slices. The learning rate was explored in a log-grid fashion in the range $[10^{-5}, 0.1]$, and the best was selected upon the Dice score coefficient computed in the validation partition and using a threshold of 0.9 on the network output. In the federated experiments, two different numbers of local epochs were explored (1,5), For β, three values were explored: $(0.9, 0.99, 0.999)$. All the centralized experiments used a learning rate of 0.00132, while 0.000932 was used for the federated experiments. Once the best learning rate was selected, each experiment run of [federated/centralized, modality, $f(n_k)$] was performed five times to reduce the effect of random initialization. All experiments were implemented in the PyTorch deep learning framework[3] with standard data augmentation (90,180,270 rotations and flip w.r.t. to the y-axis) using the TorchIO library[4]. We aim to know if there is a particular advantage in changing the aggregation of the networks' weights and not optimizing a specific architecture. Therefore, we opted only to explore the learning rate until a stable convergence for each method is obtained, leaving the rest of the hyper-parameters as default (Table 3).

Table 1. Vendor-wise partitions distribution for the ISLES challenge dataset.

ISLES	General Electric	Philips	Toshiba	Siemens
Train	15	39	9	1
Validation	3	7	2	0
Test	4	11	2	1
Total	22	57	13	2

---

[2] https://monai.io/.
[3] https://pytorch.org/.
[4] https://torchio.readthedocs.io/index.html.

Table 2. Centre distribution for the BraTS19 challenge dataset.

BraTS19	2013	CBICA	TCIA	TMC
Train	14	90	71	5
Validation	2	14	11	1
Test	4	25	20	2
Total	20	129	102	8

Table 3. Data partitions of the synthetic dataset in three centers separated by number of spheres and cubes in the dataset.

[#spheres][#cubes]	Center 1	Center 2	Center 3
Train	[20][0]	[10][0]	[0][15]
Test	[5][0]	[5][0]	[0][5]
Validation	[5][0]	[5][0]	[0][5]
Total	[30][0]	[20][0]	[0][25]

4 Results

Table 4 shows the average Dice coefficient of the synthetic data test set, the 18 ISLES and the 51 BraTS test volumes. Overall, centralized training outperforms federated learning strategies. We observed a marked performance drop between the centralized and the FedAvg approach in all cases. The β-Weighting strategy improves performance compared to the standard weight average of the FedAvg approach across all input map types. As reference, the best segmentation method submitted to the ISLES challenge using all the modalities and more training data reached a Dice score of 0.558. In the synthetic case the difference between the centralized and the β average performances suggest that they are closer than with the other FL weightings; despite the high Dice across all the models.

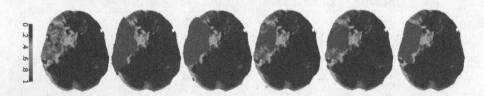

Fig. 2. Tmax slice from a test-set volume. From the left: Input image, ground truth overlay (red), centralized, FedAvg, β and softmax predictions, respectively. (Color figure online)

Dice coefficient alone is not a sufficient metric to evaluate the segmentation performance of the strategies. We reported it to align with existing literature

Table 4. Segmentation results in the synthetic, ISLES and BraTS test sets. For each entry the mean of 5 runs is reported with standard deviation.

Dataset	Centralized	FedAvg [13]	β weighting	Softmax
Synthetic	0.984 ± 0.066	0.964 ± 0.122	0.982 ± 0.092	0.969 ± 0.059
CBF	0.454 ± 0.093	0.446 ± 0.090	0.450 ± 0.008	0.4078 ± 0.020
MTT	0.450 ± 0.103	0.481 ± 0.014	0.4863 ± 0.016	0.377 ± 0.031
Tmax	0.475 ± 0.103	0.462 ± 0.097	0.476 ± 0.101	0.463 ± 0.082
CBV	0.331 ± 0.048	0.353 ± 0.050	0.362± 0.051	0.309 ± 0.033
BraTS	0.729 ± 0.039	0.688 ± 0.0021	0.692 ± 0.003	0.593 ± 0.010

and with the challenge metrics. Because of this, we also computed the overall test-set Hausdorff distance for the Tmax map, and the results confirm that the performance is better for the beta strategy: FedAvg obtained an average Hausdorff distance of 49.3 ± 9.5, while β-Weighting obtained 39.1 ± 8.3 and 24.5 ± 19.3 for the centralized training. We have also computed the precision and recall scores for all modalities in Table 5.

Table 5. Precision and recall scores for the ISLES test set.

Input	Prec. FedAvg	Prec. β	Prec. Cent.	Rec. FedAvg	Rec. β	Rec. Cent.
CBF	0.514 ± 0.19	0.516 ± 0.13	0.347 ± 0.15	0.564 ± 0.25	0.668 ± 0.18	0.580 ± 0.24
MTT	0.568 ± 0.05	0.677 ± 0.09	0.795 ± 0.11	0.423 ± 0.11	0.802 ± 0.14	0.392 ± 0.21
Tmax	0.567 ± 0.06	0.629 ± 0.05	0.818 ± 0.17	0.452 ± 0.28	0.443 ± 0.12	0.364 ± 0.26
CBV	0.627 ± 0.04	0.536 ± 0.09	0.553 ± 0.13	0.325 ± 0.23	0.290 ± 0.28	0.106 ± 0.07

For the ISLES test set, in Fig. 2 a randomly selected slice is shown with a large infarct area to better compare across methods. The centralized column shows a large high-probability connected component with more true positives. Compared with FedAvg, β-weighted model output has a larger predicted area with high within the infarcted lesion. Softmax has the largest area within the ground truth in this case. In the BraTS dataset, the β weighting performance is also closer to the centralized approach, driven by learning more from those centers with few data as shown in Fig. 3.

Statistical Test: To assess if there exists a statistically significant difference between the performance results of the β weighting and the FedAvg, we performed a statistical test as follows. We calculate the average Dice for each test volume over the five runs for a single modality, then all the modalities results vectors (β, FedAvg) are concatenated. With these two result vectors, we compute the Wilcoxon signed-rank test (scipy 1.8) to assess the null hypothesis that the results difference distribution is symmetric about zero. The test results indicated the null hypothesis was rejected, with a p-value of 0.0048. We also

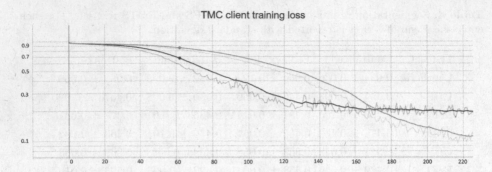

Fig. 3. Training loss on BRaTS for the TMC client in the federated approach. Orange is β-weighting and blue is FedAvg. (Color figure online)

confirmed that the median of the differences can be assumed to be positive with a p-value of 0.0024. We observe that this difference seems to be driven by an increase in the performance of centers with little available training data. Nevertheless, the center-wise test distribution (4,11,2,1) leaves very few samples to compute center-wise tests with sufficient power.

5   Discussion and Conclusion

The use of (unweighted) Federated Average for federated training of a segmentation model suffers from an important decrease in model performance if data is unbalanced and heterogeneous. We showed that simple re-weighting procedures can improve almost to the level of the centralized baseline, opening the possibility for creating large federations of medical institutions for training segmentation models regardless of the dataset size of each center's contribution.

We showed that the re-weighting strategies are useful for both 2D (ISLES18) and 3D (BraTS) standard segmentation networks, in both cases approaching closer to the centralized performance than the FedAvg baseline. We hypothesize that similar conclusions might arise using the recently proposed 3D U-nets and transformer-based segmentation networks such as Swin-UNETRs [22].

Interestingly, for CBF in Table 5 the centralized approach has lower volume-wise precision (but higher recall) than the federated approaches, suggesting that the centralized training might drift the performance towards those centers over represented in the training set, while the federated approaches retrieve more relevant voxels.

We will continue addressing these challenges in future work by using larger heterogeneous clinical datasets and comparing the re-weightings with gradient correction methods such as SCAFFOLD [9] and using multi-channel Unet and transformer-based segmentation networks.

Acknowledgements. This work was co-financed by Innosuisse (grant 43087.1 IP-LS).

References

1. Bakas, S., et al.: Advancing the cancer genome atlas glioma MRI collections with expert segmentation labels and radiomic features. Sci. Data **4**(1), 1–13 (2017)
2. Chang, K., et al.: Distributed deep learning networks among institutions for medical imaging. J. Am. Med. Inform. Assoc. **25**(8), 945–954 (2018)
3. Chen, X., et al.: Recent advances and clinical applications of deep learning in medical image analysis. Med. Image Anal. 102444 (2022)
4. Cui, Y., Jia, M., Lin, T.Y., Song, Y., Belongie, S.: Class-balanced loss based on effective number of samples. In: Proceedings of the IEEE/CVF Conference on Computer Vision and Pattern Recognition, pp. 9268–9277 (2019)
5. Diao, E., Ding, J., Tarokh, V.: Heterofl: computation and communication efficient federated learning for heterogeneous clients. arXiv preprint arXiv:2010.01264 (2020)
6. Hakim, A., et al.: Predicting infarct core from computed tomography perfusion in acute ischemia with machine learning: lessons from the isles challenge. Stroke **52**(7), 2328–2337 (2021)
7. Kairouz, P., et al.: Advances and open problems in federated learning. arXiv preprint arXiv:1912.04977 (2019)
8. Karimireddy, S.P., et al.: Mime: mimicking centralized stochastic algorithms in federated learning. arXiv preprint arXiv:2008.03606 (2020)
9. Karimireddy, S.P., Kale, S., Mohri, M., Reddi, S., Stich, S., Suresh, A.T.: SCAFFOLD: stochastic controlled averaging for federated learning. In: III, H.D., Singh, A. (eds.) Proceedings of the 37th International Conference on Machine Learning. Proceedings of Machine Learning Research, vol. 119, pp. 5132–5143. PMLR (2020). https://proceedings.mlr.press/v119/karimireddy20a.html
10. Kerfoot, E., Clough, J., Oksuz, I., Lee, J., King, A.P., Schnabel, J.A.: Left-ventricle quantification using residual U-Net. In: Pop, M., et al. (eds.) STACOM 2018. LNCS, vol. 11395, pp. 371–380. Springer, Cham (2019). https://doi.org/10.1007/978-3-030-12029-0_40
11. Li, W., et al.: Privacy-preserving federated brain tumour segmentation. In: Suk, H.-I., Liu, M., Yan, P., Lian, C. (eds.) MLMI 2019. LNCS, vol. 11861, pp. 133–141. Springer, Cham (2019). https://doi.org/10.1007/978-3-030-32692-0_16
12. Liu, Q., Chen, C., Qin, J., Dou, Q., Heng, P.A.: FEDDG: federated domain generalization on medical image segmentation via episodic learning in continuous frequency space. In: Proceedings of the IEEE/CVF Conference on Computer Vision and Pattern Recognition, pp. 1013–1023 (2021)
13. McMahan, B., Moore, E., Ramage, D., Hampson, S., Arcas, B.A.: Communication-efficient learning of deep networks from decentralized data. In: Artificial Intelligence and Statistics, pp. 1273–1282. PMLR (2017)
14. Menze, B.H., et al.: The multimodal brain tumor image segmentation benchmark (brats). IEEE Trans. Med. Imaging **34**(10), 1993–2024 (2014)
15. Minaee, S., Boykov, Y.Y., Porikli, F., Plaza, A.J., Kehtarnavaz, N., Terzopoulos, D.: Image segmentation using deep learning: a survey. IEEE Trans. Pattern Anal. Mach. Intell. **44**(7), 3523–3542 (2021)
16. Myronenko, A.: 3D MRI Brain tumor segmentation using autoencoder regularization. In: Crimi, A., Bakas, S., Kuijf, H., Keyvan, F., Reyes, M., van Walsum, T. (eds.) BrainLes 2018. LNCS, vol. 11384, pp. 311–320. Springer, Cham (2019). https://doi.org/10.1007/978-3-030-11726-9_28

17. Pati, S., et al.: Federated learning enables big data for rare cancer boundary detection. arXiv preprint arXiv:2204.10836 (2022)

18. Remedios, S.W., Butman, J.A., Landman, B.A., Pham, D.L.: Federated gradient averaging for multi-site training with momentum-based optimizers. In: Albarqouni, S., et al. (eds.) DART/DCL -2020. LNCS, vol. 12444, pp. 170–180. Springer, Cham (2020). https://doi.org/10.1007/978-3-030-60548-3_17

19. Rieke, N., et al.: The future of digital health with federated learning. NPJ Digit. Med. **3**(1), 1–7 (2020)

20. Roth, H.R., et al.: Federated learning for breast density classification: a real-world implementation. In: Albarqouni, S., et al. (eds.) DART/DCL -2020. LNCS, vol. 12444, pp. 181–191. Springer, Cham (2020). https://doi.org/10.1007/978-3-030-60548-3_18

21. Sheller, M.J., et al.: Federated learning in medicine: facilitating multi-institutional collaborations without sharing patient data. Sci. Rep. **10**(1), 1–12 (2020)

22. Tang, Y., et al.: Self-supervised pre-training of swin transformers for 3D medical image analysis. In: Proceedings of the IEEE/CVF Conference on Computer Vision and Pattern Recognition, pp. 20730–20740 (2022)

Temporally Adjustable Longitudinal Fluid-Attenuated Inversion Recovery MRI Estimation / Synthesis for Multiple Sclerosis

Jueqi Wang, Derek Berger, Erin Mazerolle, Othman Soufan, and Jacob Levman[✉]

Department of Computer Science, St Francis Xavier University, Antigonish, Canada
{x2019cwn,dberger,emazerol,osoufan,jlevman}@stfx.ca

Abstract. Multiple Sclerosis (MS) is a chronic progressive neurological disease characterized by the development of lesions in the white matter of the brain. T_2-fluid-attenuated inversion recovery (FLAIR) brain magnetic resonance imaging (MRI) provides superior visualization and characterization of MS lesions, relative to other MRI modalities. Longitudinal brain FLAIR MRI in MS, involving repetitively imaging a patient over time, provides helpful information for clinicians towards monitoring disease progression. Predicting future whole brain MRI examinations with variable time lag has only been attempted in limited applications, such as healthy aging and structural degeneration in Alzheimer's Disease. In this article, we present novel modifications to deep learning architectures for MS FLAIR image synthesis / estimation, in order to support prediction of longitudinal images in a flexible continuous way. This is achieved with learned transposed convolutions, which support modelling time as a spatially distributed array with variable temporal properties at different spatial locations. Thus, this approach can theoretically model spatially-specific time-dependent brain development, supporting the modelling of more rapid growth at appropriate physical locations, such as the site of an MS brain lesion. This approach also supports the clinician user to define how far into the future a predicted examination should target. Accurate prediction of future rounds of imaging can inform clinicians of potentially poor patient outcomes, which may be able to contribute to earlier treatment and better prognoses. Four distinct deep learning architectures have been developed. The ISBI2015 longitudinal MS dataset was used to validate and compare our proposed approaches. Results demonstrate that a modified ACGAN achieves the best performance and reduces variability in model accuracy. Public domain code is made available at https://github.com/stfxecutables/Temporally-Adjustable-Longitudinal-MRI-Synthesis.

Keywords: Image Synthesis · Longitudinal Prediction · Generative Adversarial Networks · Multiple Sclerosis

1 Introduction

Multiple sclerosis (MS) is a chronic progressive neurological disease with a variable course [1] and has become a major cause of disability among young adults [2]. MS patients develop lesions in the white matter (WM) of the brain. Medical imaging plays

S. Bakas et al. (Eds.): BrainLes 2022, LNCS 13769, pp. 57–67, 2023.
https://doi.org/10.1007/978-3-031-33842-7_5

an essential role as a diagnostic tool, where magnetic resonance imaging (MRI) is widely used for diagnosing MS because structural MRI can be used to image white matter (WM) lesions [3], and T_2-fluid-attenuated inversion recovery (FLAIR) MRI typically provides superior assessment of WM lesions than other commonly acquired sequences [2]. The development of WM lesions on follow-up MRI can be used to monitor disease progression and towards informing clinicians' treatment plans for MS patients [1]. Accurate prediction of future rounds of imaging in MS can warn clinicians as to unhealthy growth trajectories of patients with MS. Since prognoses are generally improved the earlier on in which the treatment begins, image prediction techniques have the potential to warn clinicians as to potential MS progression, and so, once highly accurate image prediction techniques are developed, they can inform clinicians and potentially form a critical component towards early treatment and improvement of clinical outcomes. Therefore, predicting future FLAIR MRI examinations could provide helpful information for clinicians in charge of managing patient care.

Recent studies have shown that deep generative models have the ability to predict future brain degeneration using MRI [4–7, 22–24]. Wegmayr et al. [4] proposed to use the Wasserstein-GAN model to generate synthetically aged brain images given a baseline scan. Their method needed to be applied recursively in order to predict different future time points, and could only predict into the future by multiples of a predefined time interval. In contrast, our model only requires one prediction and is supported by a single time lag input variable that can predict at any user-defined future point in time. Ravi et al. [5] proposed a 4D deep learning model, which could generate several future 3D scans from different time points at once. However, this method needs several time points across many participants, and requires an expanded architecture to produce multiple time point outputs. Wang et al. [7] proposed using several previous scans to predict the neurological MRI examination of a patient with Alzheimer's Disease (AD) using a U-Net. However, their method could only predict images at a fixed point in the future (6 months). Some studies [22, 24] require longitudinal images from two timepoints to predict future MRI scans.

Similar to our study, Xia et al. [6] proposed a 2D conditional GAN (cGAN) method, which also employs user-defined time as an input parameter alongside the subject scans into both the generator and discriminator, and predicts future scans at the target time point. They use an ordinal encoding of age with a 100×1 vector, which can only represent time information at discrete time intervals (such as annually). This ordinal encoding was incorporated into their novel deep learning architecture with a small bottleneck layer, which many common convolution neural network (CNN) models do not normally contain. Alternatively, our method supports a more flexible interval for temporal prediction, by simply providing the normalized time lag value, encoded in days between exams, into the learner. In our proposed approach, time information is first expanded using transposed convolutions, which is concatenated with internal feature maps in any CNN layer. In real-world clinical practice, the time between longitudinal exams for a central nervous system disorder (e.g., MS) is quite variable, and MS lesions have the potential to develop actively. We will distinguish their methods from ours more clearly in the methods section. Thus, the developments outlined in this paper have the potential to help extend image estimation / synthesis technologies to real-world clinical use. Additionally, several approaches have been proposed to use existing scans to predict future MS lesion progression [8–11], where the output of these models is lesion feature information instead of whole images. More recently, Kumar et al. [25] proposed a cGAN to generate counterfactual images to aid data-driven biomarker discovery and validated their method in a longitudinal MS dataset.

Despite those methods having shown great performance, most are concerned with predicting the healthy aging brain, as well as predicting AD MRI examinations. Predicting future brain FLAIR MRI examinations for MS patients is a topic that has not yet been fully explored. Thus, we are proposing deep learning models that can predict FLAIR images for MS patients at any user-defined amount of time into the future, while modelling time as a spatially distributed feature map, which allows for variable growth rate trajectories across different tissues, notably for brain lesions, which often progress / develop at different rates from healthy parenchyma. Our method could also be used as a novel data augmentation method for generating new samples for training deep neural networks.

Our work has four main contributions. First, we modify existing deep learning architectures with transposed convolutions to parameterize the time lag to prediction, which governs how far into the future to predict the next image. Second, the transposed convolution supports the modelling of time as a spatially distributed array of temporal variables, allowing the learning machine to model variable rates of growth distributed across brain tissues. Thus, the approach presented herein can support clinicians to estimate a patient's disease progression at multiple points in the future, and can model spatially variable tissue growth, atrophy and remission. The architecture modifications presented in this paper support the use of real-world longitudinal data whereby the time between scans is variable. Third, we developed modifications to 4 different deep learning architectures to add user-defined time lag using transposed convolutions: a modified U-Net, a generator-induced time GAN (gt-GAN), a discriminator-induced time GAN (dt-GAN) and a modified auxiliary classifier GAN (ACGAN). Fourth, we add an auxiliary classifier [15] in the discriminator in order to produce a performance improvement when compared with providing time lag information into both the discriminator and generator, as in a previous study [6].

2 Materials and Methods

2.1 Modeling Time Information by Transposed Convolution

This section illustrates our approach to providing time information into a CNN by transposed convolutions in order to predict future brain changes continuously.

We use transposed convolutions, instead of one-hot vectors [12] or ordinal binary vectors [6] used in previous studies, to expand the user selected time lag prediction variable to the same size as the input images, which theoretically supports the modelling of spatially-specific time-dependent brain development. Then we concatenate the learned spatially distributed feature map with the first layer of feature maps in the 3D U-Nets. We normalize the time information by using days between studies divided by 365, creating a floating point decimal number in years, which is more consistent with the nature of time as a continuous variable. Note that in [6], they also did an ablation study comparing normalized time information as one continuous variable (between 0 and 1) with their ordinal binary vector approach, which resulted in a network that would generate similar images to one another. In contrast, in our method, we first expand the time information by transposed convolution and then concatenate the result with our standard feature maps, while their method concatenated the continuous value with the image embedding directly. Our method also has the potential to flexibly add time information into any CNN model, while in [6], their ordinal binary vectors cannot be applied to every CNN model.

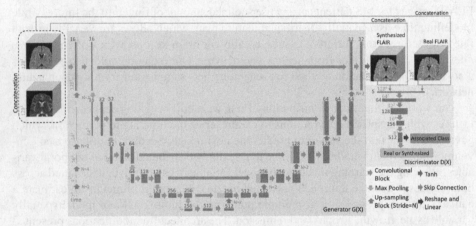

Fig. 1. Detailed architecture for modified ACGAN. Batch normalization and LeakyReLU with slope of 0.2 are used in the convolution block. Batch normalization was not used in the first blocks and last blocks of the Discriminator (D). The last convolution blocks in D used a sigmoid activation function.

2.2 Proposed Architectures

Generative adversarial networks (GANs) are widely used for image synthesis. Conditional GANs (cGANs) [13] are more suitable for image-to-image translation problems by learning the condition of the input images. To this aim, we explored 4 different architectures for this application.

3D U-Net. As shown in Fig. 1, a 6-level 3D U-Net is utilized for all methods, acting as a baseline comparative model as well as the generator in the three subsequently developed GANs. We use the L1 distance as the loss function. The expanded time information is concatenated with feature maps after the first convolution block.

Generator-Induced Time GAN (Gt-GAN). The second approach combined a discriminator and the L1 distance function for better perceptual performance and less blurring. The objective of the generator G can be expressed as:

$$L_{gt-GAN}^{G} = E_{x,t}\big[log(1 - D(x, G(x, t)))\big] + \lambda_{l1}E_{x,y,t}\big[||y - G(x, t)||_1\big] \qquad (1)$$

where E is the maximum likelihood estimation, x, y denotes the input images and x's corresponding target image after time t, separately. λ_{l1} is a non-negative trade-off parameter, which is used to balance the adversarial and L1 loss. By minimizing this objective function, the generated image will not only fool the discriminator but also approximate the ground truth output at the pixel level [13]. As in Pix2pix [13], cGANs are trained by conditioning the learning model on the source image data. The discriminator D takes both the source images and either a real target image or a synthesized one as input, and is tasked with predicting whether the image is real or not. The discriminator D is trained to maximize the following objective:

$$L_{gt-GAN}^{D} = E_{x,y}\big[logD(x, y)\big] + E_{x,t}\big[log(1 - D(x, G(x, t)))\big] \qquad (2)$$

Discriminator-Induced Time GAN (Dt-GAN). In dt-GAN, the time lag parameter is incorporated into both the generator and the discriminator D using transposed convolutions. In this way, the time lag information is also learned by the discriminator, which could possibly help the discriminator to distinguish between the real images y and synthesized images $G(x)$, towards potentially improving the generator's performance. The objective of the generator G in dt-GAN is the same as gt-GAN. The objective of the discriminator D in dt-GAN is as follows:

$$L_{gt-GAN}^{D} = E_{x,y,t}\big[logD(x, y, t)\big] + E_{x,t}\big[log(1 - D(x, G(x, t), t))\big] \qquad (3)$$

Modified Auxiliary Classifier GAN (ACGAN). Instead of providing the time information directly into the discriminator, the discriminator can potentially learn how to distinguish the difference between different time lags itself. Thus, the discriminator would learn to identify differences (i.e., the size of lesion areas) between different time lags to force the generator to generate better images. Based on this hypothesis, in the fourth approach, we used a modified auxiliary classifier GAN (ACGAN) [15]. For each given sample, there is input image x and target image y, associated with the time lag t. In addition to that, we also classify each sample into a class label c based on having similar time t. We add an auxiliary classifier on discriminator D. Figure 1 demonstrates our proposed modified ACGAN architecture. The objective of the discriminator D is:

$$\begin{aligned}L_{ACGAN}^{D} =&E_{x,y}\big[logD(x, y)\big] + E_{x,t}\big[log(1 - D(x, G(x, t)))\big] \\ &+ E_{x,y,c}\big[logp(c|x, y)\big] + E_{x,c,t}\big[logp(c|x, G(x, t))\big]\end{aligned} \qquad (4)$$

where c is an associated label with each sample classified, based on the time lag input parameter. By maximizing this objective function, D learns not only to distinguish whether this sample is a real one or not, but also to classify each sample into its corresponding class c. Simultaneously, G tries to generate images that can be classified into the target class c, to enhance the accuracy of image synthesis [21].

2.3 Dataset and Evaluation Metrics

To validate our method, we used the ISBI2015 longitudinal MS dataset [16], which consists of 19 participants. Among them, 14 participants had scans at four time points, 4 participants had scans at five time points, and one had scans at six time points. All were acquired on the same MRI scanner. The first time-point MPRAGE was rigidly registered into 1 mm isotropic MNI template space and used as a baseline for the remaining images from the same time-point, as well as from each of the follow-up time-points. Consecutive time-points are separated by approximately one year for all participants in this dataset. The following modalities are provided for each time point: T1-w MPRAGE, T2-w, PD-w, and FLAIR. Our models predict images at varying time lags into the future, as such 139 samples are available in this dataset at varying time intervals. For instance, there are 6 samples from one participant with 4 time points ($1 \rightarrow 2$, $1 \rightarrow 3$, $1 \rightarrow 4$, $2 \rightarrow 3$, $2 \rightarrow 4$, $3 \rightarrow 4$). All modalities from the early time-point and the user-defined time lag parameter were included to predict future FLAIR scans.

Three popular metrics are used in this study: peak signal-to-noise ratio (PSNR), normalized mean squared error (NMSE), and the structural similarity index (SSIM) [17].

2.4   Implementation Details

We cropped out an image size of (150, 190, 150) to reduce the background region. Each volume was linearly scaled to [-1, 1] from the original intensity values for normalization. To fit the 3D image into the generator and make the whole model fit into GPU memory, we split them into eight overlapping patches of size (128, 128, 128). The overlapped regions are averaged to aggregate those patches. A data augmentation of rotation with random angle $[-12°, 12°]$ and a random spatial scaling factor [0.9, 1.1] was employed during training. Batch size was 3 for all methods. 5-fold cross validation was applied at the participant level to effectively evaluate different methods (2 folds have 4 4-time-point participants; one fold has 3 4-time-point and one 5-time-point participants; one fold has 2 4-time-point and one 5-time-point participant with the last fold having one 4-time-point, 2 5-time-point and 1 6-time-point participants). Samples are grouped into different classes c based on rounding off the time between the input exams and the target predicted exams to a whole year value in modified ACGAN. We use the Adam optimizer [18] with momentum parameters $\beta_1 = 0.5$ and $\beta_2 = 0.999$ and weight decay $\lambda = 7 \times 10^{-8}$ to optimize all the networks. PatchGAN [13] was used for penalizing each patch to be real or fake to support the discriminator in the GAN to encourage high quality image generation. As in [19], λ_{l1} was set to 300 for all cGANs during training. To balance the generator and discriminator in GANs, we use label smoothing [20] to improve the stability of training GANs. The learning rate was set to 0.0002 for both the generator and discriminator in all the GANs during the first 150 epochs, then, linearly decaying to 0 for the following 50 epochs. For the baseline modified U-Net, the learning rate was set to 7×10^{-5} for the first 150 epochs, then linearly decaying to 0 for the following 50 epochs. Experiments were performed on 4 Nvidia A100 GPUs with 40 GBs of RAM using distributed data in parallel via the PyTorch framework. Training took around 5 h for each fold for each model.

3 Results and Discussion

Table 1 shows the quantitative results obtained by different methods that we investigated in terms of mean PSNR, NMSE, and SSIM values and their corresponding standard deviation. All the metrics are computed on the aggregated 3D volume instead of patches to represent the performance on the whole scans. We linearly scaled each volume to [0, 1] before computing all the metrics to ensure a fair comparison. First, we observe that all the GANs provide better results than the baseline modified U-Net. Nevertheless, by integrating the time lag parameter into both the generator G and the discriminator D, dt-GAN does not achieve better performance in all the three metrics as compared with gt-GAN, which only integrates the time lag parameter t into the generator G. This might confirm that integration of the time lag into both the generator and the discriminator cannot improve image synthesis performance in this situation. The modified ACGAN achieves the best results and the smallest standard error across all three performance metrics.

Table 1. Quantitative Evaluation Results of Different Methods (mean $\pm$ standard deviation), obtained by evaluated methods on the validation folds.[1]

Methods	PSNR ↑	NMSE ↓	SSIM ↑
Modified ACGAN	**28.8721 ± 2.709**	**0.2006 ± 0.080**	**0.9148 ± 0.024**
dt-GAN	27.4969 ± 2.851	0.2368 ± 0.095	0.9068 ± 0.026
gt-GAN	28.4069 ± 3.136	0.2160 ± 0.099	0.9089 ± 0.027
Modified U-Net	22.9473 ± 3.655	0.4296 ± 0.195	0.8931 ± 0.031

Qualitative results of the proposed modified ACGAN are illustrated in Fig. 2. With respect to participant A, the source image's expanded region-of-interest (ROI) exhibits three subtle lesions that are changing temporally between the source and target acquisitions, which in this examination were 3 years apart. Note that both lesions marked by a red circle appear to have gone into remission and are extremely difficult to visually identify on the target image. Also noteworthy is that the subtle lesion on the source exam, marked by a red arrow, developed into a more prominent lesion by the target image acquisition. Our proposed modified ACGAN approach to image prediction has resulted in a reduction of visual lesion prominence for both lesions exhibiting remission (marked by red circles), as well as increased visual prominence for the expanding lesion marked by a red arrow. With respect to participant B, the red circled lesion exhibits a hypointensity on the target image which likely implies the development of regional atrophy not present in the original source image. Our modified ACGAN approach was able to partially model this hypointensity's developmental trajectory, potentially reflective of tissue atrophy. These results from both participants imply that our proposed approach is

---

[1] We cannot report the metrics only based on the lesion area, since no lesion labels were provided to 14 participants in this ISBI2015 dataset.

capable of modeling subtle lesion growth, lesion remission, as well as a limited amount of lesion atrophy.

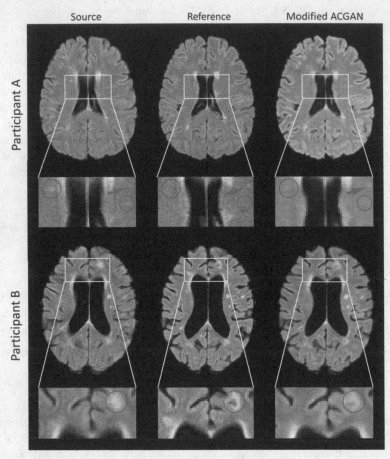

Fig. 2. Example predicted images in the validation fold from the leading modified ACGAN. Participant A: Source is FLAIR scan from time point 1, Target is FLAIR from time point 4, ACGAN is predicting images using modalities from time point 1 and the user-defined time lag parameter was set to predict time point 4 FLAIR. Participant B: Source is time point 1 FLAIR, Target is time point 5 FLAIR, ACGAN is predicting images using modalities from time point 1 and the user-defined time lag parameter was set to predict time point 5 FLAIR.

Future work could involve the use of ROI specific weighted loss, in order to increase the ability of the network to focus on small lesion areas. Although Fig. 2 demonstrates small changes to existing lesions or the appearance of new lesions, our overall loss function is expected to be dominated by whole brain factors. Thus, a model with ROI specific weighted loss could be more valuable for clinical interest, and combining ROI specific loss with the approach presented herein is the subject of future work. One of the limitations of the leading modified ACGAN is an associated class needed to be assigned to each sample, for which it is difficult to find a priority solution, when there is large variability between time intervals. A potential solution to this problem is to use clustering algorithms (i.e., K-nearest neighbors algorithm, etc.) to define the respective class labels. Future work will also examine additional datasets with more variability in the time between examinations, as this dataset largely consists of examinations acquired at yearly intervals. This dataset did not include gold-standard ROIs for most of the MS lesions, as such, we were unable to report lesion specific performance metrics in Table 1. Future work will involve evaluating the proposed approach on datasets with provided gold-standard ROIs, as well as evaluating the proposed approach on datasets such as the one we have used in this study with additional segmentation technology to automatically define the lesion ROIs, to assist in evaluating lesion-specific predictive performance.

4 Conclusion

In this work, we propose a new way to integrate time lag information into deep learning models by transposed convolutions, to predict future brain FLAIR MRI examinations for MS patients. We also compared 4 different approaches to provide time lag input parameters into cGANs and the U-Net. By using transposed convolutions, the time lag information has the potential to be spatially distributed and concatenated into any CNN architecture layer. Our method could also create a more flexible interval in a continuous way, which is more suitable for MS to help extend image estimation / synthesis technologies to real-world clinical use. We also propose to use an auxiliary classifier in the discriminator, which has potential to boost predictive accuracy. A longitudinal MS dataset with larger participant size and more timepoints with each participant will be more valuable for validating of this method.

Acknowledgements. This work was supported by an NSERC Discovery Grant to JL. Funding was also provided by a Nova Scotia Graduate Scholarship and a StFX Graduate Scholarship to JW. Computational resources were provided by Compute Canada.

References

1. McGinley, M.P., Goldschmidt, C.H., Rae-Grant, A.D.: Diagnosis and treatment of multiple sclerosis: a review. JAMA **325**, 765–779 (2021)
2. Wei, W., et al.: Fluid-attenuated inversion recovery MRI synthesis from multisequence MRI using three-dimensional fully convolutional networks for multiple sclerosis. J Med Imaging (Bellingham). **6**, 14005 (2019). https://doi.org/10.1117/1.JMI.6.1.014005
3. Salem, M., et al.: Multiple sclerosis lesion synthesis in MRI using an encoder-decoder U-NET. IEEE Access. **7**, 25171–25184 (2019). https://doi.org/10.1109/ACCESS.2019.2900198
4. Wegmayr, V., Hörold, M., Buhmann, J.M.: Generative aging of brain MRI for early prediction of MCI-AD conversion. In: 2019 IEEE 16th International Symposium on Biomedical Imaging (ISBI 2019), pp. 1042–1046 (2019). https://doi.org/10.1109/ISBI.2019.8759394
5. Ravi, D., Blumberg, S.B., Ingala, S., Barkhof, F., Alexander, D.C., Oxtoby, N.P.: Degenerative adversarial neuroimage nets for brain scan simulations: application in ageing and dementia. Med. Image Anal. **75**, 102257 (2022). https://doi.org/10.1016/j.media.2021.102257

6. Xia, T., Chartsias, A., Wang, C., Tsaftaris, S.A.: Learning to synthesise the ageing brain without longitudinal data. Med. Image Anal. **73**, 102169 (2021). https://doi.org/10.1016/J. MEDIA.2021.102169

7. Wang, J., Berger, D., Mattie, D., Levman, J.: Multichannel input pixelwise regression 3D U-Nets for medical image estimation with 3 applications in brain MRI. In: International Conference on Medical Imaging with Deep Learning (2021)

8. Doyle, A., Precup, D., Arnold, D.L., Arbel, T.: Predicting future disease activity and treatment responders for multiple sclerosis patients using a bag-of-lesions brain representation. In: Descoteaux, M., Maier-Hein, L., Franz, A., Jannin, P., Collins, D.L., Duchesne, S. (eds.) MICCAI 2017. LNCS, vol. 10435, pp. 186–194. Springer, Cham (2017). https://doi.org/10. 1007/978-3-319-66179-7_22

9. Tousignant, A., et al. (eds.): Proceedings of The 2nd International Conference on Medical Imaging with Deep Learning, pp. 483–492. PMLR (2019)

10. Sepahvand, N.M., Hassner, T., Arnold, D.L., Arbel, T.: CNN prediction of future disease activity for multiple sclerosis patients from baseline MRI and lesion labels. In: Crimi, A., Bakas, S., Kuijf, H., Keyvan, F., Reyes, M., van Walsum, T. (eds.) BrainLes 2018. LNCS, vol. 11383, pp. 57–69. Springer, Cham (2019). https://doi.org/10.1007/978-3-030-11723-8_6

11. Durso-Finley, J., Falet, J.-P.R., Nichyporuk, B., Arnold, D.L., Arbel, T.: Personalized prediction of future lesion activity and treatment effect in multiple sclerosis from baseline MRI. In: International Conference on Medical Imaging with Deep Learning, pp. 1–20 (2022)

12. Zhang, Z., Song, Y., Qi, H.: Age progression/regression by conditional adversarial autoencoder. In: Proceedings of the IEEE Conference on Computer Vision and Pattern Recognition, pp. 5810–5818 (2017)

13. Isola, P., Zhu, J.-Y., Zhou, T., Efros, A.A.: Image-to-image translation with conditional adversarial networks. In: 2017 IEEE Conference on Computer Vision and Pattern Recognition (CVPR), pp. 5967–5976 (2017)

14. Goodfellow, I.J.: NIPS 2016 Tutorial: Generative Adversarial Networks (2016). arXiv preprint arXiv:1701.00160

15. Odena, A., Olah, C., Shlens, J.: Conditional image synthesis with auxiliary classifier GANs. In: ICML'17 Proceedings of the 34th International Conference on Machine Learning – **70**, pp. 2642–2651 (2017)

16. Carass, A., et al.: Longitudinal Multiple Sclerosis Lesion Segmentation: Resource and Challenge. Neuroimage. **148**, 77–102 (2017)

17. Wang, Z., Bovik, A.C., Sheikh, H.R., Simoncelli, E.P.: Image quality assessment: from error visibility to structural similarity. IEEE Trans. Image Process. **13**, 600–612 (2004). https://doi. org/10.1109/TIP.2003.819861

18. Kingma, D.P., Ba, J.L.: Adam: a method for stochastic optimization. In: ICLR 2015: International Conference on Learning Representations 2015 (2015)

19. Yu, B., Zhou, L., Wang, L., Shi, Y., Fripp, J., Bourgeat, P.: Ea-GANs: edge-aware generative adversarial networks for cross-modality MR image synthesis. IEEE Trans. Med. Imaging **38**, 1750–1762 (2019). https://doi.org/10.1109/TMI.2019.2895894

20. Salimans, T., Goodfellow, I., Zaremba, W., Cheung, V., Radford, A., Chen, X.: Improved techniques for training GANs. In: NIPS'16 Proceedings of the 30th International Conference on Neural Information Processing Systems, pp. 2234–2242 (2016)

21. Choi, Y., Choi, M., Kim, M., Ha, J.-W., Kim, S., Choo, J.: Stargan: Unified generative adversarial networks for multi-domain image-to-image translation. In: Proceedings of the IEEE Conference on Computer Vision and Pattern Recognition, pp. 8789–8797 (2018)

22. Fu, J., Tzortzakakis, A., Barroso, J., Westman, E., Ferreira, D., Moreno, R.: Generative Aging of Brain Images with Diffeomorphic Registration (2022). arXiv preprint arXiv:2205.15607

23. Bowles, C., Gunn, R., Hammers, A., Rueckert, D.: Modelling the progression of Alzheimer's disease in MRI using generative adversarial networks. SPIE (2018)

24. Kim, S.T., Küçükaslan, U., Navab, N.: Longitudinal brain MR image modeling using personalized memory for alzheimer's disease. IEEE Access **9**, 143212–143221 (2021)

25. Kumar, A., et al.: Counterfactual image synthesis for discovery of personalized predictive image markers. In: Medical Image Assisted Biomarkers' Discovery (2022)

Leveraging 2D Deep Learning ImageNet-trained Models for Native 3D Medical Image Analysis

Bhakti Baheti[1,2,3] , Sarthak Pati[1,2,3,4] , Bjoern Menze[4,5] ,
and Spyridon Bakas[1,2,3(✉)]

[1] Center for Biomedical Image Computing and Analytics (CBICA),
University of Pennsylvania, Philadelphia, PA, USA
sbakas@upenn.edu

[2] Department of Pathology and Laboratory Medicine, Perelman School of Medicine,
University of Pennsylvania, Philadelphia, PA, USA

[3] Department of Radiology, Perelman School of Medicine,
University of Pennsylvania, Philadelphia, PA, USA

[4] Department of Informatics, Technical University of Munich, Munich, Germany

[5] Department of Quantitative Biomedicine, University of Zurich, Zurich, Switzerland

Abstract. Convolutional neural networks (CNNs) have shown promising performance in various 2D computer vision tasks due to availability of large amounts of 2D training data. Contrarily, medical imaging deals with 3D data and usually lacks the equivalent extent and diversity of data, for developing AI models. Transfer learning provides the means to use models trained for one application as a starting point to another application. In this work, we leverage 2D pre-trained models as a starting point in 3D medical applications by exploring the concept of Axial-Coronal-Sagittal (ACS) convolutions. We have incorporated ACS as an alternative of native 3D convolutions in the Generally Nuanced Deep Learning Framework (GaNDLF), providing various well-established and state-of-the-art network architectures with the availability of pre-trained encoders from 2D data. Results of our experimental evaluation on 3D MRI data of brain tumor patients for i) tumor segmentation and ii) radiogenomic classification, show model size reduction by ∼22% and improvement in validation accuracy by ∼33%. Our findings support the advantage of ACS convolutions in pre-trained 2D CNNs over 3D CNN without pre-training, for 3D segmentation and classification tasks, democratizing existing models trained in datasets of unprecedented size and showing promise in the field of healthcare.

Keywords: Deep learning · ImageNet · Transfer learning · MRI · segmentation · classification

B. Baheti and S. Pati contributed equally for this work.

S. Bakas et al. (Eds.): BrainLes 2022, LNCS 13769, pp. 68–79, 2023.
https://doi.org/10.1007/978-3-031-33842-7_6

1   Introduction

Deep learning (DL) based approaches are continuously being developed for various medical imaging tasks, including segmentation, classification, and detection, for a wide range of modalities (i.e., MRI, CT, X-Ray), regularly outperforming earlier approaches [1,2]. However, DL is computationally expensive and requires large amounts of annotated data for model training limiting their applicability in problems where large amounts of annotated datasets are unavailable [3]. Transfer learning (TL) is a popular approach to overcome this issue by initializing a DL model with pre-trained weights, thereby reducing convergence time and concluding at a superior state, while utilizing otherwise insufficient data [4,5]. The basic idea of TL involves re-using model weights trained for a problem with a large available dataset as the initialization point for a completely different task. The foundation behind this idea is that convolutional layers extract general, lower-level features (such as edges, patterns, and gradients) that are applicable across a wide variety of images [6]. The latter layers of a convolutional neural network (CNN) learn features more specific to the image of the particular task by combining the previous lower-level features. Leveraging weights of trained models has proven to be a better initialisation point for DL model training, when compared to random initialization [4,7–10].

There are numerous pre-trained models available for applications on 2D imaging data, such as ImageNet [11], YOLO [12], and MS-COCO [13], however, universally applicable pre-trained models are not available for utilization on 3D data like medical images due to the lack of associated large and diverse data. Current application of pre-trained CNN for 3D medical image segmentation and classification can be divided in three categories depending on the dimensionality of the input data:

– **2D Approaches**
  Here, a 3D input volume is considered as a stack of 2D slices, and a multi-slice planar (2D) network is applied on each 2D slice independently [14,15]. Some earlier approaches considered 3D medical images as tri-planar representation where axial, coronal, and sagittal views are considered as 3 channels of the input data. But such 2D representation learning is fundamentally weak in capturing 3D contexts. Some DL based approaches for classification of brain cancer MRI images use representative 2D slices as the input data rather than utilizing full 3D volume [16,17].

– **3D Approaches**
  In this case, a 3D network is trained using native 3D convolution layers that are useful in capturing spatial correlations present along the 3rd dimension, in order to capture 3D contextual information [18–21]. Significant improvement in classification accuracy was observed in [22] with the use of native 3D convolutions compared to 2D convolutions. Although data in adjacent slices, across each of the three axes, are correlated and can be potentially used to yield a better model, this suffers from two weaknesses: a) reduced model stability due to random weight initialization (since there are no available pre-trained models) and b) unnecessarily high memory consumption.

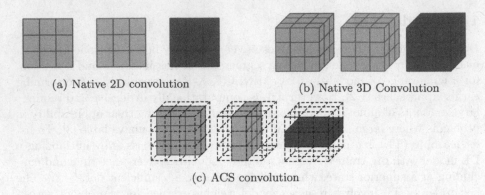

(a) Native 2D convolution   (b) Native 3D Convolution

(c) ACS convolution

Fig. 1. Comparison of various types of convolution for 3D medical data (Figure adapted from [28]).

- **Hybrid Approaches**

  There are few studies using a hybrid of the two aforementioned approaches, i.e. 2D & 3D. An ensemble-based learning framework built upon a group of 2D and 3D base learners was designed in [23]. Another strategy is to train multiple 2D networks on different viewpoints and then generate final segmentation results by 3D volumetric fusion net [24]. A similar approach was proposed in [25], which consists of a 2D DenseUNet for intra-slice feature extraction and its 3D counterpart for aggregating volumetric contexts. Finally, Ni *et al.* trained a 2D deep network for 3D medical image segmentation by introducing the concept of elastic boundary projection [26].

Current literature shows inadequate exploration on the application of 2D pre-trained models in native 3D applications. As medical datasets are limited when compared with those from the computer vision domain, TL of models trained in the latter can be beneficial in medical applications.

In this paper, we explore the concept of Axial-Coronal-Sagittal (ACS) convolution to utilize pre-trained weights of models trained on 2D datasets to perform natively 3D operations. This is achieved by splitting the 2D kernels into 3 parts by channels and convolving separately across Axial-Coronal-Sagittal views to enable development of native 3D CNNs for both classification and segmentation workloads. This way, we can take advantage of the 3D spatial context, as well as the available pre-trained 2D models to pave the way towards building better models for medical imaging applications. Multiple options of pre-trained models for use in 3D datasets have been made publicly available through the Generally Nuanced Deep Learning Framework (GaNDLF) [27][1].

2   Methods

In this work, we leverage the concept of Axial-Coronal-Sagittal (ACS) proposed in [28] and incorporate it into the Generally Nuanced Deep Learning Framework

---

[1] https://github.com/CBICA/GaNDLF.

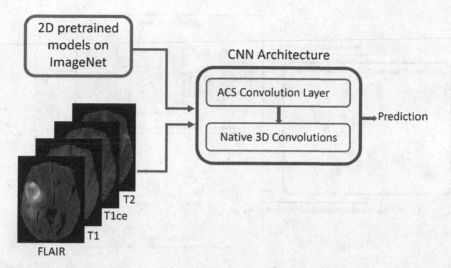

Fig. 2. Idea of integrating ACS convolutions with pre-trained 2D model weights to enable native 3D convolutions on 3D medical data (e.g., MRI)

(GaNDLF) [27]² which supports a wide variety of model architectures, loss functions, pre-processing, and training strategies.

2.1 ACS Convolutions

Convolution operations in CNNs can be classified as either 2D or 3D. The 2D convolutional layers use 2D filter kernels ($K \times K$) and capture 2D spatial correlation, whereas 3D convolutional kernels ($K \times K \times K$) are used in native 3D convolutional layers capturing 3D context (Fig. 1). As mentioned earlier, each of these approaches have their own advantages and disadvantages.

Yang *et al.* [28] introduced the concept of Axial-Coronal-Sagittal (ACS) convolutions to learn the spatial representation of three dimensions from the combination of each of the three (A-C-S) views (Fig. 1(c)). The basic concept of the ACS convolutions is to split the kernel into three parts ($K \times K \times 1$), ($K \times 1 \times K$) and ($1 \times K \times K$) and run multiple 2D convolution filters across the three views (axial, coronal, and sagittal). For any convolution layer, let us consider the number of input channels as C_i and number of output channels as C_o. The number of output channels in ACS convolution are then set as:

$$C_o^{Axial} \approx C_o^{Coronal} \approx C_o^{Sagittal} \approx \lfloor \frac{C_o}{3} \rfloor \tag{1}$$

Thus 2D convolutions are transformed into 3 dimensions by simultaneously performing computations across axial, coronal, and sagittal axes. The final output

---

² https://github.com/CBICA/GaNDLF.

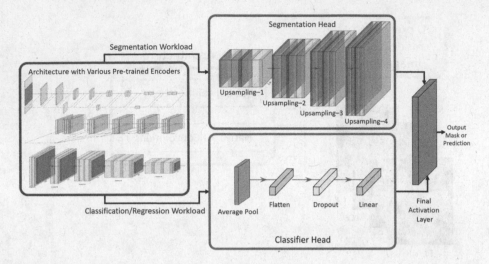

Fig. 3. The architecture that allows using different pre-trained encoders with either a segmentation or classifier head for specific workloads.

is then obtained by the concatenation of three convolved feature maps without any additional fusion layer.

The concept of ACS convolutions can be used as a generic plug-and-play replacement of 3D convolution enabling development of native 3D CNNs using 2D pre-trained weights as illustrated in Fig. 2.

2.2   Architecture Design

We have incorporated the concept of ACS convolutions in GaNDLF, which is a framework for training models for segmentation, classification, and regression in a reproducible and deployable manner [27]. GaNDLF has several architectures for segmentation and classification, as well as a wide range of data pre-processing and augmentation options along with the choice of several training hyper parameters and loss functions. We integrated several encoders from [29], pre-trained on ImageNet [11] into this framework, including variants of VGG [30], ResNet [31], DenseNet [32], and EfficientNet [33]. We have created a mechanism to combine the outputs of these encoders with either a segmentation or a classification head depending on the task, as shown in Fig. 3. The segmentation head consists of a set of upsampling layers similar to the decoder mechanism of the UNet network topology/architecture [34], where the user has the flexibility to choose the number of upsampling layers and the number of feature maps in each layer. The classification head consists of a average pooling layer applied on the top of feature maps obtained from the encoder. Dropout can be set between range 0 to 1 to reduce overfitting to the training data before the final classification layer.

While the 2D pre-trained weights could be directly loaded for applications on 2D data, we have replaced the usual convolution layer with an ACS convolution layer in GaNDLF, enabling their use for training on 3D medical data in a native manner, regardless of the number of input modalities. In comparison with the 2D models, ACS convolution layers do not introduce any additional computation cost, memory footprint, or model size.

2.2.1   Design for Segmentation Gliomas are among the most common and aggressive brain tumors and accurate delineation of the tumor sub-regions is important in clinical diagnosis. We trained two different architectures for segmentation through GaNDLF. UNet [34] with residual connections (ResUNet) is one of the famous architectures for 2D and 3D medical segmentation. It consists of encoder and decoder modules and feature concatenation pathways. The encoder is a stack of convolutional and downsampling layers for feature extraction from the input images, and the decoder consists of a set of upsampling layers (applying transpose convolutions) to generate the fine-grained segmentation output.

We trained two different models using the publicly available multi-parametric magnetic resonance imaging (mpMRI) data of 369 cases from training set of the International Brain Tumor Segmentation [35–37] (BraTS2020) challenge. This dataset consists of four multi-parametric magnetic resonance imaging (mpMRI) scans per subject/case, with the exact modalities being: a) native (T1) and b) post-contrast T1-weighted (T1-Gd), c) T2-weighted (T2), and d) T2 fluid attenuated inversion recovery (T2-FLAIR). These models are evaluated on 125 unseen cases from the BraTS2020 validation dataset. We first trained a standard ResUNet architecture of depth = 4 and base filters = 32 such that weights of all the layers were randomly initialized. We then built another architecture by using pre-trained ResNet50 as an encoder with depth = 4 and the standard UNet decoder. For each of these experiments, 40 patches of $64 \times 64 \times 64$ were extracted from each subject. Various training parameters were also kept constant, like the choice of optimizer (we used SGD), scheduler (modified triangular) with learning rate of 0.001, and loss function based on the Dice similarity coefficient (DSC) [38]. Maximum number of epochs was set to 250 with patience of 30 for early stopping. The performance is evaluated on clinically-relevant tumor regions, i.e., whole tumor (considered for radiotherapy), tumor core (considered for surgical resection) as well as enhancing tumor.

2.2.2   Design for Classification Glioblastoma (GBM) is the most aggressive and common adult primary malignant brain tumor and epidermal growth factor receptor variant III (EGFRvIII) mutation is considered a driver mutation and therapeutic target in GBM [39–41]. Usually, the presence of EGFRvIII is determined by the analysis of actual tissue specimens and is stated as positive or negative. We focus on non-invasive prediction of EGFRvIII status by analysis of these pre-operative and pre-processed MRI data. Residual Networks (ResNets) [31] introduced the idea of skip connections which enabled design of much deeper CNNs. GaNDLF supports variants of ResNet, including ResNet18,

ResNet34, ResNet50, ResNet101, and ResNet152, each having different number of layers.

We use an internal private cohort of 146 patients containing four structural mpMRI modalities (T1, T2, T1-Gd and T2-FLAIR) such that the positive and negative classes were equally distributed. These 146 cases were distributed in Training (80%) and Validation (20%) sets for experimentation. We used cross entropy loss function, adam optimiser and cosine annealing scheduler with learning rate of 0.0001. As the dataset is smaller, we set the maximum number epochs to 100 and patience of 30 epochs for early stopping.

3   Results

In this section we present the quantitative results of the segmentation and classification workloads described above, to showcase the feasibility and performance of ACS convolutions on 3D medical imaging data. Specifically, we compare the 2D pre-training approach with the random initialization to evaluate the superiority of the ACS convolutions over usual 3D convolution operations.

3.1   Brain Tumor Segmentation Workload

The segmentation model is trained on the publicly available training data of BraTS2020 challenge. We then quantitatively evaluate the performance of the final models on the unseen BraTS2020 validation data by submitting results to the online evaluation platform (CBICA Image Processing Portal). Table 1 lists the number of parameters of each model, as well as the comparative performance, in terms of Dice Similarity Coefficient (DSC) and the 95th percentile of the Hausdorff distance between the predicted ground truth labels.

3.2   Binary Classification of Brain Tumor Molecular Status

For the performance evaluation of the classification workload, we have used the structural mpMRI scans in-tandem as input (i.e., passing all the scans together at once as separate channels) similar to the segmentation workload. The classification model performance on training and validation data is summarized in Table 2, illustrating the effectiveness of pre-trained weights.

4   Discussion

In this work, we have assessed the functionality of transfer learning for 3D medical data based on the available 2D models pre-trained on ImageNet for segmentation and classification. The framework that this functionality is evaluated is designed such that deep learning network architecture's first and last layers are flexible to be able to process input images of any size with varying number of channels or modalities, and provide the final prediction based on the relevant

Table 1. Results on Brain Tumor Segmentation (BraTS2020) validation dataset

Metric	Region	Standard ResUNet	ResNet50+UNet (Random init.)	ResNet50+UNet (Pre-trained)
DSC	Whole Tumor	0.8771	0.8775	0.8736
	Tumor Core	0.7735	0.7458	0.7719
	Enhancing Tumor	0.7138	0.69508	0.7017
Hausdorff95	Whole Tumor	13.2425	7.6747	9.5384
	Tumor Core	14.7492	8.6579	15.4840
	Enhancing Tumor	34.8858	41.00332	40.2053
#Parameters	-	33.377 Million	25.821 Million	25.821 Million
#Epochs for convergence	-	104 epochs	250 epochs	95 epochs

number of classes for the specified task. The rest of the layers are initialized with pre-trained weights from the ImageNet models and are further fine-tuned.

The results of brain tumor segmentation using i) 3D U-Net with residual connections, ii) randomly initialized ResNet50 encoder & UNet decoder, and iii) pre-trained ResNet50 encoder & UNet decoder are shown in Table 1. In these architectures, the obvious difference was in the encoders being randomly initialised in the former i) 3DUNet and ii) ResNet50 and pre-trained in the latter ResNet50-UNet (iii). As the pre-trained decoders are not available from ImageNet, the decoder was initialised with random weights in all the three architectures. We hypothesize that this might be the reason for comparable segmentation performance in terms of dice and hausdorff95 scores, while the difference in number of parameters is significant. It should be observed that the ResNet50-UNet (ii and iii) has only 25.821 Million parameters, which is around 22% less compared to 33.377 Million parameters of the standard ResUNet (i), with the same encoder-decoder depth. The randomly initialised ResNet50-UNet model oscillates around the same performance and did not converge in the specified maximum number of epochs (250). On the other hand, the same model initialised with pre-trained weights converged within 95 epochs. Thus models initialized with pre-trained weights have advantage of better convergence speed as well as smaller model size. Importantly, smaller models are more preferable in the clinical setting due to their higher feasibility for deployment in low-resource environments.

Baseline results of binary classification for the determination of the EGFRvIII mutational status are reported in Table 2, with ResNet50 architecture. We did not use any additional data augmentation techniques. As the data in this task were limited, the effect of pre-trained weights are clearly observed resulting in better accuracy. Figure 4 shows the plots of cross entropy loss and accuracy in training with respect to epochs. Similar performance is observed for validation set as well. The weights of the model with lowest validation loss are stored for reproducibility and the accuracy and loss values reported in Table 2 are for the saved model with lowest validation loss.

Table 2. Results on EGFR Classification

	ResNet50 (Random initialization)	ResNet50 (Pre-trained on ImageNet)
Training Accuracy	0.7203	0.9915
Training Loss	0.5736	0.3292
Val Accuracy	0.5357	0.7142
Val Loss	0.6912	0.5758

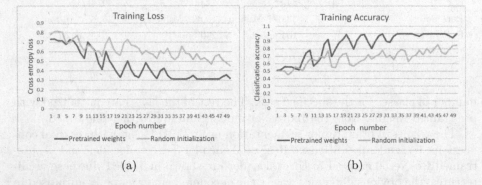

(a)   (b)

Fig. 4. Comparison plots of training loss and accuracy for binary classification of EGFRvIII mutation status. These plots are for ResNet50 architecture with and without use of 2D pre-trained weights from ImageNet

Our findings support the incorporation of 2D pre-trained models towards improving the performance on 3D medical image segmentation and classification workloads, with demonstrably smaller model size (Table 1). Large increase in accuracy is specially observed in those applications where sufficient labelled data are not available. Incorporating this functionality in GaNDLF provides a readily available solution to researchers towards an end-to-end solution for several computational tasks, along with support for pre-trained encoders, making it a robust application framework for deployment and integration in clinical workflows. Future studies can explore this mechanism by applying it to compare randomly initialized and pre-trained models for convergence speed (in both centralized and federated learning settings [8,9,42,43]), performance gains in applications requiring 3D datasets, model optimization allowing deployment in low-resource environments, and privacy analysis.

Acknowledgments. Research reported in this publication was partly supported by the National Institutes of Health (NIH) under award numbers NIH/NCI:U01CA242871 and NIH/NINDS:R01NS042645. The content of this publication is solely the responsibility of the authors and does not represent the official views of the NIH.

References

1. Zhou, S.K., et al.: A review of deep learning in medical imaging: imaging traits, technology trends, case studies with progress highlights, and future promises. Proc. IEEE **109**(5), 820–838 (2021)
2. Chen, X., et al.: Recent advances and clinical applications of deep learning in medical image analysis. Med. Image Anal. 102444 (2022)
3. Varoquaux, G., Cheplygina, V.: Machine learning for medical imaging: methodological failures and recommendations for the future. NPJ Digit. Med. **5**(1), 1–8 (2022)
4. Yosinski, J., Clune, J., Bengio, Y., Lipson, H.: How transferable are features in deep neural networks? In: Advances in Neural Information Processing Systems, vol. 27 (2014)
5. Goodfellow, I., Bengio, Y., Courville, A.: Deep Learning. MIT Press, Cambbridge (2016)
6. Aloysius, N., Geetha, M.: A review on deep convolutional neural networks. In: 2017 International Conference on Communication and Signal Processing (ICCSP), pp. 0588–0592. IEEE (2017)
7. Pan, S.J., Yang, Q.: A survey on transfer learning. IEEE Trans. Knowl. Data Eng. **22**(10), 1345–1359 (2010)
8. Pati, S., et al.: Federated learning enables big data for rare cancer boundary detection. arXiv preprint arXiv:2204.10836 (2022)
9. Sheller, M.J., et al.: Federated learning in medicine: facilitating multi-institutional collaborations without sharing patient data. Sci. Rep. **10**(1), 1–12 (2020)
10. Baid, U., et al.: NIMG-32. The federated tumor segmentation (FETS) initiative: the first real-world large-scale data-private collaboration focusing on neuro-oncology. Neuro-Oncology. **23**, pp. vi135–vi136 (2021)
11. Deng, J., Dong, W., Socher, R., Li, L.-J., Li, K., Fei-Fei, L.: Imagenet: a large-scale hierarchical image database. In: 2009 IEEE Conference on Computer Vision and Pattern Recognition, pp. 248–255. IEEE (2009)
12. Redmon, J., Farhadi, A.: Yolov3: An incremental improvement. arXiv preprint arXiv:1804.02767 (2018)
13. Lin, T.-Y., et al.: Microsoft COCO: common objects in context. In: Fleet, D., Pajdla, T., Schiele, B., Tuytelaars, T. (eds.) ECCV 2014. LNCS, vol. 8693, pp. 740–755. Springer, Cham (2014). https://doi.org/10.1007/978-3-319-10602-1_48
14. Chen, J., Yang, L., Zhang, Y., Alber, M., Chen, D.Z.: Combining fully convolutional and recurrent neural networks for 3d biomedical image segmentation. In: Advances in Neural Information Processing Systems, vol. 29 (2016)
15. Yu, Q., Xie, L., Wang, Y., Zhou, Y., Fishman, E.K., Yuille, A.L.: Recurrent saliency transformation network: incorporating multi-stage visual cues for small organ segmentation. In: Proceedings of the IEEE Conference on Computer Vision and Pattern Recognition, pp. 8280–8289 (2018)
16. Díaz-Pernas, F.J., Martínez-Zarzuela, M., Antón Rodríguez, M., González-Ortega, D.: A deep learning approach for brain tumor classification and segmentation using a multiscale convolutional neural network. In: Healthcare, vol. 9, p. 153, MDPI (2021)
17. Ismael, S.A.A., Mohammed, A., Hefny, H.: An enhanced deep learning approach for brain cancer MRI images classification using residual networks. Artif. Intell. Med. **102**, 101779 (2020)

18. Çiçek, Ö., Abdulkadir, A., Lienkamp, S.S., Brox, T., Ronneberger, O.: 3D U-Net: Learning dense volumetric segmentation from sparse annotation. In: Ourselin, S., Joskowicz, L., Sabuncu, M.R., Unal, G., Wells, W. (eds.) MICCAI 2016. LNCS, vol. 9901, pp. 424–432. Springer, Cham (2016). https://doi.org/10.1007/978-3-319-46723-8_49

19. Zhao, W., et al.: 3d deep learning from CT scans predicts tumor invasiveness of subcentimeter pulmonary adenocarcinomas. Cancer Res. **78**(24), 6881–6889 (2018)

20. Milletari, F., Navab, N., Ahmadi, S.-A.: V-net: fully convolutional neural networks for volumetric medical image segmentation. In: 2016 Fourth International Conference on 3D Vision (3DV), pp. 565–571. IEEE (2016)

21. Baid, U., et al.: A novel approach for fully automatic intra-tumor segmentation with 3d u-net architecture for gliomas. Front. Comput. Neurosci. 10 (2020)

22. Trivizakis, E., et al.: Extending 2-d convolutional neural networks to 3-d for advancing deep learning cancer classification with application to mri liver tumor differentiation. IEEE J. Biomed. Health Inform. **23**(3), 923–930 (2019)

23. Zheng, H., et al.: A new ensemble learning framework for 3d biomedical image segmentation. Proc. AAAI Conf. Artif. Intell. **33**, 5909–5916 (2019)

24. Xia, Y., Xie, L., Liu, F., Zhu, Z., Fishman, E.K., Yuille, A.L.: Bridging the gap between 2D and 3D organ segmentation with volumetric fusion net. In: Frangi, A.F., Schnabel, J.A., Davatzikos, C., Alberola-López, C., Fichtinger, G. (eds.) MICCAI 2018. LNCS, vol. 11073, pp. 445–453. Springer, Cham (2018). https://doi.org/10.1007/978-3-030-00937-3_51

25. Li, X., Chen, H., Qi, X., Dou, Q., Fu, C.-W., Heng, P.-A.: H-DenseUNet: hybrid densely connected UNet for liver and tumor segmentation from CT volumes. IEEE Trans. Med. Imaging **37**(12), 2663–2674 (2018)

26. Ni, T., Xie, L., Zheng, H., Fishman, E.K., Yuille, A.L.: Elastic boundary projection for 3d medical image segmentation. In: Proceedings of the IEEE/CVF Conference on Computer Vision and Pattern Recognition, pp. 2109–2118 (2019)

27. Pati, S., et al.: GandLF: a generally nuanced deep learning framework for scalable end-to-end clinical workflows in medical imaging. arXiv preprint arXiv:2103.01006 (2021)

28. Yang, J., et al.: Reinventing 2d convolutions for 3d images. IEEE J. Biomed. Health Inform. **25**(8), 3009–3018 (2021)

29. Yakubovskiy, P.: Segmentation models Pytorch. https://github.com/qubvel/segmentation_models.pytorch (2020)

30. Simonyan, K., Zisserman, A.: Very deep convolutional networks for large-scale image recognition. arXiv preprint arXiv:1409.1556 (2014)

31. He, K., Zhang, X., Ren, S., Sun, J.: Deep residual learning for image recognition. In: Proceedings of the IEEE Conference on Computer Vision and Pattern Recognition, pp. 770–778 (2016)

32. Huang, G., Liu, Z., Van Der Maaten, L., Weinberger, K.Q.: Densely connected convolutional networks. In: Proceedings of the IEEE Conference on Computer Vision and Pattern Recognition, pp. 4700–4708 (2017)

33. Tan, M., Le, Q.: Efficientnet: Rethinking model scaling for convolutional neural networks. In: International Conference on Machine Learning, pp. 6105–6114. PMLR (2019)

34. Ronneberger, O., Fischer, P., Brox, T.: U-Net: convolutional networks for biomedical image segmentation. In: Navab, N., Hornegger, J., Wells, W.M., Frangi, A.F. (eds.) MICCAI 2015. LNCS, vol. 9351, pp. 234–241. Springer, Cham (2015). https://doi.org/10.1007/978-3-319-24574-4_28

35. Menze, B.H., et al.: The multimodal brain tumor image segmentation benchmark (brats). IEEE Trans. Med. Imaging **34**(10), 1993–2024 (2014)

36. Bakas, S., et al.: Advancing the cancer genome atlas glioma MRI collections with expert segmentation labels and radiomic features. Sci. Data **4**(1), 1–13 (2017)

37. Bakas, S., et al.: Identifying the best machine learning algorithms for brain tumor segmentation, progression assessment, and overall survival prediction in the brats challenge. arXiv preprint arXiv:1811.02629 (2018)

38. Zijdenbos, A.P., Dawant, B.M., Margolin, R.A., Palmer, A.C.: Morphometric analysis of white matter lesions in MR images: method and validation. IEEE Trans. Med. Imaging **13**(4), 716–724 (1994)

39. Binder, Z.A., et al.: Epidermal growth factor receptor extracellular domain mutations in glioblastoma present opportunities for clinical imaging and therapeutic development. Cancer cell **34**(1), 163–177 (2018)

40. Bakas, S., et al.: In vivo detection of EGFRVIII in glioblastoma via perfusion magnetic resonance imaging signature consistent with deep peritumoral infiltration: The ϕ-indexin vivo EGFRVIII detection in glioblastoma via MRI signature. Clin. Cancer Res. **23**(16), 4724–4734 (2017)

41. Akbari, H., et al.: In vivo evaluation of EGFRVIII mutation in primary glioblastoma patients via complex multiparametric MRI signature. Neuro-oncology **20**(8), 1068–1079 (2018)

42. Rieke, N., et al.: The future of digital health with federated learning. NPJ Digit. Med. **3**(1), 1–7 (2020)

43. Baid, U., et al.: Federated learning for the classification of tumor infiltrating lymphocytes. arXiv preprint arXiv:2203.16622 (2022)

Probabilistic Tissue Mapping for Tumor Segmentation and Infiltration Detection of Glioma

Selene De Sutter[1]([envelope])[iD], Wietse Geens[2][iD], Matías Bossa[1][iD],
Anne-Marie Vanbinst[3][iD], Johnny Duerinck[2][iD],
and Jef Vandemeulebroucke[1,3,4][iD]

[1] Department of Electronics and Informatics (ETRO), Vrije Universiteit Brussel
(VUB), Brussels, Belgium
selene.de.sutter@vub.be
[2] Department of Neurosurgery, Vrije Universiteit Brussel (VUB),
Universitair Ziekenhuis Brussel (UZ Brussel), Brussels, Belgium
[3] Department of Radiology, Vrije Universiteit Brussel (VUB),
Universitair Ziekenhuis Brussel (UZ Brussel), Brussels, Belgium
[4] imec, Leuven, Belgium

Abstract. Segmentation of glioma structures is vital for therapy planning. Although state of the art algorithms achieve impressive results when compared to ground-truth manual delineations, one could argue that the binary nature of these labels does not properly reflect the underlying biology, nor does it account for uncertainties in the predicted segmentations. Moreover, the tumor infiltration beyond the contrast-enhanced lesion – visually imperceptible on imaging – is often ignored despite its potential role in tumor recurrence. We propose an intensity-based probabilistic model for brain tissue mapping based on conventional MRI sequences. We evaluated its value in the binary segmentation of the tumor and its subregions, and in the visualisation of possible infiltration. The model achieves a median Dice of 0.82 in the detection of the whole tumor, but suffers from confusion between different subregions. Preliminary results for the tumor probability maps encourage further investigation of the model regarding infiltration detection.

Keywords: Glioma · Segmentation · Infiltration · Probabilistic · Magnetic resonance imaging (MRI)

1 Introduction

Gliomas are the most common malignant primary tumors of the brain [1]. High-grade gliomas (HGG) are commonly considered to consist of three components: the contrast-enhanced (CE) tumor, a necrotic part (NEC), and adjacent vasogenic edema containing tumorous infiltration (ED) [2]. These allow to define tumor subregions: whole tumor (WT) = CE, NEC and ED; tumor core (TC) = CE and NEC; and enhanced tumor (ET) = CE. Standard glioma imaging practice

S. Bakas et al. (Eds.): BrainLes 2022, LNCS 13769, pp. 80–89, 2023.
https://doi.org/10.1007/978-3-031-33842-7_7

generally entails pre- and post-contrast T1, T2 and FLAIR [3], referred to as conventional MRI (cMRI) in the following. Standard treatment of HGG consists of maximum resection of the tumor, followed by combined radiochemotherapy [4]. Current practice relies on the ET for the determination of surgery and radiotherapy margins as it is clearly distinguishable on cMRI. However, HGG are characterized by infiltrative growth of tumor cells into the brain parenchyma beyond the margins of the ET [5], a phenomenon which can not be visually discerned on the scans [6]. Fast recurrence after treatment is observed in the vast majority of HGG cases, which may be related to unresected tumor infiltration [7].

Reliable segmentation of the tumoral structures is a vital step for therapy planning, or when assessing the patient's response. In clinical practice, this task is currently performed manually or interactively, which is time-consuming and prone to inter-reader variability. Latest research in computer vision leans towards the use of convolutional neural networks (CNN), with U-net architectures showing a particularly increasing popularity [8]. This tendency can be observed in the yearly BraTS challenge [9–11], where the winners of the previous two challenges achieved high performance with optimized U-net architectures, resulting in Dice scores of 0.89 (WT), 0.85 (TC) and 0.82 (ET) in 2020 [12], and a mean Dice score of 0.92 in 2021 [13].

Although constantly improving results are being reported, one could argue that the binary nature of these segmentations does not properly reflect the underlying biology of brain tissue, since it does not account for the mix of different cell types it consists of, causing some tumor subregions to gradually evolve from one type into another. This is of particular relevance for the case of infiltrative growth of tumorous cells into edema and healthy tissue [5]. In addition, authors are questioning the black-box nature of these deep learning models as they do not offer insight into why a generated prediction was made and what the uncertainty is associated with the prediction [14]. Current study describes a method that estimates the probability of a voxel pertaining to a certain tissue class, instead of a deterministic class label, and evaluates its performance compared to binary segmentations. In addition, we perform a preliminary exploration of the potential of probabilistic mapping in revealing information about tumor infiltration.

Few authors have explored the estimation of tumor probability maps. One study constructed probability maps of tumor presence based on apparent diffusion coefficient (ADC) maps and amino-acid positron emission tomography (PET) imaging combinations, which showed larger target volumes than standard ET [15]. Another synthesized tumor load images from the T1- and T2-relaxation maps, which were able to visualize amino-acid tracer uptake presented on PET [16]. Maps of infiltration probabilities have also been constructed by mining radiomic features in the vicinity of the ET from cMRI [17].

Raschke *et al.* [18] developed a model based on multimodal MRI (proton density, T2 and p and q diffusion maps) in an attempt to generates tissue heterogeneity maps that indicate tumor grade and infiltration margins. The method was based on probability density distributions for tumorous (low-grade and high-grade), healthy and edema regions. Ground-truth regions were determined through magnetic resonance spectroscopy, after which corresponding image intensities were extracted for the construction of the distributions from which tissue-type maps were derived.

Our approach bears some similarity with the latter [18], in that it also involves a statistical method in which image intensities are sampled from relevant tissue regions for the modelling of tissue probability distributions. However, we choose to focus on the use of cMRI as input images, because of their wide availability across institutes. Furthermore, we target the three main structures (CE, NEC and ED) as tumorous regions and explore the potential of the probability maps in uncovering information about infiltration.

2   Methods

2.1   Imaging Data

Data from the BraTS20 challenge [9–11] was used, including 369 low and high-grade glioma subjects, each containing cMRI scans and expert-annotated ground-truth segmentations for the CE, NEC and ED region. The data set was randomly split into a sampling, validation, and test set, respectively containing 269 (73%), 70 (19%) and 30 (8%) subjects.

2.2   Pre-processing and Normalization

Images in the BraTS dataset are co-registered, resampled to an isotropic voxel spacing of 1mm, and skull-stripped [9–11]. Since intensity distributions play a crucial role in our method, an intensity normalization step was performed. Three different techniques were compared. *Scaled normalization* involves scaling intensities linearly from $(0, P_{99.5})$ to $(0, 1)$, while values above are clipped to 1. *Z-scoring* involves centering the data using the intensity mean and scaling it to unit variance, after which the intensities are clipped and rescaled from $(-4, 4)$ to $(0, 1)$. In the case of *masked normalization*, an approximate tumor mask is automatically generated by thresholding the hyperintense region present on FLAIR, which is used to exclude the pathological region from the calculation of intensity mean and standard deviation. Z-score values are calculated, then scaled and clipped from $(-4, 4)$ to $(0, 1)$.

2.3   Region Selection

Our method is based on modelling the probability distributions of the multi-parametric intensities on cMRI of six different regions. Three tumorous regions are considered: CE, NEC and ED; the ground-truth segmentations of which are contained in the BraTS data set [9–11]. Additionally, three healthy regions were included: white matter (WM), grey matter (GM) and cerebrospinal fluid (CSF). Segmentations for these regions were acquired by applying FAST by FSL [19], while masking the tumorous regions.

2.4   Prior Region Probability Distributions

We used a subset of 269 subjects containing 1076 images to compute the prior distributions (PD). We started from images of a given subject and the corresponding ground-truth segmentation for a given region. We assumed increased uncertainty in the segmentations at the edges, and therefor eroded the ground-truth segmentation using a kernel radius of 1 prior to sampling. From the resulting regions, the intensities were extracted from each of the four modalities and repeated for each of the subjects in the sampling set. A probability density function was fitted on this set of samples through kernel density estimation using Gaussian kernels, leading to a 4D (one dimension for each modality) PD for the given region. The PD are regularly spaced between 0 and 1 along each dimension, and spacings of 0.1 and 0.05 were investigated.

2.5   Supervoxels

Before predicting brain tissue regions for an input image, the multimodal input intensities are first simplified using supervoxels, calculated based on the combination of the four modalities using simple iterative clustering (SLIC) [20]. Then, the mean intensity for each of the modalities is derived, creating a vector of 4 features for each of the supervoxels. Supervoxels are defined by two parameters: the number of segments and their compactness. For evaluation of the normalization and spacing, these were set to 10000 and 100, respectively. Subsequently, different values for both parameters were explored in combination with the optimized normalization and spacing setting, namely 1000, 5000, 10000, 15000, 20000, 25000 and 0.01, 0.1, 1, 10, 100, 1000, respectively.

2.6   Inference

For each supervoxel, the probability for each of the regions is predicted by extracting the prior probabilities for each region from the PD based on the intensities in the feature vector, and calculating the posterior probability of the supervoxel belonging to a certain region according to Bayes' theorem,

$$P(C_i|X) = \frac{P(C_i)p(X|C_i)}{\sum_j P(C_j)p(X|C_j)} ,$$
(1)

where $p(X|C_i)$ is the likelihood of having a voxel with intensities X in tissue class C_i, which can be derived from the PD. $P(C_i)$ is the prior probability of tissue class C_i, which was defined as the average volume fraction of that tissue type over the training subjects, with values of 0.45, 0.41, 0.06, 0.05, 0.02 and 0.01 for WM, GM, CSF, ED, CE and NEC, respectively.

By associating each supervoxel with their posterior probabilities, we can visualize probability maps for each of the considered regions. To obtain binary segmentations which are comparable to the available ground truth and state of the art, a supervoxel is assigned to the segmentation of one of the 6 regions (CE,

NEC, ED, GM, WM or CSF) when its probability is the maximum probability between all regions. After, the binary segmentations are combined into subregions (WT, TC and ET) for evaluation. Presuming tumor cells are most present within the tumor core, we derive the tumor probability map from the probabilities of the CE and NEC regions in accordance with $P_{tumor} = P_{CE} + P_{NEC}$.

3   Results

3.1   Tumor Segmentation

The predicted binary tumor segmentations were quantitatively compared to the available ground truth: Dice score and average Hausdorff distance (AHD) were calculated for subregions WT, TC and ET. Evaluation on the validation set was used to asses the optimal normalization technique and spacing of the distributions, for which corresponding results are summarized in Table 1 and Fig. 1. Inferior results for scaled normalization were found. Differences between the Z-score and masked technique were small, yet Z-score provided the best mean Dice and lowest variance. Results for a spacing of 0.05 consistently exceeded those for 0.1. Subsequently, Z-score normalization and a spacing of 0.05 were used for further evaluation. Different values for supervoxel parameters were explored, for which results are visualized in Fig. 2. Optimal values, based on Dice scores for WT and subregions, for these parameters were found to be 1000 and 0.1 for number of segments and compactness, respectively, and were chosen for evaluation on the test set (see Table 2).

Three segmentation cases of the test set were selected for qualitative assessment of the results, visualized in Fig. 3. Selection was based on the Dice score averaged over the three subregions (WT, TC and ET) and correspond to the 5th percentile, median and 95th percentile cases.

Table 1. Median and mean values of Dice score and AHD for validation set results. Metrics are averaged over the different subregions (WT, TC and ET).

	median Dice		mean Dice		median AHD (mm)		mean AHD (mm)	
Spacing	0.1	0.05	0.1	0.05	0.1	0.05	0.1	0.05
Scaled	0.458	0.448	0.448	0.433	3.217	3.123	6.499	6.792
Z-score	0.615	0.615	0.571	0.579	2.926	2.481	6.256	6.182
Masked	0.602	0.623	0.556	0.576	3.145	2.526	6.371	5.892

Table 2. Median and mean values of Dice score and AHD for test set results.

	median Dice	mean Dice	median AHD (mm)	mean AHD (mm)
WT	0.816	0.736	1.170	3.139
TC	0.623	0.605	2.171	6.179
ET	0.767	0.641	0.768	6.190

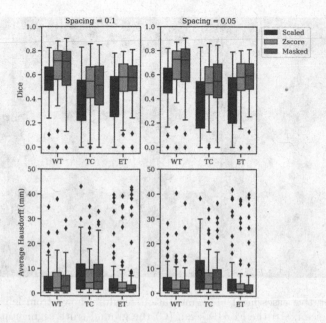

Fig. 1. Boxplots of Dice score and AHD for validation set results. Different normalization techniques and different spacings are compared.

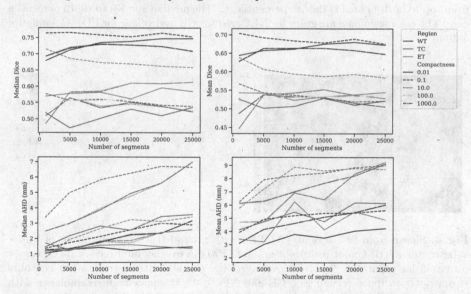

Fig. 2. Median and mean values of Dice score and AHD for evaluation of the influence of different values for supervoxel parameters (compactness and number of segments) on the validation set.

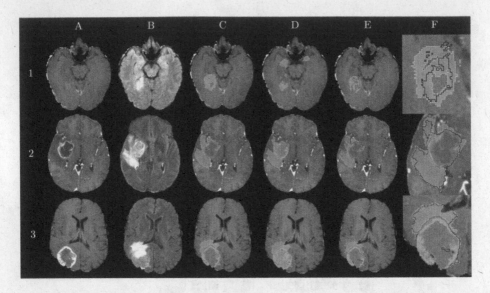

Fig. 3. Qualitative assessment of segmentation results. Shown from left to right are (A) the T1ce scan, (B) the FLAIR scan, (C) the ground-truth segmentation, (D) the predicted segmentation, (E) the ground-truth segmentation (color segments) compared to the predicted WT delineation (black line) with (F) its zoomed-in version. Shown from top to bottom are (1) the 5th percentile, (2) the median and (3) the 95th percentile case. The color segments are green for NEC, red for CE and yellow for ED. (Color figure online)

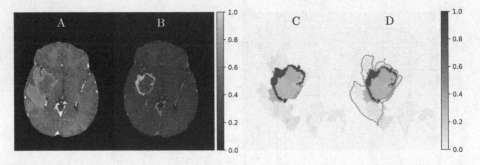

Fig. 4. Shown from left to right: (A) T1ce with ground-truth segmentations of tumor substructures, (B) tumor probability map (TPM) in overlay on T1ce scan, (C) tumor probabilities separately and (D) overlayed by ground-truth segmentation contours (from outer to inner region: ED, CE and NEC). TPM shows high resemblance with ground-truth TC segmentation. High probabilities are found in CE region, lower values bleed into the ED region.

3.2   Tumor Probability Mapping

To demonstrate the potential of the tumor probability map, we visualize the median case based on the performance in the segmentation task. The generated tumor probability map is shown in Fig. 4.

4   Discussion and Conclusion

Automated binary segmentations of glioma regions can be time-saving for clinicians by abating the need for manual delineations. The proposed model derives such segmentations from the estimated tissue probability maps and was evaluated for segmentations of WT, TC and ET. While evaluating on the validation set, different normalization techniques were compared. The Z-score and masked technique, with little difference in performance, exceeded scaled normalization. Z-score was found to be more robust than masked normalization. We believe this is the case because scaling is more sensitive to intensity outliers compared to Z-scoring, while masking introduces an extra step which might give rise to more variance. Two different spacings for the distributions were investigated, which were empirically determined as a good initial compromise between accuracy and computational time during preliminary experiments. A spacing of 0.05 yielded the best results, yet further investigation of this hyperparameter is recommended.

The performance on the validation set was evaluated for different values for the supervoxel parameters. Their values were chosen as an initial exploration, thus further refinement of these values will be required. A superior performance in terms of Dice scores was observed for a compactness value of 0.1, which provided a good balance between the evenness of the segments while still respecting the natural edges of the brain anatomy. Maximum Dice scores were found for all subregions in combination with a number of segments equal to 1000. While a low value for this parameter has the advantage of low computational complexity – the number of supervoxels linearly influences the computation time in current implementation – such a rough parcellization limits achievable accuracies in possible further optimizations. In addition, our approach currently lacks spatial awareness of a supervoxel for its surroundings. This limitation should be addressed in future research, and may partially remedy the need for large supervoxels.

We report a mean Dice score over the three subregions of 0.66, which implies that the model performs less accurately than the state of the art (mean Dice $= 0.92$). However, the model performs substantially better in detecting the WT compared to subregions, for which a median Dice of 0.82 was obtained. Visualizations in Fig. 3 show that the P_5-case (1) contains merely a subtle lesion on FLAIR in addition to a small TC, where Dice is known to strongly penalize small errors. The P_{50}-case (2) shows reasonable segmentations for WT and subtypes, while the P_{95}-case (3) shows a very good match for WT and ET. Difficulty in correctly identifying necrosis is observed, particularly due to confusion with edema, which could partly be attributed to the low average volume fraction of this region, serving as prior probability during inference, indicating further optimization of these values might be necessary.

Tumor probability maps can visualize tumor presence from a combination of modalities, providing additional insight over the mere visual interpretation of the clinician. Awareness of infiltrating tumor cells could motivate the treatment of highly probable infiltrated tissue beyond the CE lesion and potentially prevent recurrence. The proposed model aims to generate such probability maps in an interpretable manner from cMRI. An alternative interpretation of the probabilities relate to the density of cell types. Given this interpretation, we expect high probabilities in the middle of a tissue region and descending at the edges where it transitions into another type. The most significant usage of this concept is in the case of tumor cell densities, where the transitional region into healthy tissue is referred to as infiltration. Visualization of tumor probability maps (Fig. 4) demonstrate high values within the CE region, where it is known to have a high tumor cell density, while low values bleed into the edema region, possibly suggesting tumor infiltration. However, due to a lack of ground truth, it is not yet possible to ascertain if the probability maps indicate tissue type proportions, uncertainty or other. Hence, further validation of this statement with strong ground truth will be necessary.

In this work, we explored an intensity-based probabilistic model for brain tissue probability mapping. Although binary tumor segmentations from such probability maps underperform compared to state of the art, the probabilistic nature of the maps provide additional, possibly valuable information and encourages further investigation of their use for possible tumor and infiltration visualization.

References

1. Hanif, F., et al.: Glioblastoma multiforme: a review of its epidemiology and pathogenesis through clinical presentation and treatment. Asian Pac. J. Cancer Prevent. APJCP. **18**(1), 3 (2017)
2. Menze, B.H., et al.: The multimodal brain tumor image segmentation benchmark (BRATS). IEEE Trans. Med. Imaging. **34**(10), 1993–2024 (2014)
3. Thust, S.C., et al.: Glioma imaging in Europe: a survey of 220 centres and recommendations for best clinical practice. Eur. Radiol. **28**(8), 3306–3317 (2018)
4. Wolfgang, W., et al.: Treatment of glioblastoma in adults. Therapeut. Adv. Neurol. Disorders. **11**, 1756286418790452 (2018)
5. Ferrer, V.P., Neto, V.M., Mentlein, R.: Glioma infiltration and extracellular matrix: key players and modulators. Glia. **66**(8), 1542–1565 (2018)
6. Rudie, J.D., et al.: Emerging applications of artificial intelligence in neuro-oncology. Radiology. **290**(3), 607 (2019)
7. Senft, C., et al.: Intraoperative MRI guidance and extent of resection in glioma surgery: a randomised, controlled trial. The Lancet Oncol. **12**(11), 997–1003 (2011)
8. van Kempen, E.J., et al.: Performance of machine learning algorithms for glioma segmentation of brain MRI: a systematic literature review and meta-analysis. Eur. Radiol. **31**(12), 9638–9653 (2021). https://doi.org/10.1007/s00330-021-08035-0

9. Menze, J., et al., A comparison of random forest and its GINI importance with standard chemometric methods for the feature selection and classification of spectral data. BMC Bioinform. **10**(1) (2009)

10. Lloyd, C.T., Sorichetta, A., Tatem, A.J.: High resolution global gridded data for use in population studies. Sci. Data. **4**(1), 1–17 (2017)

11. Bakas, S., et al.: Identifying the best machine learning algorithms for brain tumor segmentation, progression assessment, and overall survival prediction in the BRATS challenge. arXiv preprint arXiv:1811.02629 (2018)

12. Isensee, F., Jäger, P.F., Full, P.M., Vollmuth, P., Maier-Hein, K.H.: nnU-net for brain tumor segmentation. In: Crimi, A., Bakas, S. (eds.) BrainLes 2020. LNCS, vol. 12659, pp. 118–132. Springer, Cham (2021). https://doi.org/10.1007/978-3-030-72087-2_11

13. Futrega, M.l., et al.: Optimized U-Net for Brain Tumor Segmentation. arXiv preprint arXiv:2110.03352 (2021)

14. Daisy, P.S., Anitha, T.S.: Can artificial intelligence overtake human intelligence on the bumpy road towards glioma therapy? Med. Oncol. **38**(5), 1–11 (2021). https://doi.org/10.1007/s12032-021-01500-2

15. Verburg, N., et al.: Improved detection of diffuse glioma infiltration with imaging combinations: a diagnostic accuracy study. Neuro-oncology **22**(3), 412–422 (2020)

16. Kinoshita, M., et al.: Magnetic resonance relaxometry for tumor cell density imaging for glioma: an exploratory study via 11C-methionine PET and its validation via stereotactic tissue sampling. Cancers **13**(16), 4067 (2021)

17. Rathore, S., et al.: Radiomic signature of infiltration in peritumoral edema predicts subsequent recurrence in glioblastoma: implications for personalized radiotherapy planning. J. Med. Imaging **5**(2), 021219 (2018)

18. Raschke, F., et al.: Tissue-type mapping of gliomas. NeuroImage Clin. **21**, 101648 (2019)

19. Zhang, Y., Brady, M., Smith, S.: Segmentation of brain MR images through a hidden Markov random field model and the expectation-maximization algorithm. IEEE Trans. Med. Imaging. **20**(1), 45–57 (2001)

20. Achanta, R., et al.: SLIC superpixels compared to state-of-the-art superpixel methods. IEEE Trans. Pattern Anal. Mach. Intell. **34**(11), 2274–2282 (2012)

Robustifying Automatic Assessment of Brain Tumor Progression from MRI

Krzysztof Kotowski[1], Bartosz Machura[1], and Jakub Nalepa[1,2]

[1] Graylight Imaging, Gliwice, Poland
kotowski.polsl@gmail.com, {bmachura,jnalepa}@graylight-imaging.com
[2] Department of Algorithmics and Software, Silesian University of Technology, Gliwice, Poland
jnalepa@ieee.org

Abstract. Accurate assessment of brain tumor progression from magnetic resonance imaging is a critical issue in clinical practice which allows us to precisely monitor the patient's response to a given treatment. Manual analysis of such imagery is, however, prone to human errors and lacks reproducibility. Therefore, designing automated end-to-end quantitative tumor's response assessment is of pivotal clinical importance nowadays. In this work, we further investigate this issue and verify the robustness of bidimensional and volumetric tumor's measurements calculated over the delineations obtained using the state-of-the-art tumor segmentation deep learning model which was ranked 6th in the BraTS21 Challenge. Our experimental study, performed over the Brain Tumor Progression dataset, showed that volumetric measurements are more robust against varying-quality tumor segmentation, and that improving brain extraction can notably impact the calculation of the tumor's characteristics.

Keywords: Brain tumor · Segmentation · RANO · Brain extraction

1 Introduction

Glioblastoma (GBM) is the most common of malignant brain tumors in adults and despite decades of research, it remains one of the most feared of all cancers due to its poor prognosis. Thus, accurate evaluation of the therapy response in GBM presents considerable challenges and is of high clinical importance. It is commonly based on the use of the Response Assessment in Neuro-Oncology (RANO) criteria and the measurement of two perpendicular diameters of the

This work was supported by the National Centre for Research and Development (POIR.01.01.01-00-0092/20). JN was supported by the Silesian University of Technology funds through the grant for maintaining and developing research potential. This paper is in memory of Dr. Grzegorz Nalepa, an extraordinary scientist, pediatric hematologist/oncologist, and a compassionate champion for kids at Riley Hospital for Children, Indianapolis, USA, who helped countless patients and their families through some of the most challenging moments of their lives.

S. Bakas et al. (Eds.): BrainLes 2022, LNCS 13769, pp. 90–101, 2023.
https://doi.org/10.1007/978-3-031-33842-7_8

contrast-enhancing tumor (ET) [9], as well as a qualitative evaluation of abnormalities in magnetic resonance imaging (MRI) sequences, which correspond to regions of edema with or without tumor cell infiltration. Radiological evaluation is complex as the tumor appearance is heterogeneous, with an irregular shape associated with the infiltrative nature of the disease. Also, manual analysis suffers from intra- and inter-rater variability which negatively impacts its reproducibility, thus making the tracking of the disease progression difficult.

There are techniques which automate the process of brain tumor segmentation. They range across classic and deep learning algorithms, with the former techniques exploiting hand-crafted feature extractors, commonly followed by feature selectors [1,20]. In deep learning, we benefit from automated representation learning to capture the tumor characteristics which may not be visible to the naked eye [18]. Such techniques have established the state of the art in medical image segmentation tasks through delivering the winning solutions in the biomedical competitions [11,22]. Segmentation of brain tumors is, however, virtually never the final step in the analysis chain—once the tumor is delineated, we extract the tumor's characteristics which allow us to track its progression (or regression). To precisely track the disease, accurate delineation of the brain tumor is pivotal, as its inaccurate segmentation would directly influence the extracted metrics, such as bidimensional or volumetric measurements [6].

Automated end-to-end quantitative tumor's response assessment, encompassing its segmentation, further quantification and extraction of additional image-based features [21], has been gaining research attention to overcome the inherent limitations of manual assessment of tumor burden [26]. In [14], Kickingereder et al. compiled a single-institution MRI set from patients with brain tumors, and exploited it for training a U-Net. The model was later validated over single- and multi-institutional longitudinal sets. The authors showed that the deep model enabled objective assessment of tumor response in neuro-oncology at high throughput which would not be achievable with manual analysis. Interestingly, several works showed that there is no clear evidence that volumetric measurement methods could provide more accurate progression tracking, hence suggest that bidimensional and volumetric measurements could be used interchangeably [5,10].

In this work, we aim at further investigating this issue, as indeed performing bidimensional measurements is much easier in practice. We utilize a fully-automated deep learning-powered approach for the tumor response assessment in longitudinal studies which includes separate algorithms for (i) brain extraction (skull stripping), (ii) segmenting the enhancing tumor (as two perpendicular diameters of the contrast-enhancing tumor are used in RANO), and (iii) extracting bidimensional and volumetric measurements of the resulting volume of interest (Sect. 2). Here, we hypothesize that improving brain extraction may influence other analysis steps, and that it can be assessed indirectly through verifying the quality of segmentation, hence the quality of extracted quantifiable tumor's measurements. The experimental study performed over the recent Brain Tumor Progression dataset revealed that improving the widely-used brain extraction method may notably enhance the segmentation models operating on such skull-stripped MRI data, therefore can improve the quantifiable tumor's measures which are tracked in the progression analysis (Sect. 3). Additionally, we showed that bidimensional measurements are much more sensitive to any changes in the segmentation pipeline when compared to the volumetric measurements, and can be even completely misleading for (even slightly) modified segmentation masks. It indicates that the volumetric measurements can be more robust metrics, even though it was not that evident in previous studies [5,10].

2   Materials and Methods

In this section, we discuss the dataset exploited in our study (Sect. 2.1), together with the approaches utilized for extracting brain (this step is commonly referred to as skull stripping) from multi-modal MRI, segmenting brain tumors, and performing automated bidimensional tumor measurements (Sect. 2.2).

2.1   Dataset Description

We used the Brain Tumor Progression (BTP) dataset [23] from The Cancer Imaging Archive (TCIA) [7] containing 20 patients with newly diagnosed primary glioblastoma. For each patient, two MRI studies are included, one acquired within 90 days after surgery and chemo-radiation therapy, and one captured at the tumor's progression determined clinically (in average, 178 days after the first examination; minimum: 29 days, maximum: 966 days). Each study contains the pre- and post-contrast T1-weighted (T1), T2-weighted (T2), and fluid-attenuated inversion recovery (FLAIR) sequences, among others. The enhancing-tumor ground-truth masks were generated by the authors of the set using T1 images for both time points, therefore this dataset can be used to validate automated brain tumor progression techniques through comparing the calculated and ground-truth change in tumor's characteristics (e.g., bidimensional or volumetric). The details of this ground-truth elaboration procedure were, however, not disclosed—we may observe that the quality of the ground-truth masks can be questionable in some cases, as there exist "noisy" delineations, as in an example rendered in Fig. 1.

2.2   Bidimensional and Volumetric Tumor Measurements

Our analysis pipeline encompasses five pivotal steps. First, (1) we apply MRI preprocessing from BraTS21 Challenge using Cancer Imaging Phenomics Toolkit (CaPTK) [8,19] (omitting the final brain extraction step). Then, (2) we pre-process the input MRI sequences to remove all non-brain tissue from further processing (brain extraction). Such skull-stripped MRI sequences are fed into (3) the brain tumor segmentation pipeline to delineate its contrast-enhancing region, for which we (4) calculate its bidimensional (RANO) and volumetric measurements. Those measurements are finally used to (5) quantify the disease progression through evaluating the difference between RANO and the tumor's volume

Original image (first examination)   Original image (second examination)

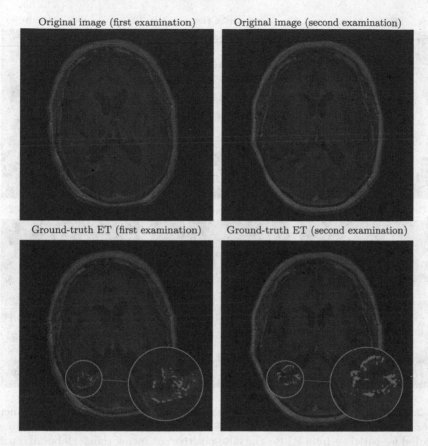

Ground-truth ET (first examination)   Ground-truth ET (second examination)

Fig. 1. Ground-truth enhancing-tumor masks for the first and second examination of patient 15 from BTP, overlaid on the T1w post-contrast slices.

in two consecutive time points (Δ_{RANO} and Δ_V, respectively). The details of each step are given in the sections below.

Brain Extraction. The original BraTS21 preprocessing pipeline in CaPTK implements brain extraction with DeepMedic [24], being a 3D convolutional neural network with the fully-connected conditional random field [13,24]. However, we observed many false positives (being the voxels of the skull marked as the brain) in the predictions of this network over the BraTS21 and BTP datasets. We hypothesize that such incorrect brain extraction may negatively impact the brain tumor segmentation step—it is indeed shown in Fig. 4, where the DeepMedic skull stripping "fooled" the deep learning brain tumor segmentation model leading to false-positive enhancing tumor detection. Therefore, to improve the quality of automated brain extraction in the BTP dataset (hence, the quality of tumor's delineation), we replaced DeepMedic with the HD-BET network based on a 3D U-Net [12] which was previously validated over various MRI scans, and was shown to be delivering accurate skull stripping [17] (Fig. 2).

Original image   Brain extraction (DeepMedic)   Brain extraction (HD-BET)

Original image (zoomed)   ET segmentation (DeepMedic)   ET segmentation (HD-BET)

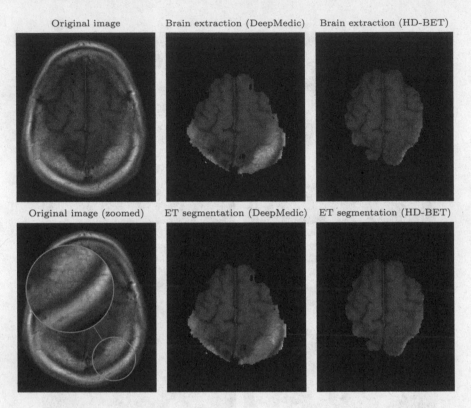

Fig. 2. Brain tumor extraction (top row) may easily influence the quality of enhancing tumor segmentation (bottom row). We present an example T1w post-contrast image captured for patient 1 from BTP—the false-positive enhancing tumor elaborated using our tumor segmentation model is rendered in red. (Color figure online)

Segmenting Brain Tumors from MRI. For segmenting the brain tumor, we utilize our deep learning algorithm [15] which was ranked 6th in the recent BraTS21 Challenge [2]. It was trained on BraTS21 training set that captures 1251 multi-institutional routine clinically-acquired multi-parametric MRI (mpMRI) scans accompanied with the ground-truth multi-class brain tumor delineations [2,3,16]. The model is based on the nnU-Net architecture [11] and produces predictions of three tumor subregions: enhancing tumor (ET), necrotic tumor core, and edema. However, we focus only on the ET subregion to quantify the tumor progression. This deep learning model achieved the mean DICE of 0.86 and mean Hausdorff of 13.09 over the BraTS21 testing set. The segmentation model was originally trained on the BraTS21 data pre-processed as described in [4], including reorientation and resampling of the original image data, followed by brain extraction, denoising, bias correction and co-registration. We applied the very same pre-processing pipeline to the BTP data using Cancer Imaging Phenomics Toolkit (CaPTK) [8,19]. The predictions generated for such pre-processed data were transformed back to the original coordinates of the ground truth by reverting coregistration, resampling, and reorientation. Additionally, we investigated if improving the brain extraction step with HD-BET over the unseen test set (here, BTP) may positively impact brain tumor segmentation (note that the training MRI scans was never changed, hence it included the scans skull-stripped with DeepMedic).

Automatic Bidimensional and Volumetric Measurements. To automatically calculate the bidimensional measurements according to the Response Assessment in Neuro-Oncology (RANO) criteria [25], we utilize the AutoRANO algorithm [6]. For each detected ET region in the input scan, the algorithm exhaustively searches for the longest segment (major diameter) over all axial slices, and then for the corresponding longest perpendicular diameter, with the tolerance of $5°$ inclusive. Such segments are valid if they (i) are fully included in ET, and (ii) are both at least 10 mm long (otherwise, the lesion is not measurable). Finally, the product of the perpendicular diameters is calculated. If there are more measurable ET regions, the sum of up to five largest products is returned. Additionally, to calculate the "full ET volume" for of all ET regions (measurable and non-measurable), we count all non-zero voxels in the resulting binary ET mask and multiply this number by a voxel size of the scan. On the other hand, in the "measurable ET volume", we calculate the volume of the measurable (in terms of RANO criteria) ET regions only.

3   Experimental Results

The objectives of our experimental study are two-fold: to (i) investigate the impact of improving the brain extraction algorithm on the quality of brain tumor segmentation, hence on the quality of bidimensional and volumetric tumor measurements used for tumor response assessment, and to (ii) verify the robustness of bidimensional and volumetric tumor measurements against varying segmentation quality. The deep learning tumor segmentation model was trained over the BraTS21 training data, therefore the entire BTP dataset is used as the unseen test set. To quantify the segmentation quality, we exploit DICE. The inter-algorithm agreements for bidimensional and volume measurements were evaluated using the Intraclass Correlation Coefficient (ICC) calculated on a single measurement, absolute-agreement, two-way random-effects model. The R package IRR (Inter Rater Reliability, version 0.84.1) was used for ICC, whereas GraphPad Prism 9.4.0 for calculating the Spearman's correlation coefficients.

In Fig. 3, we present the distribution of the metrics obtained using the deep learning model deployed for the BTP patients skull-stripped with the DeepMedic (DM) and HD-BET algorithms, together with the Bland-Altman plots for DICE, RANO and measurable ET volume (in mm^3). For DM, the mean and median DICE amounted to 0.72 and 0.77, respectively (with the lower and upper 95% confidence interval [CI] of mean: 0.66 and 0.79), whereas for HD-BET, we obtained the mean and median DICE of 0.73 and 0.79 (lower/upper 95% CI: 0.67 and 0.80). It is worth mentioning that the results are comparable to those

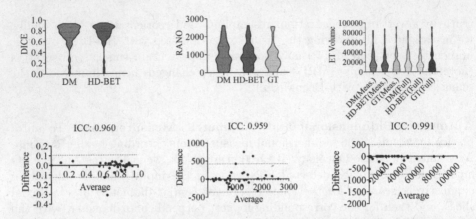

Fig. 3. Distribution of the metrics (DICE, RANO, ET volume) obtained for all BTP patients (first row), and the Bland-Altman plots (second row) for DICE, RANO, and measurable ET volume (for DM vs. HD-BET brain extraction).

reported over the BraTS21 dataset—interestingly, although the brain tumor deep learning segmentation model was trained solely over the pre-operative glioma patients, it was capable of delivering high-quality post-treatment ET delineations. There was no statistically significant difference between DICE and RANO calculated for DM, HD-BET and the ground-truth ET masks (GT) according to the Wilcoxon tests ($p < 0.05$), but the differences in volume are indeed statistically significant across only measurable and all lesions (annotated as Full in Fig. 3) for GT ($p < 0.01$). It confirms that there exist small ET regions in GT, possibly related to "noisy" areas (as in Fig. 1), which do not affect the bidimensional measurements. The visual examples rendered in Fig. 4 not only show that utilizing different brain extraction techniques can easily lead to selecting different MRI images for which RANO is calculated, but also indicates that the lesion's shape characteristics within the longitudinal study can drastically change, hence being able to accurately delineate both large and small ET regions using the same model is pivotal to ensure high-quality progression analysis.

To quantify the brain tumor progression, we calculated the change in the bidimensional and volumetric characteristics of the tumor for each BTP patient (Fig. 5a). Here, the differences across DM, HD-BET and GT are more visible for all metrics (RANO and volume), showing that the brain extraction step does influence the progression analysis. It is further confirmed in Fig. 5b, where the largest Spearman's correlation coefficient values were obtained for the HD-BET skull stripping: 0.68, 0.93, 0.93 for RANO, volume of measurable and volume of all ET regions, respectively (the correlation coefficient amounted to 0.58, 0.90, and 0.89 for DM). For all segmentation methods (deep learning-powered with DM and HD-BET, and GT), we can observe high RANO and measurable ET volume correlations: 0.73, 0.77, 0.80, with the correlation obtained by the model operating on the MRI data skull-stripped by HD-BET approaching the correlation obtained for GT. Volumetric measurements are, however, more robust against inaccurate segmentation, as bidimensional measurements are significantly affected by the

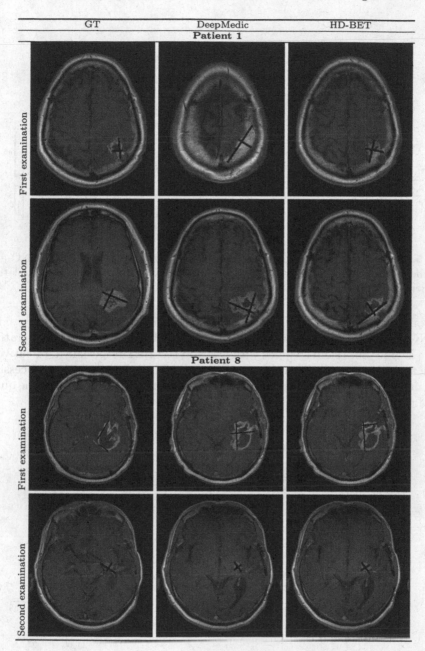

Fig. 4. AutoRANO measurements (red segments) and ET masks (yellow overlays) for patient 1 and 8 in the first (top row) and second (bottom row) timepoint. (Color figure online)

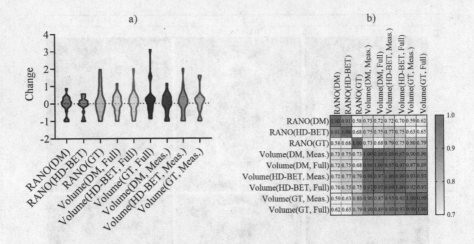

Fig. 5. Brain tumor progression assessed as the a) change in the metric (RANO and volumetric measurements, Δ_{RANO} and Δ_V), together with the Spearman's correlation coefficient calculated for the extracted metrics for all BTP patients.

contouring quality (Fig. 4). Finally, the Bland-Altman plots gathered in Fig. 6 for RANO and volume indicate a notable discrepancy between the models operating over the BTP data skull-stripped with DM and HD-BET (especially for relatively large tumor's changes). Therefore, revisiting the brain extraction pre-processing step in the BraTS dataset may be an interesting issue to further improve the quality of segmentation models trained from such pre-processed image data.

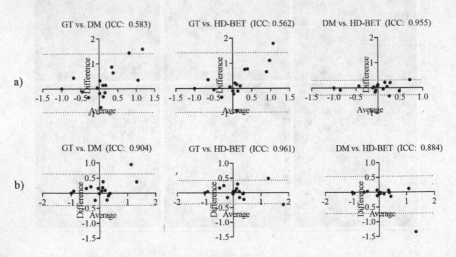

Fig. 6. Bland-Altman plots for the change in a) RANO and b) ET volume. The Bland-Altman plots show a discrepancy between the models operating over the data skull-stripped with DM and HD-BET (especially for large tumor's changes).

4 Conclusions

Accurate brain tumor progression assessment is a critical issue in clinical practice which allows us to precisely monitor the patient's response to a given treatment. Manual analysis of acquired MRI data is, however, an important obstacle in quantifiable and reproducible disease's tracking, as it suffers from significant inter- and intra-rater disagreement. In this work, we tackled this issue and utilized an automated end-to-end approach for extracting bidimensional and volumetric measures which are commonly used in the tumor response assessment. In the experimental study performed over the BTP dataset, we investigated the impact of updating the skull-stripping algorithm on the brain tumor segmentation and quantification steps. Interestingly, the model trained over pre-operative MRI scans allowed us to obtain accurate enhancing-tumor contouring for post-treatment patients. We showed that improving brain extraction (assessed indirectly through investigating the brain tumor segmentation quality) can help enhance the following steps of the analysis chain, as inaccurate skull stripping results in many false positives in enhancing tumor prediction, especially for tumors close to the skull where the bone can be interpreted as the contrast enhancement. Additionally, bidimensional measurements were more sensitive to any changes in the segmentation pipeline than the volumetric measurements. They can be completely misleading when the delineations are "noisy", e.g., like the GT of the BTP set—automating the process of volumetric ET measurements is of utmost clinical relevance to ensure robust assessment of disease's progression. The results presented in this work may be an interesting point of departure for further research, and may lead to revisiting the MRI scans skull-stripped in various datasets (e.g., in BraTS), in order to improve the quality of skull stripping which can directly influence the quality of brain tumor segmentation delivered by the automatic algorithms trained from such pre-processed image data.

References

1. Abbas, H.K., Fatah, N.A., Mohamad, H.J., Alzuky, A.A.: Brain tumor classification using texture feature extraction. J. Phys. Conf. Ser. **1892**(1), 012012 (2021)
2. Baid, U., et al.: The RSNA-ASNR-MICCAI BraTS 2021 Benchmark on Brain Tumor Segmentation and Radiogenomic Classification (2021). https://doi.org/10.48550/arXiv.2107.02314. http://arxiv.org/abs/2107.02314, number: arXiv:2107.02314
3. Bakas, S., et al.: Advancing the cancer genome atlas glioma MRI collections with expert segmentation labels and radiomic features. Sci. Data **4**(1), 170117 (2017). https://doi.org/10.1038/sdata.2017.117. https://www.nature.com/articles/sdata2017117
4. Bakas, S., et al.: Advancing the cancer genome atlas glioma MRI collections with expert segmentation labels and radiomic features. Nat. Sci. Data **4**, 1–13 (2017). https://doi.org/10.1038/sdata.2017.117

5. Berntsen, E.M., et al.: Volumetric segmentation of glioblastoma progression compared to bidimensional products and clinical radiological reports. Acta Neurochir. **162**(2), 379–387 (2020)

6. Chang, K., et al.: Automatic assessment of glioma burden: a deep learning algorithm for fully automated volumetric and bidimensional measurement. Neuro Oncol. **21**(11), 1412–1422 (2019)

7. Clark, K., et al.: The cancer imaging archive (TCIA): maintaining and operating a public information repository. J. Digit. Imaging **26**(6), 1045–1057 (2013)

8. Davatzikos, C., et al.: Cancer imaging phenomics toolkit: quantitative imaging analytics for precision diagnostics and predictive modeling of clinical outcome. J. Med. Imaging **5**(1), 011018 (2018)

9. Ellingson, B.M., Wen, P.Y., Cloughesy, T.F.: Modified criteria for radiographic response assessment in glioblastoma clinical trials. Neurotherapeutics **14**(2), 307–320 (2017)

10. Gahrmann, R., et al.: Comparison of 2D (RANO) and volumetric methods for assessment of recurrent glioblastoma treated with bevacizumab-a report from the BELOB trial. Neuro Oncol. **19**(6), 853–861 (2017)

11. Isensee, F., Jaeger, P.F., Kohl, S.A.A., Petersen, J., Maier-Hein, K.H.: nnU-Net: a self-configuring method for deep learning-based biomedical image segmentation. Nat. Methods **18**(2), 203–211 (2021)

12. Isensee, F., et al.: Automated brain extraction of multisequence MRI using artificial neural networks. Hum. Brain Mapp. **40**(17), 4952–4964 (2019)

13. Kamnitsas, K., et al.: Efficient multi-scale 3D CNN with fully connected CRF for accurate brain lesion segmentation. Med. Image Anal. **36**, 61–78 (2017)

14. Kickingereder, P., et al.: Automated quantitative tumour response assessment of MRI in neuro-oncology with artificial neural networks: a multicentre, retrospective study. Lancet Oncol. **20**(5), 728–740 (2019)

15. Kotowski, K., Adamski, S., Machura, B., Zarudzki, L., Nalepa, J.: Coupling nnU-nets with expert knowledge for accurate brain tumor segmentation from MRI. In: Crimi, A., Bakas, S. (eds.) Brainlesion: Glioma, Multiple Sclerosis, Stroke and Traumatic Brain Injuries. LNCS, vol. 12963, pp. 197–209. Springer, Cham (2022). https://doi.org/10.1007/978-3-031-09002-8_18

16. Menze, B.H., et al.: The multimodal brain tumor image segmentation benchmark (BRATS). IEEE Trans. Med. Imaging **34**(10), 1993–2024 (2015)

17. Nalepa, J., et al.: Fully-automated deep learning-powered system for DCE-MRI analysis of brain tumors. Artif. Intell. Med. **102**, 101769 (2020)

18. Naser, M.A., Deen, M.J.: Brain tumor segmentation and grading of lower-grade glioma using deep learning in MRI images. Comput. Biol. Med. **121**, 103758 (2020)

19. Pati, S., et al.: The cancer imaging phenomics toolkit (CaPTk): technical overview. In: Crimi, A., Bakas, S. (eds.) BrainLes 2019. LNCS, vol. 11993, pp. 380–394. Springer, Cham (2020). https://doi.org/10.1007/978-3-030-46643-5_38

20. Poernama, A.I., Soesanti, I., Wahyunggoro, O.: Feature extraction and feature selection methods in classification of brain MRI images: a review. In: Proceedings of IEEE IBITeC, vol. 1, pp. 58–63 (2019)

21. Rucco, M., Viticchi, G., Falsetti, L.: Towards personalized diagnosis of glioblastoma in fluid-attenuated inversion recovery (FLAIR) by topological interpretable machine learning. Mathematics **8**(5), 770 (2020)

22. Saleem, H., Shahid, A.R., Raza, B.: Visual interpretability in 3D brain tumor segmentation network. Comput. Biol. Med. **133**, 104410 (2021)

23. Schmainda, K., Prah, M.: Data from Brain-Tumor-Progression (2019). https://doi.org/10.7937/K9/TCIA.2018.15QUZVNB. https://wiki.cancerimagingarchive.net/x/1wEGAg. Version Number: 1 Type: dataset

24. Thakur, S., et al.: Brain extraction on MRI scans in presence of diffuse glioma: multi-institutional performance evaluation of deep learning methods and robust modality-agnostic training. Neuroimage **220**, 117081 (2020)

25. Wen, P.Y., et al.: Updated response assessment criteria for high-grade gliomas: response assessment in neuro-oncology working group. J. Clin. Oncol. **28**(11), 1963–1972 (2010)

26. Zegers, C., et al.: Current applications of deep-learning in neuro-oncological MRI. Physica Med. **83**, 161–173 (2021)

MidFusNet: Mid-dense Fusion Network
for Multi-modal Brain MRI Segmentation

Wenting Duan[1][(✉)], Lei Zhang[1], Jordan Colman[1,2], Giosue Gulli[2], and Xujiong Ye[1]

[1] Department of Computer Science, University of Lincoln, Lincoln, UK
wduan@lincoln.ac.uk
[2] Ashford and St Peter's Hospitals NHS Foundation Trust, Surrey, UK

Abstract. The fusion of multi-modality information has proved effective at improving the segmentation results of targeted regions (e.g., tumours, lesions or organs) of medical images. In particular, layer-level fusion represented by DenseNet has demonstrated a promising level of performance for various medical segmentation tasks. Using stroke and infant brain segmentation as example of ongoing challenging applications involving multi-modal images, we investigate whether it is possible to create a more effective of parsimonious fusion architecture based on the state-of-art fusion network - HyperDenseNet. Our hypothesis is that by fully fusing features throughout the entire network from different modalities, this not only increases network computation complexity but also interferes with the unique feature learning of each modality. Nine new network variants involving different fusion points and mechanisms are proposed. Their performances are evaluated on public datasets including iSeg-2017 and ISLES15-SSIS and an acute stroke lesion dataset collected by medical professionals. The experiment results show that of the nine proposed variants, the 'mid-dense' fusion network (named as MidFusNet) is able to achieve a performance comparable to the state-of-art fusion architecture, but with a much more parsimonious network (i.e., 3.5 million parameters less compared to the baseline network for three modalities).

Keywords: Multi-Modal Fusion · Dense Network · Brain Segmentation

1 Introduction

Due to the different physical principles utilised by alternative medical imaging techniques, a screened targeted tissue in the human body can appear visually very different. Important and detailed information can be revealed in detail in one type of imaging modality but hidden in another. Therefore, the use of multiple imaging modalities is often employed to obtain abundant and complementary information about the tissues of interest in clinical practice. For example, to assess ischemic stroke lesions, the lesion area showing darker than the normal tissue in T1 appear brighter compared to the normal tissue in T2. Sometimes, hyperintense artificial signals appearing in T2/FLAIR can be ruled out using ADC [1]. For human eyes, it is quite easy to recognise the corresponding regions in different modalities. However, creating an algorithm to automatically combine complementary data and find correspondence among different modalities to infer meaningful information is a challenging task.

S. Bakas et al. (Eds.): BrainLes 2022, LNCS 13769, pp. 102–114, 2023.
https://doi.org/10.1007/978-3-031-33842-7_9

In the field of medical image segmentation, there are many approaches that have utilised multi-modal sequencing. The most common way to tackle the problem is to simply concatenate the inputs from different modalities and treat them as different channels to learn a fused feature set from the start [2–7]. These approaches are mostly deep learning based, with a strategy of early fusion applied at the input feature level and are computationally simple to implement. As demonstrated by [8], early fusion is an improvement to decision-making (or output) level fusion where each modality is learned independently and the final decision from the multi-modal scheme is made through some form of 'voting' [9–11]. However, early fusion in the form of multi-modal input concatenation also explicitly assumes the relationship between different modalities is linear which may not necessarily be correct. Subsequently, as machine learning techniques have rapidly developed in recent years, more fusion methods that perform the merging of multi-modal features within the network (different from input or output level fusion) have been developed [12–15]. A typical example of this type of fusion strategy in the field of medical segmentation is proposed by Nie et al. [16]. In their approach, each modality has an independently CNN path for feature extraction, and then multi-modal features are fused in deeper layers. This results in complementary high-level representation of image features and outperforms the early fusion strategy as demonstrated by Nie et al.'s experiment. Tseng et al. [17] explored cross-modality convolution within an encoder decoder network, where the cross-modality fusion happens in the late layers of the encoder, and connects to a convolutional LSTM before the decoder part. Together, with several other recently published methods [18–21], this body of research suggests that performing within network fusion is better than outside network fusion, and that different modalities requires unique parameters for deep learning-based segmentation. However, within network fusion can still suffer from cross modality interference and inaccurate modelling if possible non-linearity between modality is not considered. The method proposed by Dolz et al. [21] takes these factors into account. Their so called HyperDenseNet architecture is based on DenseNet [22] where feature re-use is induced by connecting each layer with all layers before it. Each modality has its own CNN path. A unique characteristic of HyperDenseNet is that dense connections are not only incorporated among layers in the same path, but also among layers across different paths. This means that although feature fusion happens early in the network, independent paths are retained for each modality, allowing more complex feature representation to be exploited. The network has performed very well when applied to multi-modal datasets of brain tissue segmentation. Nevertheless, as discussed in [22], "dense connections can introduce redundancies when early features are not needed in later layers". On top of that, the issue of cross modality interference has not been alleviated.

Based on these findings, we exploit HyperDenseNet further and investigate whether it is possible to create a more effective within network fusion strategy. Using the original architecture in [21] as a baseline, we propose nine new network variants that use different merging points and mechanisms to fuse multi-modal features. The performance of the variants is compared to the original architecture of HyperDenseNet on an acute stroke lesion dataset made available to us by Ashford and St Peter's Hospitals NHS. The best performing network is also tested on ISLES2015 SISS – the public evaluation benchmark for sub-acute ischemic stroke lesion segmentation [23] and iSeg17 – MICCAI grand challenge on 6-month infant brain MRI segmentation [24].

2 Method

2.1 Baseline Architecture

In this section, we briefly describe the baseline architecture – HyperDenseNet and its key features. For more details about this network, please refer to the original paper [20, 21] and its architecture layout is presented in the Appendix A. The network comprises of 9 convolutional blocks and 4 fully convolutional layers with a $1 \times 1 \times 1$ kernel. Each imaging modality has its own stream for the propagation of the features until it reaches the fully convolutional layer. The network expects a 3D input patch of $27 \times 27 \times 27$ for each modality stream. The first convolutional block with a $3 \times 3 \times 3$ kernel simply processes the input of different modality independently. Starting from the second block, the input for each convolutional block is the concatenation of outputs along the 4th dimension from all preceding blocks of all streams. The concatenation of feature maps from different modalities is shuffled and linked differently for each stream to provide regularization effect and enhance modeling performance. The 3D convolutional block typically applies batch normalization, PReLU activation, and convolution with no spatial pooling. The outputs of the 9th layer are of size $9 \times 9 \times 9$ along each stream. All streams are then concatenated together before being fed into the fully convolutional layers where the multi-modal merging occurs. After four layers of fully convolutional layers, the length of the feature channel is reduced to the number of classes associated with the dataset. The output from the network is fed into a softmax function to generate the probabilistic label map. The highest softmax probability for each class is computed to yield the final segmentation result. The Adam optimiser is used to optimise the parameters associated with the network. The cost function employed is cross entropy loss.

2.2 Proposed Architecture

To investigate ways of reducing computation complexity and to alleviate cross modality interference, we propose nine new ways of interleaving the feature maps from different modalities. The baseline architecture can be considered as a full dense fusion network where the linking of layers from different streams happens immediately after the first convolutional block. Hence the first two variants we explore are dense networks that leave the concatenation of the feature maps from other modalities until a deeper layer is reached. We define these two variants as mid-dense and late-dense fusion networks, respectively. The design allows dense connections to be established between modalities, but only lets the deeper layers of the network learning the complex relationship amongst various modalities. The feature maps for each modality are learned independently until the 4th convolutional block for the mid-dense variant (as indicated by the dashed arrow in Fig. 1) and the 7th convolutional block for the late-dense variant. Compared to the mid-dense fusion network, the late-dense fusion design allows more convolutional blocks for independent learning and less layers for cross-modality dense connection. Both variants significantly reduce the number of computational operations involved in the network. The third variant we investigated is a so-called skip-dense fusion, where feature mixing happens in every other layer of the dense convolutional network (i.e., a layer is skipped after each fusion). Our experiment first compares these three variants and found that mid-dense fusion network outperforms the other two. Therefore, we put particular focus on exploring mid-dense fusion variants and investigate if it is possible to reduce the parameters even further.

The fourth variant we investigate allows fusion to occur on the 5th convolutional block and is denoted as mid5-dense. As we demonstrated in the experiment section, this network performed worse when fusion is left to occur on the 5th layer. From experiments, we concluded that there should be at least six out of nine consecutive convolutional blocks to conduct feature fusion in the network. Then we investigate two more variants to search the optimal location of the six convolution blocks. Compared to the mid-dense network which performs the fusion from 4th to 9th layer, the fifth variant – mid2-dense, allows fusion to happen between 2nd to 7th layer. Similarly, the sixth variant – mid3-dense, fuses features between 3rd to 8th layer. Please note dense connections only occur after the first layer, so there is not a variant for starting from the 1st layer. Figure 2 illustrates the overall involvement of convolutional blocks for all the variants proposed so far.

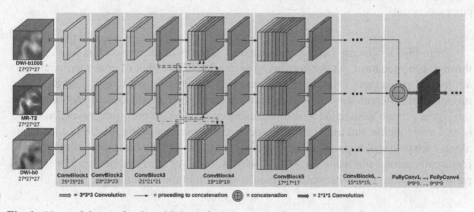

Fig. 1. Network layout for the mid-dense fusion strategy. Dense connections are propagated along each modality stream independently until the 4th convolutional block. Multi-modal fusion happens from the 4th convolutional block and continues until fully merged at the first fully connected layer.

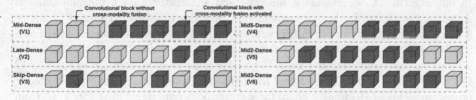

Fig. 2. The location layout of convolutional blocks for different proposed fusion networks.

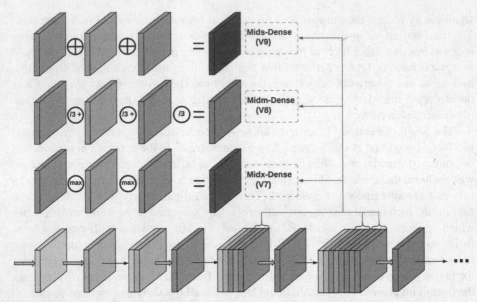

Fig. 3. Different fusion operations implemented to replace concatenation in the other three proposed variants.

From Fig. 1, we can see that the fusion of features in the network is implemented through concatenation. As the network goes deeper, the number of computational operations and parameters relating to concatenated features grows larger. Therefore, we investigated different ways of fusing features from other modalities to each path. For this, three variants associated with three fusing operations are proposed, named as midx-dense, midm-dense and mids-dense, respectively. As shown in Fig. 3, dense connection along each path still happens to facilitate feature reuse, but the cross-modality fusion of features is carried out using element-wise max, mean or sum operations. The detailed parameter setting for all proposed networks is given in the Appendix B.

3   Experiment

3.1   Datasets

In our experiment, we evaluated the proposed architectures on a hospital-collected dataset on acute stroke lesion segmentation, the iSeg17 MICCAI Grand Challenge dataset on 6-month infant brain MRI segmentation, as well as the dataset of ISLES15-SISS on segmentation of sub-acute stroke lesion. The hospital-collected dataset contains 90 training cases and 30 testing cases. There are three modalities in each case, i.e., T2, DWI-b1000, DWI-b0 and the ground truth of stroke lesion segmentation annotated by physicians. These MRI images are of three dimensions with size $256 \times 256 \times 32$. Comparably, ISLES15 SISS contains images of sub-acute stroke lesions and has much less data for training (i.e., 28 cases). Image slice number is not uniform; being either 230 $\times$ 230 $\times$ 154 or 230 $\times$ 230 $\times$ 153. This does not need cropping since our networks take patched based input. The MRI modalities included are T1, T2, FLAIR and DWI. All four modalities are used in our experiment. The ground truth for both stroke related datasets has two labels: lesion and non-lesion. The iSeg17 dataset contains even less images. There are 10 available volumes with two modalities, T1- and T2- weighted. To be consistent with the experiment conducted in the baseline paper [21], we also split the dataset into training, validation and testing sets, each having 6, 1, and 3 subjects, respectively. There are four classes involved in iSeg17 dataset, i.e., background, cerebrospinal fluid (CSF), grey matter (GM) and white matter (WM).

3.2 Implementation Details

The model is implemented in PyTorch and trained on NVIDIA 1080Ti GPU, with a batch size of 10 for the outsourced dataset, 5 for the iSeg17 dataset and 4 for the ISLES15 dataset. Images from each modality are skull stripped and normalized by subtracting the mean value and dividing by the standard deviation. For Adam optimisation, the parameters involved are empirically set with a learning rate of 0.0002 for both the outsourced dataset and the ISLES15, $\beta1 = 0.9$, and $\beta2 = 0.999$. For iSeg17, the learning rate is initially set to be 0.001 and is halved every 100 epochs (same setting as the baseline paper). To tackle with the data imbalance issue that typically occurs in lesion image data where the lesion region can be very small, the $27 \times 27 \times 27$ patches are randomly extracted and only the ones with lesion voxels will be used for training. The model implemented for the outsourced dataset with larger number of images are trained for 900 epochs, whereas the model for ISLES15 and iSeg17 with smaller number of images are trained for 600 epochs. The validation accuracy is measured every 10 epochs. For the inference of the models, we first normalize the testing image sequence and then extract the $27 \times 27 \times 27$ 3D patches with extraction step of 9 incrementally along each dimension. The output, which is the $9 \times 9 \times 9$ classification obtained from the prediction at the centre of the patch, is used to reconstruct the full image volume by reversing the extraction procedure. The code for this paper will be made publicly available on GitHub[1] in due course.

4 Results and Discussion

The proposed networks are first evaluated by assessing their performance using dice similarity coefficient (DSC) on segmenting acute stroke lesions from the outsourced dataset. The testing results are shown in Table 1. From this experiment, we observed that the late-dense fusion strategy performs the worst out of all in terms of both training and testing. The big gap in accuracy between the performance of the late-dense fusion network and the rest of the networks further demonstrates that it is important not to leave fusion of information late in the network. The skip-dense fusion network shows a slightly weaker learning ability than the mid-dense and the baseline networks with lower testing accuracy and occasional large drops in training performance. This implies that skipping layers during fusion can lead to information loss and so affect feature propagation. The mid2-dense and mid3-dense show the largest fluctuation and unstable learning.

---

[1] https://github.com/Norika2020/MidFusNet

As expected, mid5-dense performs slightly worse than mid-dense since fusion happens at one layer deeper into the network. The midx-dense, midm-dense and mids-dense variants, although largely reduced parameters, their testing results show that concatenation still outperforms the proposed fusion operators. The mid-dense fusion network (Mid-FusNet) is the only variant that can achieve a competitive performance comparable to the baseline fusion network. It is able to achieve similar performance with 15% (i.e., 3.5 million for three modalities) less parameters than the baseline network. The reduction of parameter numbers is reflected in Table 2. The MidFusNet model is also compared to another state-of-art network - 3D U-Net [25], the results are shown in Table 3. For the 3D U-Net, we concatenate the volume data from different modalities at input level and used the code provided by DLTK[2] [26]. Both HyperDenseNet and the proposed Mid-FusNet show better performance on DSC than the 3D U-Net, suggesting the importance of exploiting fusion between modalities within the network. However, 3D U-Net shows clear advantage when distance-based metric - average Hausdorff distance is used to measure the network performance. By observing the qualitative results (Fig. 4), we can see this is mainly caused by some fractional outliers detected by the patch input-based networks (which typically lacks global context of the image).

Table 1. The testing results measured by DSC (%) for the experimented networks. The best performing network is highlighted in bold.

Network	DSC	Network	DSC
Baseline	65.6 ± 18.0	Mid2-dense	60.9 ± 17.1
Mid-dense	**65.8 ± 16.2**	Mid3-dense	58.4 ± 19.7
Late-dense	55.9 ± 19.5	Midx-dense	57.0 ± 12.1
Skip-dense	62.4 ± 16.3	Midm-dense	58.7 ± 13.5
Mid5-dense	62.2 ± 12.0	Mids-desne	55.8 ± 23.4

We also tested the MidFusNet on the ISLES15 public dataset to investigate its performance on MRI multi-modal sequences of sub-acute stroke lesions. Since the training set provided is very small (n = 28), we used all modalities and evaluated with leave-one-out cross validation. The mean and standard deviation score for DSC is calculated. The results (as presented in Table 4) show that the proposed mid-dense fusion architecture was able to perform well on the sub-acute stroke cases and managed to achieve training results comparable to the top three ranked participants on the online league table. Although it appears to have performed not as well as the top ranked networks, there was not any post-processing (such as non-maximal suppression or conditional random field) used in the algorithm which are proved to improve the network performance. The MidFusNet is further tested on the iSeg17 dataset to investigate its performance on infant brain segmentation from an even smaller dataset with two modalities and four classes. The results for the baseline are reproduced using the authors' published code

---

[2] https://github.com/DLTK/DLTK

Table 2. Number of parameters (convolutional blocks, fully convolutional layers, and total) associated with the baseline and mid-dense network.

Network	No. Parameters			% Reduced
	Conv	Fully-Conv	Total	
Baseline for two mods	9.52 M	0.83 M	10.32 M	11%
Mid-dense for two mods	8.41 M	0.79 M	9.20 M	
Baseline for three mods	21,42 M	1.73 M	23.15 M	15%
Mid-dense for three mods	18.08 M	1.61 M	19.69 M	
Baseline for four mods	38.07 M	2.99 M	41.07 M	17%
Mid-dense for four mods	31.39 M	2.75 M	34.14 M	

Table 3. Comparing our network to other state-of-art segmentation networks on the acute stroke dataset.

Network	DSC mean	DSC std	HD mean	HD std
3D U-Net	63.3	24.8	30.3	30.8
HyperDenseNet	65.6	18.0	87.8	20.7
MidFusNet	65.8	16.2	85.4	15.0

written in PyTorch[3] to compare results under the same experimental setting. Results in Table 5 shows the proposed network yields better segmentation results than the baseline. Although there is not a significant improvement in the averaged Dice score, the results are achieved using about 1.2 million less parameters than the state-of-art network.

---

[3] https://github.com/josedolz/HyperDenseNet

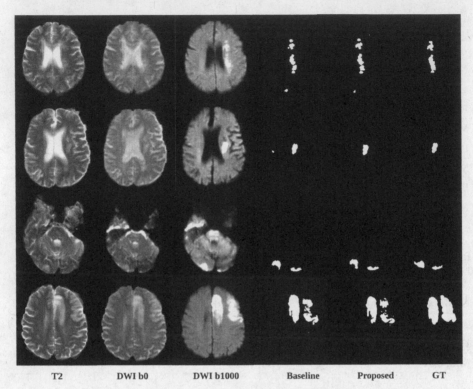

T2   DWI b0   DWI b1000   Baseline   Proposed   GT

Fig. 4. Qualitative results on acute stroke lesion segmentation.

Table 4. Comparing our network's DSC to the training evaluation results of the top three systems ranked on the ISLES15-SISS league table.

Network author	Mean DSC	DSC Std
Kamnitsas et al. [27]	66	24
Feng et al. [28]	63	28
Halme et al. [29]	61	24
Ours	63	25

Table 5. The performance comparison on the testing set of the iSeg17 brain segmentation measured in DSC (%).

Architecture	CSF	WM	GM
Baseline	93.4 ± 2.9	89.6 ± 3.5	87.4 ± 2.7
MidFusNet	93.7 ± 2.6	90.2 ± 2.9	87.7 ± 2.5

5 Conclusion

We have proposed nine new ways of applying feature fusion on a multi-modal dense network for the task of brain and stroke segmentation. Compared to the baseline architecture – HyperDenseNet, we exploit an efficient fusion strategy in order to reduce the computation complexity involved in the baseline network and alleviate the cross-modality interference. The experiment results show that the proposed MidFusNet reduced parameters from the baseline in millions without degrading the segmentation performances. The other fusion strategies did not perform well, but on the other hand demonstrated that features for each modality in early layers can be learned more efficiently if left independent, leaving fusion to too deep layers, or skipping layers during fusion can prevent complex multi-modal feature learning. We also found that applying feature fusion through element-wise max, mean and sum operations, although largely reduced parameters, does not perform better than concatenated fusion. For future work, we plan to exploit better aggregation of feature maps from different modalities and integrate global context into the network (Fig. 5 and Table 6).

Appendix A. Architecture Layout of the Baseline Network

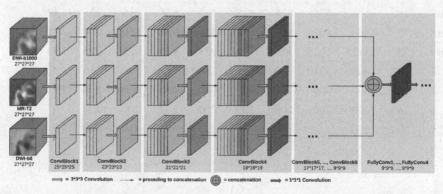

Fig. 5. Baseline architecture layout in the case of three imaging modality. The feature map generated by each convolutional block is colour coded. Top stream is represented using shades of blue; middle stream is colour coded using shades of red; and shades of green are used for the bottom stream. As the layer goes deeper the feature map's colour goes deeper too. The stacked feature maps show how the dense connection happens and the unique shuffling for concatenation along each modality path. (Architecture drawing adapted and modified from [21])

Appendix B. Detailed Parameter Setting of Proposed Networks

Table 6. The parameters associated with each convolutional layer in the baseline and proposed networks. The number of kernels and processed 3D image output are kept the same for all networks. Major difference occurs when interleaving concatenation happens which leads to varying input size along the feature channels. Notations: CB - convolutional block; FC - fully convolutional layer; No. k – Number of kernels; No. c – Number of classes; v1 - mid-dense; v2 - late-dense; v3 - skip-dense; v4 - mid5-dense; v5 - mid2-dense; v6 - mid3-dense; v7 - midx-dense; v8 - midm-dense; and v9 - mids-dense.

Layer	No. k	Input size along the feature channel								Output size
		v0	v1	v2	v3	v4	v5	v6	v7-v9	
CB1	25	1	1	1	1	1	1	1	1	25^3
CB2	25	75	25	25	75	25	75	25	25	23^3
CB3	25	150	50	50	100	50	150	100	50	21^3
CB4	50	225	125	75	175	75	225	175	75	19^3
CB5	50	375	275	125	225	225	375	325	125	17^3
CB6	50	525	425	175	375	375	525	475	175	15^3
CB7	75	675	575	325	425	525	675	625	225	13^3
CB8	75	900	800	550	650	750	750	850	300	11^3
CB9	75	1125	1025	775	725	975	825	925	375	9^3
FC1	400	4050	3750	3000	2850	3600	3150	3450	1350	9^3
FC2	200	400	400	400	400	400	400	400	400	9^3
FC3	150	200	200	200	200	200	200	200	200	9^3
FC4	No. c	150	150	150	150	150	150	150	150	9^3

References

1. Oppenheim, C., et al.: Tips and traps in brain mri: applications to vascular disorders. Diagnostic Inter. Imaging **93**(12), 935–948 (2012)
2. Havaei, M., et al.: Brain tumor segmentation with deep neural networks. Med. Image Anal. **35**, 18–31 (2017)
3. Kamnitsas, K., et al.: Efficient multi-scale 3d CNN with fully connected CRF for accurate brain lesion segmentation. Med. Image Anal. **36**, 61–78 (2017)
4. Lavdas, I., et al.: Fully automatic, multiorgan segmentation in normal whole body magnetic resonance imaging (MRI), using classification forests (CFs), convolutional neural networks (CNNs), and a multi-atlas (MA) approach. Med. Phys. **44**(10), 5210–5220 (2017)
5. Moeskops, P., Viergever, M.A., Mendrik, A.M., de Vries, L.S., Benders, M.J., Išgum, I.: Automatic segmentation of mr brain images with a convolutional neural network. IEEE Trans. Med. Imaging **35**(5), 1252–1261 (2016)

6. Valverde, S., et al.: Improving automated multiple sclerosis lesion segmentation with a cascaded 3d convolutional neural network approach. Neuroimage **155**, 159–168 (2017)
7. Zhang, W., et al.: Deep convolutional neural networks for multi-modality isointense infant brain image segmentation. Neuroimage **108**, 214–224 (2015)
8. Guo, Z., Li, X., Huang, H., Guo, N., Li, Q.: Deep learning-based image segmentation on multimodal medical imaging. IEEE Trans. Radiation Plasma Med. Sci. **3**(2), 162–169 (2019)
9. Cai, H., Verma, R., Ou, Y., Lee, S., Melhem, E.R., Davatzikos, C.: Probabilistic segmentation of brain tumors based on multi-modality magnetic resonance images. In: 4th IEEE International Symposium on Biomedical Imaging, pp. 600–603 (2007)
10. Klein, S., van der Heide, U.A., Lips, I.M., van Vulpen, M., Staring, M., Pluim, J.P.: Automatic segmentation of the prostate in 3d mr images by atlas matching using localized mutual information. Med. Phys. **35**(4), 1407–1417 (2008)
11. Menze, B.H., et al.: The multimodal brain tumor image segmentation benchmark. IEEE Trans. Med. Imaging **34**(10), 1993–2024 (2015)
12. Bhatnagar, G., Wu, Q.M.J., Liu, Z.: Directive contrast based multimodal medical image fusion in nsct domain. IEEE Trans. Multimedia **15**(5), 1014–1024 (2013)
13. Singh, R., Khare, A.: Fusion of multimodal medical images using daubechies complex wavelet transform — a multiresolution approach. Inf. Fusion **19**, 49–60 (2014)
14. Yang, Y.: Multimodal medical image fusion through a new dwt based technique. In: Proceeding of 4th International Conference on Bioinformatatics and Biomedical Engineering, pp. 1–4 (2010)
15. Zhu, X., Suk, H.I., Lee, S.W., Shen, D.: Subspace regularized sparse multitask learning for multiclass neurodegenerative disease identification. IEEE Trans. Biomed. Eng. **63**(3), 607–618 (2016)
16. Nie, D., Wang, L., Gao, Y., Shen, D.: Fully convolutional networks for multi-modality isointense infant brain image segmentation. In: Biomedical Imaging (ISBI). IEEE 13th International Symposium on, pp. 1342–1345 (2016)
17. Tseng, K.L., Lin, Y.L., Hsu, W., Huang, C.Y.: Joint sequence learning and cross-modality convolution for 3d biomedical segmentation. In: IEEE Computer Society Conference on Computer Vision and Pattern Recognition (CVPR 2017), pp. 3739–3746 (2017)
18. Aygun, M., Sahin, Y.H., Unal, G.: Multimodal Convolutional Neural Networks for Brain Tumor Segmentation (2018). arXiv preprint:1809.06191
19. Chen, Y., Chen, J., Wei, D., Li, Y., Zheng, Y.: Octopusnet: a deep learning segmentation network for multi-modal medical images. In: Multiscale Multimodal Medical Imaging (MMMI 2019), Lecture Notes in Computer Science **11977** (2019)
20. Dolz, J., Ben Ayed, I., Yuan, J., Desrosiers, C.: Isointense infant brain segmentation with a hyper-dense connected convolutional neural network. In: IEEE 15th International Symposium on Biomedical Imaging (ISBI), pp. 616–620 (2018)
21. Dolz, J., Gopinath, K., Yuan, J., Lombaert, H., Desrosiers, C., Ben Ayed, I.: Hyperdensenet: a hyper-densely connected cnn for multi-modal image segmentation. IEEE Trans. Med. Imaging **38**(5), 1116–1126 (2019)
22. Huang, G., Liu, Z., van der Maaten, L., Weinberger, K.Q.: Densely connected convolutional networks. In: Computer Vision and Pattern Recognition. CVPR 2017. IEEE Computer Society Conference on, pp. 2261–2269 (2017)
23. Maier, O., et al.: ISLES 2015 - a public evaluation benchmark for ischemic stroke lesion segmentation from multispectral mri. Med. Image Anal. **35**, 250–269 (2017)
24. Wang, L., et al.: Benchmark on au-tomatic 6-month-old infant brain segmentation algorithms: the iseg-2017 challenge. IEEE Trans. Med. Imaging **38**, 2219–2230 (2019)
25. Çiçek, Ö., Abdulkadir, A., Lienkamp, S.S., Brox, T., Ronneberger. O.: 3d u-net: learning dense volumetric segmentation from sparse annotation.In: Ourselin, S., Joskowicz, L., Sabuncu, M.,

Unal, G., Wells, W. (eds): Medical Image Computing and Computer-Assisted Intervention – MICCAI 2016. Lecture Notes in Computer Science, p. 9901 (2016). https://doi.org/10.1007/978-3-319-46723-8_49

26. Pawlowski, N., et al.: Dltk: State of the Art Reference Implementations for Deep Learning on Medical Images (2017). arXiv preprint arXiv:1711.06853

27. Kamnitsas, K., Chen, L., Ledig, C., Rueckert, D., Glocker, B.: Multi-scale 3d convolutional neural networks for lesion segmentation in brain mri. In: Ischemic Stroke Lesion Segmentation - MICCAI, pp. 13–16 (2015)

28. Feng, C., Zhao, D., Huang, M.: Segmentation of stroke lesions in multi-spectral mr images using bias correction embedded fcm and three phase level sets. In: Ischemic Stroke Lesion Segmentation – MICCAI (2015)

29. Halme, H., Korvenoja, A., Salli, E.: Segmentation of stroke lesion using spatial normalisation, random forest classification and contextual clustering. In: Ischemic Stroke Lesion Segmentation - MICCAI (2015)

Semi-supervised Intracranial Aneurysm Segmentation with Selected Unlabeled Data

Shiyu Lu[1], Hao Wang[2], and Chuyang Ye[1(✉)]

[1] School of Integrated Circuits and Electronics, Beijing Institute of Technology, Beijing, China
chuyang.ye@bit.edu.cn
[2] Deepwise AI Lab., Beijing, China

Abstract. The intracranial aneurysm is a common life-threatening disease, and its rupture can lead directly to subarachnoid haemorrhage, with a mortality rate of up to one-third. Therefore, the diagnosis of intracranial aneurysms is of great significance. The widespread use of advanced imaging techniques, such as computed tomography angiography (CTA) and magnetic resonance angiography (MRA), has made it possible to diagnose intracranial aneurysms at an early stage. However, manual annotation of intracranial aneurysms is very time-consuming and labour-intensive, making it difficult to obtain a sufficient amount of labeled data. For deep learning, it is difficult to train reliable segmentation models with only a small amount of labeled data. On this basis, semi-supervised aneurysm segmentation can be used to better exploit the small amount of labeled data and abundant unlabeled data. In practice, the unlabeled data may comprise both images with or without aneurysms, yet existing semi-supervised learning methods do not filter the training data to remove the data aneurysms, which may negatively impact model training as the data is purely negative. Therefore, we propose a semi-supervised approach to intracranial aneurysm segmentation with unlabeled data selection, where negative data is excluded from model training. Specifically, we train a 2D image classification network to filter negative samples without aneurysms and then a 3D image segmentation network based on the filtered data for semi-supervised aneurysm segmentation. The proposed method was evaluated on an MRA dataset, and the results show that our method performs better than the vanilla semi-supervised learning that does not exclude negative unlabeled data.

Keywords: Aneurysm segmentation · semi-supervised learning · incomplete annotation

1 Introduction

Intracranial aneurysm (IA) is an aneurysmal dilatation disease due to abnormal local changes in cerebral blood vessel. It is a relatively common cerebrovascular

S. Bakas et al. (Eds.): BrainLes 2022, LNCS 13769, pp. 115–123, 2023.
https://doi.org/10.1007/978-3-031-33842-7_10

disease with an incidence of about 3%–5% in the general population and 80–85% in patients with spontaneous subarachnoid hemorrhage (SAH). The majority (approximately 90%) of patients with unruptured IAs (UIAs) usually have no obvious clinical manifestations, with only about 10% of patients presenting specific manifestations such as headache and unilateral facial numbness. The rate of death and disability caused by ruptured IAs is high, with approximately 12% of patients dying before treatment and 40% dying within one month after treatment. Approaching 30% of patients have residual neurological deficits and only a small proportion having a slightly better prognosis [17]. Early and accurate detection of IAs is important for the clinical management and prognosis of patients with intracranial aneurysms. Medical imaging plays an increasingly important role in the diagnosis and treatment of disease, which is an important tool for physicians in screening, clinical diagnosis, treatment guidance and efficacy assessment. In recent years, with the development of medical imaging technology, the detection rate of IAs has also been increasing. Magnetic resonance angiography (MRA), computed tomography angiography (CTA) and digital subtracted angiography (DSA) are common methods for detecting IAs. In particular, MRA uses the flow effect of blood to obtain good vascular contrast images and is increasingly popular among radiologists because it is radiation-free, non-invasive, does not require the introduction of any contrast agent and is easier to perform compared to CTA [7,11].

Computer-aided diagnosis (CAD) systems, which use machine learning algorithms to analyse medical images and make probabilistic judgements, are a major branch of artificial intelligence technology. The deep learning (DL) approach is generally referred to as a deep segmentation network model based on convolutional neural networks (CNN), which can automatically learn features from a large amount of input data layer by layer and perform target tasks such as classification and recognition, forming an "end-to-end" structure with strong robustness and generalisation capability [12]. Since 2017, several studies have evaluated the value of DL-based CAD systems for the detection of IAs [1,5,14,15]. Nakao et al [9] used a 2D CNN combined with a maximal intensity projection algorithm to develop a CAD system for aneurysms, achieving a sensitivity of 90% in a single-centre study. Ueda et al [15] developed an IAs detection system based on 3D CNN combined with multi-centre data and achieved a sensitivity of 91%, but the high false-positive rate has limited the dissemination and further application of the model in clinical practice. However, manual annotation of medical image data is costly and requires specialised skills, especially in labeling aneurysm, resulting in only a small amount of labeled data and a large amount of unlabeled data. It is challenging to train a reliable segmentation model with only a limited amount of labeled data.

In this work, to address the shortage of labeled data and to make effective use of the large amount of unlabeled data, we propose a semi-supervised approach to intracranial aneurysm segmentation. Motivated by the fact that existing semi-supervised learning methods do not filter the training samples sufficiently, resulting in training being affected by negative samples which do not contain foreground information, a 2D image classification network was designed to filter negative samples without aneurysms, where is the main difference between us and other semi-supervised learning methods. For demonstration, DA-ResUNet was used as our aneurysm segmentation network, while ResNet was used as a secondary filtering network to help filter the training data. Experimental results show that our method leads to improved aneurysm segmentation compared to the vanilla semi-supervised learning that does not exclude negative unlabeled data.

2   Methods

Our goal is to expand the positive training data with a negative data filter while reducing the negative impact of the negative data on the semi-supervised training. As shown in Fig. 1, our proposed method consists of two major modules: 1)Negative data filtering, 2)Semi-supervised IA segmentation. In the negative data filtering module, we use a residual network to train a slice-level positive and negative sample classifier to determine the classification results for each individual slice and then a threshold-comparison method was used to convert the slice-level predictions into image-level predictions. In Semi-supervised IA segmentation module, we use the potential positive images selected in the previous module as finely selected supplementary training data to train our semi-supervised segmentation network, which is also trained in two steps. Based on this, the selected training samples are fed into our semi-supervised learning model together with expert-labeled positive data and trained to produce our final segmentation model.

2.1   Negative Data Filtering Method

Previous research has shown that adding too much purely negative data for segmentation model training can negatively affect the training result [8]. In order to exclude negative data for training from a large amount of unlabeled data, we designed a two-dimensional slice level classifier that slices each MRA image, feeds them into the classification network and get prediction results of each slice. Finally, a threshold method was used to determine the image level prediction results from the slice prediction results i.e. if there are multiple consecutive levels of slices are classified as positive, then the whole image is classified as positive.

The slice level classification network was designed with ResNet34 [3] and experimentally, the threshold for determining positive MRA images for aneurysms, i.e. the number of consecutive positive slices, was set to 15, which have the best classification performance according to the experiment results.

2.2   Semi-supervised IA Segmentation

Our work is inspired by the recent success in semi-supervised learning (SSL) for image classification [18] and semantic segmentation [16], demonstrating promising performance given very limited labeled data and a sufficient amount of unlabeled data. In this work, we propose a simple method to improve segmentation

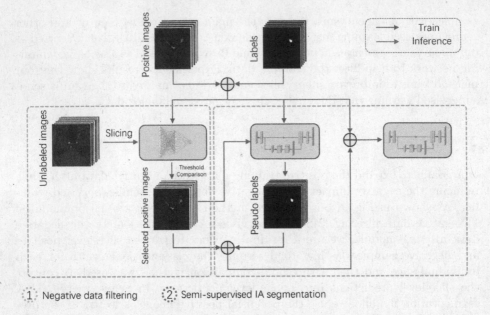

Fig. 1. Overview of method pipeline.

performance by using a limited amount of pixel-labeled data and sufficient unlabeled data. First, we build the model using a small amount of labeled data which can predict the pseudo-labels of the unlabeled data from the previously trained model, and then the reliable pseudo-labels of unlabeled data will be applied to subsequent semi-supervised learning.

The network we use for training segmentation model is called DA-ResUNet [13], its architecture is shown in Fig. 2. DA-ResUNet is a 3D CNN with an encoder-decoder architecture similar to 3D U-Net, which contains an encoder module for abstracting contextual information and a symmetric decoder module for expanding the encoded features into a full-resolution map of the same size and dimensionality as the input volume. It employed a residual block instead of the original convolutional block of U-Net [10] to ensure stable training when the network depth increases significantly. To improve the performance of the network by exploring contextual information over long distances, a dual-attention [2] module is added between the encoder and decoder. Before being sampled and fed into the network, input images were normalized to $[-1, 1]$ using Z-score normalization, and a series of data augmentation methods such as rotation, mirroring and flipping were applied.

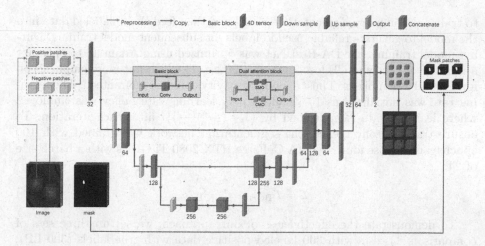

Fig. 2. Overview of segmentation framework for semi-supervised segmentation based on DA-ResUNet. During training, it learns not only expert-labeled aneurysm-positive data, but also pseudo-labeled data from unlabeled data.

3   Results

3.1   Overview of Dataset and Experimental Setting

We retrieved the data collection from October 2010 to September 2019 of the MRA images of the intracranial arteries in the database in Jinling hospital. The dataset contained a total of 1800 patient images, out of all MRA data, only 800 cases were available with a definitive diagnosis, including 400 positive and 400 negative cases. Those data containing annotations are labeled by three experienced radiologists. On this basis, we divided the 800 labeled data into three parts, where training data: validation data: test data = 6:1:1. In addition, we ensure that the proportion of positive and negative data is the same in each part of the data to prevent the negative effects of data imbalance. The remaining 1000 images are not labeled by experts i.e. unlabeled data.

Our proposed semi-supervised approach consists of two cascaded neural network models. First is 2D classification network based on slicing, where we slice each 3D image along the axial position on the basis of 600 sets of training data. To keep the number of samples in different categories of the training data consistent, the positive data are sliced at the level with aneurysms and each negative data is sliced randomly by 11 slices, while the validation data are generated in the same way as the 2D validation data to help us determine the experimental parameters. Once we have filtered the negative data from the unlabeled data using negative data filter, we start to train the 3D MRA image aneurysm segmentation model by DA-ResUNet. Although some of the unlabeled data in the model training don't have expert annotations, we rely on the expert-labeled data to train a preliminary segmentation model and then feed the unlabeled data into the model to generate reliable pseudo-labels for subsequent model training. During model training, the DA-ResUNet was optimized using Adam [6] to optimize a mixture of Dice and CE loss function (see Eq. 1) which put more emphasis on foreground lesion pixels. Thus, a high sensitivity could be guaranteed. The learning rate was initialized as 10^{-4}, and a poly learning rate policy was employed where learning rate is multiplied by $\left(1 - \left(\frac{iter}{totaliter}\right)\right)^2$ after each iteration. To ensure training convergence, the segmentation network was trained with 100 epochs, and we use four NVIDIA GeForce RTX 2080 Ti GPUs with a batch size of 24.

$$\mathcal{L} = \mathcal{L}_{\text{BCE}} + \mathcal{L}_{\text{DICE}}. \tag{1}$$

To demonstrate the effectiveness of our approach, we set up three sets of comparison: 1) tests with 300 labeled positive data with true labels (300 LP), 2) 300 labeled positive data and all unlabeled data with pseudo-labels (300 LP + all UL), 3) 300 labeled positive data and selected positive data with pseudo-labels (300 LP + selected UL). The visualisation of the segmentation results under different training conditions are shown in Fig. 3. It can be seen that our proposed method works best for voxel segmentation of aneurysms.

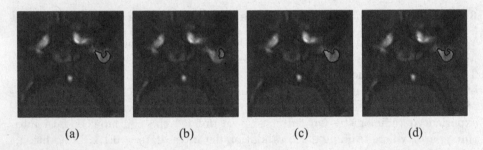

(a)   (b)   (c)   (d)

Fig. 3. Examples of segmentation results on test images. From left to right: (a) Result of ground truth label; (b) Result of training with only 300 expert-labeled positive data; (c) Result of training with 300 expert-labeled positive data and all unlabeled data with pseudo-labels; (d) Result of training with 300 expert-labeled positive data and selected unlabeled data with pseudo-labels.

3.2   Slice Level Classifier Results

We used different structures of the residual network and selected ResNet34 as the final 2D image classification network based on comparing the F1-score of the classification results under the different networks, and the results are shown in Table 1.

To control the false positive rate on image level's prediction, we used a thresholding method where a patient will be predicted to be aneurysm-positive case when the count of consecutive predicted positive slices for an image is greater

Table 1. Comparison of classification performance using different ResNet backbones on slice level.

Architecture	Precision	Recall	F1-Score
ResNet18	0.7933	0.9324	0.8572
ResNet34	**0.7829**	**0.9635**	**0.8639**
ResNet50	0.8013	0.8832	0.8403

than a certain number. According to the result (See in Table 2), we set the threshold-parameter at 15.

Table 2. Comparison of classification performance under different thresholds.

Threshold	Precision	Recall	F1-score
10	0.84	0.72	0.7754
15	**0.94**	**0.68**	**0.7891**
20	0.98	0.6	0.7443
25	1	0.54	0.7013

3.3   Segmentation Results Under Different Training Settings

For the different training settings (see Sect. 3.1), we first trained the segmentation models using DA-ResUNet and expert-labeled data separately and do inference on the test set, calculating the relevant metrics at lesion-level and compare dice coefficients to do model selection. The results show that the inclusion of the pseudo-labeled samples which are selected by the slice-level classifier performs better than the vanilla semi-supervised learning that does not exclude negative unlabeled data.

To verify the performance of the method on other segmentation models, we used the nnUNet architecture [4] to train the segmentation models, and the findings remain the same as before, the results are shown in Table 3. It can be seen that the segmentation results of nnUNet is not as good as DA-ResUNet because of its low precision but the results show that our proposed method which is based on the unlabeled data selection does improve model performance. Also, we investigate the effectiveness of the method for different dataset sizes by varying the data partition and find that our proposed training method based on filtering negative data improves the model the most. The comparison experiment is based on DA-ResUNet for 3D segmentation model training and ResNet34 for 2D image classification for filtering negative samples without aneurysms, the results can be seen in Table 4, which indicates that our method is equally effective under different data partition.

Table 3. Performance comparison when training with only 300 expert-labeled positive data, with 300 expert-labeled positive data and all unlabeled data with pseudo-labels, with 300 expert-labeled positive data and selected unlabeled data with pseudo-labels.

Framework	Dataset setup	Precision	Recall	F1-Score	Dice
DA-ResUNet	300 LP	0.3443	0.7273	0.4673	0.4090
	300 LP + all UL	0.3721	0.8727	0.5217	0.6020
	300 LP + selected UL	**0.4404**	0.8727	**0.5853**	**0.6243**
nnUNet	300 LP	0.1	0.7273	0.1758	0.4261
	300 LP + all UL	0.1512	0.7455	0.2514	0.4421
	300 LP + selected UL	**0.1938**	**0.8**	**0.3121**	**0.4861**

Table 4. Evaluation on test data under different experimental data partition settings.

Dataset setup	Precision	Recall	F1-Score	Dice
300 LP	0.3443	0.7273	0.4673	0.4090
300 LP + all UL	0.3721	0.8727	0.5217	0.6020
300 LP + selected UL	**0.4404**	0.8727	**0.5853**	**0.6243**
200 LP	0.2821	0. 8181	0.4196	0.3603
200 LP + all UL	0.2604	0.8181	0.3953	0.3318
200 LP + selected UL	**0.3087**	**0.8346**	**0.4509**	**0.3848**
100 LP	0.2088	0. 7091	0.3226	0.3143
100 LP + all UL	0.1822	0.6727	0.2867	0.2982
100 LP + selected UL	**0.2253**	**0.7455**	**0.346**	**0.3475**

4   Conclusion

In this work, we introduce a simple and effective method which seeks to address the problem of network training with limited labeled data and make full use of unlabeled data. It is inappropriate to include too many negative samples in training, so we propose to apply data filtering using 2D slice classifier to select potential positive data which can enrich our limited labeled-positive data. In that case, we can train a reliable segmentation model using semi-supervised learning method. The experimental results on MRA dataset show that our method performs better on aneurysm segmentation than the vanilla semi-supervised learning that do not do any filtering on data.

References

1. Faron, A., et al.: Performance of a deep-learning neural network to detect intracranial aneurysms from 3D TOF-MRA compared to human readers. Eur. Radiol. **30**, 591–598 (2020)

2. Fu, J., et al.: Dual attention network for scene segmentation. In: IEEE Conference on Computer Vision and Pattern Recognition, pp. 3146–3154 (2019)
3. He, K., Zhang, X., Ren, S., Sun, J.: Deep residual learning for image recognition. In: IEEE Conference on Computer Vision and Pattern Recognition, pp. 770–778 (2016)
4. Isensee, F., Jaeger, P.F., Kohl, S.A.A., Petersen, J., Maier-Hein, K.H.: nnu-net: a self-configuring method for deep learning-based biomedical image segmentation. Nat. Methods 18(2), 203–211 (2021)
5. Joo, B., et al.: A deep learning algorithm may automate intracranial aneurysm detection on MR angiography with high diagnostic performance. Eur. Radiol. 30, 5785–5793 (2020)
6. Kingma, D.P., Ba, J.: Adam: a method for stochastic optimization. arXiv preprint arXiv:1412.6980 (2014)
7. Li, M., et al.: Accurate diagnosis of small cerebral aneurysms <5 mm in diameter with 3.0-t MR angiography. Radiology 271(2), 553–560 (2014)
8. Maloof, M.A.: Learning when data sets are imbalanced and when costs are unequal and unknown. In: ICML Workshop on Learning from Imbalanced Data Sets (2003)
9. Nakao, T., et al.: Deep neural network-based computer-assisted detection of cerebral aneurysms in MR angiography. J. Magn. Reson. Imaging 47(4), 948–953 (2018)
10. Ronneberger, O., Fischer, P., Brox, T.: U-Net: convolutional networks for biomedical image segmentation. In: Navab, N., Hornegger, J., Wells, W.M., Frangi, A.F. (eds.) MICCAI 2015. LNCS, vol. 9351, pp. 234–241. Springer, Cham (2015). https://doi.org/10.1007/978-3-319-24574-4_28
11. Sailer, A., Wagemans, B., Nelemans, P., de Graaf R, van Zwam WH: Diagnosing intracranial aneurysms with MR angiography: systematic review and meta-analysis. Stroke 45(1), 119–126 (2014)
12. Shelhamer, E., Long, J., Darrell, T.: Fully convolutional networks for semantic segmentation. IEEE Trans. Pattern Anal. Mach. Intell. 39(4), 640–651 (2017)
13. Shi, Z., et al.: A clinically applicable deep-learning model for detecting intracranial aneurysm in computed tomography angiography images. Nat. Commun. 11(1), 6090 (2020)
14. Ueda, D., et al.: Convolutional neural networks for the detection and measurement of cerebral aneurysms on magnetic resonance angiography. J. Digit. Imaging 32(5), 808–815 (2019)
15. Ueda, D., et al.: Deep learning for MR angiography: automated detection of cerebral aneurysms. Radiology 290(1), 187–194 (2019)
16. Wang, Y., et al.: Semi-supervised semantic segmentation using unreliable pseudo-labels. In: IEEE Conference on Computer Vision and Pattern Recognition, pp. 4248–4257 (2022)
17. Westerlaan, H.E., et al.: Intracranial aneurysms in patients with subarachnoid hemorrhage: CT angiography as a primary examination tool for diagnosis; systematic review and meta-analysis. Radiology 134–145 (2010)
18. Wu, H., Prasad, S.: Semi-supervised deep learning using pseudo labels for hyperspectral image classification. IEEE Trans. Image Process. 27(3), 1259–1270 (2018)

BraTS

Multimodal CNN Networks for Brain Tumor Segmentation in MRI: A BraTS 2022 Challenge Solution

Ramy A. Zeineldin[1,2,3]([✉]), Mohamed E. Karar[2], Oliver Burgert[1], and Franziska Mathis-Ullrich[3]

[1] Research Group Computer Assisted Medicine (CaMed), Reutlingen University, Reutlingen, Germany
Ramy.Zeineldin@Reutlingen-University.DE
[2] Faculty of Electronic Engineering (FEE), Menoufia University, Menouf, Egypt
[3] Health Robotics and Automation (HERA), Karlsruhe Institute of Technology, Karlsruhe, Germany

Abstract. Automatic segmentation is essential for the brain tumor diagnosis, disease prognosis, and follow-up therapy of patients with gliomas. Still, accurate detection of gliomas and their sub-regions in multimodal MRI is very challenging due to the variety of scanners and imaging protocols. Over the last years, the BraTS Challenge has provided a large number of multi-institutional MRI scans as a benchmark for glioma segmentation algorithms. This paper describes our contribution to the BraTS 2022 Continuous Evaluation challenge. We propose a new ensemble of multiple deep learning frameworks namely, DeepSeg, nnU-Net, and DeepSCAN for automatic glioma boundaries detection in pre-operative MRI. It is worth noting that our ensemble models took first place in the final evaluation on the BraTS testing dataset with Dice scores of 0.9294, 0.8788, and 0.8803, and Hausdorf distance of 5.23, 13.54, and 12.05, for the whole tumor, tumor core, and enhancing tumor, respectively. Furthermore, the proposed ensemble method ranked first in the final ranking on another unseen test dataset, namely Sub-Saharan Africa dataset, achieving mean Dice scores of 0.9737, 0.9593, and 0.9022, and HD95 of 2.66, 1.72, 3.32 for the whole tumor, tumor core, and enhancing tumor, respectively. The docker image for the winning submission is publicly available at (https://hub.docker.com/r/razeineldin/camed22).

Keywords: BraTS · CNN · Ensemble · Glioma · MRI · Segmentation

1 Introduction

Glioma is the most common tumor type of tumor to originate in the brain and arises from the supportive tissue of the brain, called glial cells. Diagnosis of glioma is often challenging because of its invasive nature, extreme heterogeneity, its ability to occur in any part of the brain, and its sub-regions of varying shapes and sizes including the enhancing tumor (ET), peritumoral edema (ED), and the necrotic and non-enhancing tumor core (NET) [1, 2].

© The Author(s), under exclusive license to Springer Nature Switzerland AG 2023
S. Bakas et al. (Eds.): BrainLes 2022, LNCS 13769, pp. 127–137, 2023.
https://doi.org/10.1007/978-3-031-33842-7_11

Manual segmentation of gliomas is the process of manually identifying and outlining the extent of glioma on medical imaging scans, such as magnetic resonance imaging (MRI) scans [3]. This is typically done by a trained medical professional, for example, a radiologist. One of the main challenges of manual glioma segmentation is its time-consuming and labor-intensive nature, requiring the person doing the segmentation to carefully review the images and outline the tumor. Additionally, manual segmentation can be subject to human error, causing inaccuracies in the final segmentation. Consequently, it is difficult to accurately assess the size and location of the tumor, which may have a negative impact on the treatment planning procedures.

The Brain Tumor Segmentation (BraTS) Challenge is an annual competition organized by the Medical Image Computing and Computer-Assisted Interventions (MIC-CAI) [4, 5]. The BraTS challenge is designed to encourage research in the field of medical image segmentation, with a focus on segmenting brain tumors in MRI scans. The challenge participants are provided with a dataset of MRI scans and asked to develop automated algorithms that can accurately segment the tumors in the images. BraTS 2022 Continuous Evaluation (BraTSCE) utilizes the largest annotated and publicly available multi-parametric (mpMRI) dataset provided by the BraTS 2021 challenge [2, 6, 7] as a common benchmark to foster the development of algorithms that can assist doctors in the diagnosis and treatment of brain tumors.

Deep learning is a sub-field of artificial intelligence that uses neural networks to learn from data and make predictions. In the context of glioma segmentation, deep learning algorithms can be trained to analyze MRI scans of the brain and identify areas that contain tumors. More specifically, the encoder-decoder architecture with skip connections, first introduced by the U-Net [8, 9], has gained popularity in the medical field outperforming other traditional methods in brain glioma segmentation [10–12]. The use of deep learning in glioma segmentation can help to automate the process, making it faster and more efficient. By using deep learning, researchers and doctors can more quickly and accurately identify tumors in MRI scans, which can ultimately improve patient care. In the context of the BraTS challenge, the recent winning contributions of 2019 [13], 2020 [14], and 2021 [11] extend the U-Net architecture by adding two-stage cascaded U-Net [13], making significant architecture changes [14], or using ensemble predictions.

In this paper, we extend our previous work [12] by proposing a fully automated convolutional neural network (CNN) method for glioma segmentation based on an ensemble of three encoder-decoder methods, namely, DeepSeg [15], our earlier deep learning framework for automatic brain tumor segmentation using two-dimensional T2 Fluid Attenuated Inversion Recovery (FLAIR) scans, nnU-Net [14], a self-configuring method for automatic biomedical segmentation, and DeepSCAN [16] architecture which contains densely connected blocks of dilated convolutions. The remainder of the paper is organized as follows: The BraTS dataset and the encoder-decoder CNN architecture are described in Sect. 2. Section 3 presents the experimental methods of the ensemble model, whereas the paper is concluded in Sect. 4.

2   Materials and Methods

2.1   Dataset

The MRI volumes have been used for the training and evaluation of models based on the Multi-modal BraTS Challenge 2021 [2]. The BraTS 2021 training dataset contains 1251 scans along with truth annotations of tumorous regions. For each case, BraTS provide four modalities: native (T1), post-contrast T1-weighted (T1Gd), T2-weighted (T2), and FLAIR. Ground truth segmentation consists of four classes: enhancing tumor (ET) (label 4), peritumoral edema (ED) (label 2), necrotic tumor core (NCR) (label 1), and background (label 0). These sub-regions can be clustered together to compose three semantically meaningful tumor classes enhancing tumor (ET), the addition of ET and NCR represents the tumor Core (TC) region, and the addition of ED to TC represents the whole tumor (WT). The BraTS 2021 database includes also 219 cases that were used for the public leaderboard during the validation phase, in addition to 530 cases for the final ranking of the participants.

Initial preprocessing steps were performed by the BraTS including co-registration to the same anatomical template, isotropic resampling to $1mm^3$ resolution, and skull-stripping. The resultant MRI volumes and associated labels are of shape $240 \times 240 \times 155$. The provided data were further processed prior to being fed into the networks. The MRI volumes were cropped to non-zero voxels to reduce the computation with a spatial resolution of $192 \times 224 \times 160$. Since the intensity in MR images is qualitative, the voxels were normalized by their mean and standard deviation for each input MRI image.

2.2   Neural Network Architectures

DeepSeg. Figure 1 outlines our previously proposed model [12, 15], which is a modular CNN framework for fully automatic brain tumor detection and segmentation. Inspired by the U-Net, DeepSeg consists of a contracting path followed by an expansive path. The contracting path is made up of a series of $3 \times 3 \times 3$ convolutional and $2 \times 2 \times 2$ max-pooling layers, which extract hierarchical features from the input image. The expansive path, on the other hand, is made up of a series of $2 \times 2 \times 2$ deconvolutional layers, which use those hierarchical features to upsample the output of the contracting path and produce a segmentation map for the input image. DeepSeg utilizes recent advances in CNNs including dropout, batch normalization (BN), and rectified linear unit (ReLU) [17, 18]. The initial filter size of convolutional kernels is set to 8 and doubled at the following layers which allow the network to learn features at multiple scales and improve its performance on the segmentation task. Finally, a $1 \times 1 \times 1$ convolutional layer followed by a softmax function is employed for the output segmentation.

nnU-Net Is a deep-learning framework for medical image segmentation [10]. It is an extension of the U-Net architecture, which is a popular deep-learning architecture for image segmentation tasks. In contrast to DeepSeg, nnU-Net does not employ any of the recently proposed architectural advances in deep learning and is based only on plain convolutions for feature extraction. More specifically, nnU-Net uses strided convolutions for downsampling whereas transposed convolutions are applied for upsampling. Figure 2

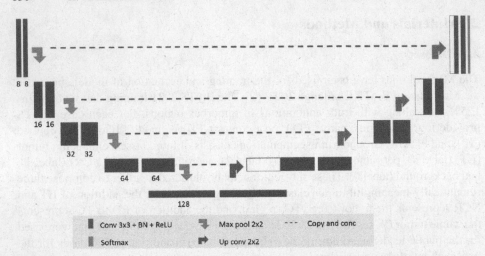

Fig. 1. DeepSeg architecture, as applied to brain tumor segmentation in BraTS 2021 challenge [12].

outlines the enhanced nnU-Net incorporating three main modifications that led to the first rank in the segmentation task of the BraTS challenge in 2021 [11]. First, the network size is asymmetrically increased by doubling the number of filters in the encoder while maintaining the same filters in the decoder. Second, group normalization layers are replaced by batch normalization which has been shown to work better for the low batch size. Third, the employment of a self-attention mechanism or transformer [19] in the decoder allows the model to focus on different parts of the input image at different times, which can be useful for identifying and segmenting complex glioma sub-structures.

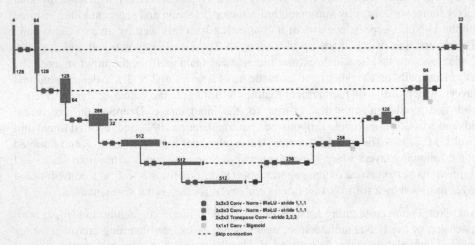

Fig. 2. Enhanced nnU-Net network, as applied to brain tumor segmentation in BraTS 2021 challenge [11].

DeepSCAN. Figure 3 shows the two DeepSCAN architectures introduced for brain tumor segmentation. Inspired by the recent Densenet architecture [20] and U-Net [8], DeepSCAN architecture was proposed for semantic segmentation. Instead of using transition layers and pooling operations, dilated convolutions are used to increase the receptive field of the encoder. Similar to Densenet, the output of each layer is concatenated with its input before passing to the next layer. Moreover, label uncertainty is applied directly to the loss function, which allows the prediction of the CNN to be involved in evaluating the network decision. This hybrid 2D/ 3D approach led to more stable results and ranked third in the BraTS 2018 challenge.

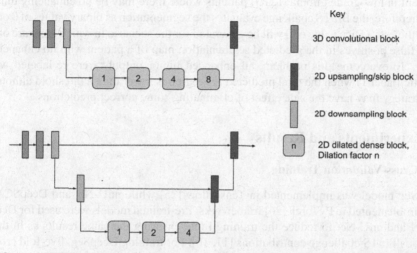

Fig. 3. DeepSCAN architectures, as applied to brain tumor segmentation in BraTS 2018 challenge [16].

2.3 Ensemble Learning

The ensemble is a technique in machine learning where multiple models are trained and combined to make a single prediction [21, 22]. In the context of glioma segmentation, an ensemble of models could be used to improve the performance of the segmentation process and provide more accurate results. For example, multiple models could be trained on different subsets of the data, and their predictions could be combined to create a more accurate segmentation of the tumor in an MRI scan.

In this paper, we used three different CNN models, namely, DeepSeg [15], nnU-Net [10], and DeepSCAN [16] which follow the U-Net pattern [8, 9] and consist of encoder-decoder architecture interconnected by skip connections (as discussed in Sect. 2.3). The final results were obtained by using the Simultaneous Truth and Performance Level Estimation (STAPLE) [23], which is an expectation-maximization ensemble method used in medical image segmentation. The STAPLE method works by estimating the truth, or ground truth, and the performance level of each model in the ensemble. It then combines the predictions of the models to create a final segmentation that is more accurate than any of the individual models.

2.4 Post-processing

Post-processing is a step in the glioma segmentation process that follows the initial segmentation of the tumor. It typically involves refining the initial segmentation to improve its accuracy and reduce any errors or inconsistencies. These methods could include techniques such as morphological operations, region growing, or level set evolution. The goal of post-processing is to produce a final segmentation that is as accurate and reliable as possible.

In the BraTS Challenge, the segmentation of the tumor core, and determining the small blood vessels (necrosis or edema), is particularly challenging. This is especially apparent in low-grade glioma (LGG) patients where there may be no enhancing tumor and, therefore, the BraTS challenge evaluates the segmentation as binary values of 0 or 1. Nevertheless, a Dice value of 0 will be generated for the scenario in which there are only small false positives in the predicted segmentation map of a patient with no enhancing tumor. To overcome this problem, all enhanced tumor outputs were re-labeled with necrotic (label 1) when the total predicted ET region is lower than a threshold although this strategy may have the side effect of eliminating some correct predictions.

3 Experiments and Results

3.1 Cross-Validation Training

DeepSeg model was implemented in Tensorflow [25] while nnU-Net and DeepSCAN were implemented in PyTorch [26] frameworks. Pre-trained models were used for Deep-SCAN and nnU-Net to reduce the training time, ensuring the same results as in their previous BraTS challenge contributions [11, 16]. For training DeepSeg, five-fold cross-validation was used for training each model on the 1251 cases of the BraTS 2021 training dataset for a maximum of 1200 epochs. This allows each model to be trained and evaluated multiple times using different combinations of training and testing data, which can provide a more accurate estimate of the performance of a model. Adam optimizer [24] has been applied with an initial learning rate of $1e^{-4}$ and a default value of $1e^{-7}$ for epsilon. All experiments were conducted on a single Nvidia GPU (RTX 2080 Ti GPU with 11 GB VRAM or RTX 3060 with 12 GB VRAM). Randomly sampled patches of $128 \times 128 \times 128$ voxels are input to our networks with batch sizes varying from 2 to 5 and the post-processing threshold is set to 200 voxels. This tiling strategy allows the model to be trained on multi-modal high-resolution MRI images with low GPU memory requirements. To overcome the effect of class imbalance between tumor labels and the brain healthy tissue, on-the-fly spatial data augmentations during training have been applied including random rotation between 0 and 30°, random 3D flipping, power-law gamma intensity transformation, or a combination of them.

3.2 Online Evaluation

Table 1 summarizes the results of the models on the BraTS 2021 validation, where the five-fold cross-validation for each model is averaged as an ensemble. Two evaluation metrics are used for the BraTS 2021 benchmark, computed by the online evaluation platform of Sage Bionetworks Synapse (Synapse)[1], which are the DSC and the Hausdorff

---

[1] The online evaluation platform synapse, https://www.synapse.org/

distance (95%) (HD95). Similarly, we computed the averages of DSC scores and HD95 values across the three evaluated tumor sub-regions and then used them to rank our methods in the final column.

By using a region-based version of DeepSeg with an input patch size of 128 × 128 × 128 voxels, batch size of 5, applied post-processing stage, and on-the-fly data augmentation, the DeepSeg model achieved good results of DSC values of 0.8356, 0.8508, and 0.9137 for the ET, TC, and WT regions, respectively. Additionally, we used two different models of nnU-Net [14], the BraTS 2020 winning approach, and DeepSCAN, one of the BraTS 2018 winning approaches. The first model, nnU-Net, is a region-based version of the standard nnU-Net, large batch size of 5, more aggressive data augmentation as described in [14], trained using batch Dice loss, and including the postprocessing stage. DeepSCAN model is similar to nnU-Net and DeepSeg model with the output layer as three logits, one for the whole tumor, tumor core, and enhancing regions rather than using a softmax layer. DeepSCAN model ranks third in our ranking (see Table 1) achieving the best average HD95 of 8.7886 while maintaining a good DSC of 0.8739.

For the BraTSCE 2022 challenge, we selected the three top-performing models to build our final ensemble: DeepSeg + nnU-Net + DeepSCAN. It is worth mentioning that our final ensemble was implemented by first predicting the validation cases individually with each model configuration, followed by averaging the softmax outputs to obtain the final cross-validation predictions. After that, the STAPLE [23] was applied to aggregate the segmentation produced by each of the individual methods using the probabilistic estimate of the true segmentation. This led to our best score of 0.8821 and 9.5440 for the mean DSC and HD95, respectively on the BraTS 2021 final validation dataset.

Table 1. Results of our five-fold cross-validation models on BraTS 2021 validation cases. All reported values were computed by the online evaluation platform Synapse. The average of DSC and HD95 scores are computed and used for ranking our methods.

Model	DSC				HD95				Rank
	ET	TC	WT	Avg	ET	TC	WT	Avg	
DeepSeg	0.8356	0.8508	0.9137	0.8667	17.75	11.56	4.15	11.15	4
nnU-Net	0.8402	0.8718	0.9213	0.8778	16.03	8.95	3.82	9.60	2
DeepSCAN	0.8306	0.8683	0.9228	0.8739	**14.50**	7.91	3.95	**8.79**	3
Ensemble	**0.8438**	**0.8753**	**0.9271**	**0.8821**	17.50	**7.53**	**3.60**	9.54	1

- Bold values correspond to higher scores

Table 2, Table 3, and Table 4 provide complete statistics of the ensemble model performance on the test datasets. All reported values were provided by the challenge organizers. Our method took first place in the BraTSCE 2022 competition on both the unseen BraTS and Sub-Saharan Africa (SSA) datasets[2]. However, the results were not so great on the third pediatric test dataset. This is particularly due to the inherent

[2] BraTSCE results dashboard, https://www.synapse.org/#!Synapse:syn27046444/wiki/617004/

variability and complexity of the tumor tissue in pediatric data which makes segmentation of pediatric brain tumors challenging. Unlike other types of tumors, which tend to be more homogeneous, pediatric brain tumors can be highly heterogeneous, with different types of tissue and abnormal cells. Additionally, the small size and delicate nature of the brain tissue in pediatric patients can make it difficult to accurately identify and segment the tumor tissue. Other challenges in the segmentation of pediatric brain tumors include the need for specialized techniques, as well as the lack of large, annotated datasets for training and validation.

Table 2. Final ensemble results on the BraTS 2021 test dataset.

	DSC			HD95		
	ET	TC	WT	ET	TC	WT
Mean	0.8803	0.8788	0.9294	12.05	13.54	5.24
StdDev	0.1765	0.2384	0.1026	59.61	59.67	23.08
Median	0.9351	0.9637	0.9602	1.00	1.41	1.57
25quantile	0.8633	0.9179	0.9210	1.00	1.00	1.00
75quantile	0.9645	0.9814	0.9791	1.73	3.00	3.61

Table 3. Final ensemble results on the SSA test dataset.

	DSC			HD95		
	ET	TC	WT	ET	TC	WT
Mean	0.9022	0.9593	0.9737	3.32	1.72	2.66
StdDev	0.1303	0.0704	0.0468	6.09	1.44	6.50
Median	0.9492	0.9841	0.9872	1.41	1.00	1.00
25quantile	0.9014	0.9725	0.9735	1.00	1.00	1.00
75quantile	0.9608	0.9893	0.9904	3.00	1.41	1.00

Table 4. Final ensemble results on the pediatric test dataset.

	DSC		HD95	
	TC	WT	TC	WT
Mean	0.2639	0.7953	181.76	24.84
StdDev	0.3535	0.2465	179.51	80.43
Median	0.0150	0.8802	68.48	4.12
25quantile	0.0000	0.8225	7.07	3.08
75quantile	0.5948	0.9049	373.13	6.48

3.3 Qualitative Output

Figure 4 depicts the qualitative performance of the segmentation predictions. It shows results generated by the final ensemble model on the BraTS 2021 validation dataset. In the three rows, the best, median, and worse segmentations are shown according to their DSC scores. It is obviously that our proposed model achieved best results with overall high quality. However, applying our post-processing strategy showed a limitation as illustrated in Sect. 2.4. Nevertheless, the WT region was detected with a good quality (DSC of 0.9606) which could be valuable for future clinical use.

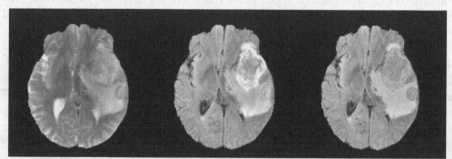

(a) **Best:** BraTS2021_Validation_01779, EC (0.9817), TC (0.9867), WT (0.9919)

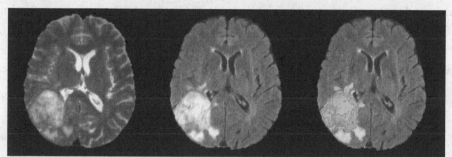

(b) **Median:** BraTS2021_Validation_01684, EC (0.8953), TC (0.9662), WT (0.9338)

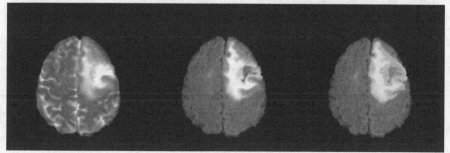

(c) **Worse:** BraTS2021_Validation_01774, EC (0), TC (0.8247), WT (0.9606)

Fig. 4. Sample qualitative validation set results of our ensemble model. The best, median and worse cases are shown in the rows. Columns display the T2, T2-FLAIR, and the overlay of our predicted segmentation on the T2-FLAIR image. WT includes all visible labels (green, yellow and red labels), TC is a union of green and red, while ET class is shown in green.

4 Conclusion

This paper presented our contribution to the segmentation task of the BraTSCE 2022 challenge. Ensemble models from multiple configurations of different state-of-the-art U-Net variants, namely, DeepSeg [12], nnU-Net [14], and DeepSCAN [16], have been explored. Based on our internal ranking strategy, the final submission was selected as the ensemble of these methods. Post-processing methods were used to improve the accuracy of the developed segmentation algorithms despite the side effects of ignoring some correct predictions. Table 1 lists the results of our methods on the validation set computed by the online evaluation platform Synapse. Remarkably, our method achieved DSC of 0.9271, 0.8753, and 0.8438 as well as HD95 of 17.5041, 7.5326, and 3.5952 for, ET, TC, and WT regions on the validation dataset, respectively.

This ensemble method won the BraTSCE 2022 competition on two unseen test datasets. On the BraTS test dataset, our submission achieved DSC scores of 0.8803, 0.8788, and 0.9294 as well as HD95 of 12.05, 13.54, and 5.24 for ET, TC, and WT, respectively. Remarkably, our model obtained DSC scores of 0.9022, 0.9593, and 0.9737 as well as HD95 of 3.32, 1.72, and 2.66 for ET, TC, and WT on the SSA test dataset, respectively. In general, qualitative evaluation supports the numerical evaluation showing a high-quality segmentation. The findings suggest that this approach can be readily employed for clinical practice.

Acknowledgments. The first author is supported by the German Academic Exchange Service (DAAD) [scholarship number 91705803].

References

1. Louis, D.N., et al.: cIMPACT-NOW update 6: new entity and diagnostic principle recommendations of the cIMPACT-Utrecht meeting on future CNS tumor classification and grading. Brain Pathol. **30**, 844–856 (2020)
2. Baid, U., et al.: The RSNA-ASNR-MICCAI BraTS 2021 Benchmark on Brain Tumor Segmentation and Radiogenomic Classification. arXiv:2107.02314 (2021)
3. Visser, M., et al.: Inter-rater agreement in glioma segmentations on longitudinal MRI. NeuroImage: Clinical **22** (2019)
4. Menze, B.H., et al.: The multimodal brain tumor image segmentation benchmark (BRATS). IEEE Trans. Med. Imaging **34**, 1993–2024 (2015)
5. Bakas, S., et al.: Advancing the cancer genome atlas glioma MRI collections with expert segmentation labels and radiomic features. Scientific Data **4** (2017)
6. Bakas, S., Akbari, H., Sotiras, A.: Segmentation labels for the pre-operative scans of the TCGA-GBM collection. The Cancer Imaging Archive (2017)
7. Bakas, S., et al.: Segmentation labels and radiomic features for the pre-operative scans of the TCGA-LGG collection. The Cancer Imaging Archive **286** (2017)
8. Ronneberger, O., Fischer, P., Brox, T.: U-net: Convolutional networks for biomedical image segmentation. Lecture Notes in Computer Science (including subseries Lecture Notes in Artificial Intelligence and Lecture Notes in Bioinformatics) **9351**, 234–241 (2015)
9. Çiçek, Ö., Abdulkadir, A., Lienkamp, S.S., Brox, T., Ronneberger, O.: 3D U-net: learning dense volumetric segmentation from sparse annotation. In: Ourselin, S., Joskowicz, L., Sabuncu, M.R., Unal, G., Wells, W. (eds.) MICCAI 2016. LNCS, vol. 9901, pp. 424–432. Springer, Cham (2016). https://doi.org/10.1007/978-3-319-46723-8_49

10. Isensee, F., Jaeger, P.F., Kohl, S.A.A., Petersen, J., Maier-Hein, K.H.: nnU-Net: a self-configuring method for deep learning-based biomedical image segmentation. Nat. Methods **18**, 203–211 (2020)

11. Luu, H.M., Park, S.-H.: Extending nn-UNet for brain tumor segmentation. Brainlesion: Glioma, Multiple Sclerosis, Stroke and Traumatic Brain Injuries, pp. 173–186 (2022)

12. Zeineldin, R.A., Karar, M.E., Mathis-Ullrich, F., Burgert, O.: Ensemble CNN Networks for GBM Tumors Segmentation using Multi-parametric MRI. Brainlesion: Glioma, Multiple Sclerosis, Stroke and Traumatic Brain Injuries (2022)

13. Jiang, Z., Ding, C., Liu, M., Tao, D.: Two-stage cascaded u-net: 1st place solution to BraTS challenge 2019 segmentation task. In: Crimi, A., Bakas, S. (eds.) BrainLes 2019. LNCS, vol. 11992, pp. 231–241. Springer, Cham (2020). https://doi.org/10.1007/978-3-030-46640-4_22

14. Isensee, F., Jäger, P.F., Full, P.M., Vollmuth, P., Maier-Hein, K.H.: nnU-Net for brain tumor segmentation. In: Crimi, A., Bakas, S. (eds.) BrainLes 2020. LNCS, vol. 12659, pp. 118–132. Springer, Cham (2021). https://doi.org/10.1007/978-3-030-72087-2_11

15. Zeineldin, R.A., Karar, M.E., Coburger, J., Wirtz, C.R., Burgert, O.: DeepSeg: deep neural network framework for automatic brain tumor segmentation using magnetic resonance FLAIR images. Int. J. Comput. Assist. Radiol. Surg. **15**(6), 909–920 (2020)

16. McKinley, R., Meier, R., Wiest, R.: Ensembles of densely-connected CNNs with label-uncertainty for brain tumor segmentation. In: Crimi, A., Bakas, S., Kuijf, H., Keyvan, F., Reyes, M., van Walsum, T. (eds.) BrainLes 2018. LNCS, vol. 11384, pp. 456–465. Springer, Cham (2019). https://doi.org/10.1007/978-3-030-11726-9_40

17. Srivastava, N., Hinton, G., Krizhevsky, A., Salakhutdinov, R.: Dropout: a simple way to prevent neural networks from overfitting. In: Journal of Machine Learning Research, pp. 1929–1958 (2014)

18. Ioffe, S., Szegedy, C.: Batch normalization: Accelerating deep network training by reducing internal covariate shift. In: 32nd International Conference on Machine Learning, ICML 2015, vol. 1, pp. 448–456. International Machine Learning Society (IMLS) (2015)

19. Vaswani, A., et al.: Attention is All You Need. Advances in Neural Information Processing Systems **30** (2017)

20. Huang, G., Liu, Z., Van Der Maaten, L., Weinberger, K.Q.: Densely connected convolutional networks. In: Proceedings of the IEEE conference on computer vision and pattern recognition, pp. 4700–4708 (2017)

21. Polikar, R.: Ensemble Learning. Ensemble Machine Learning, pp. 1–34 (2012)

22. Sagi, O., Rokach, L.: Ensemble learning: A survey. WIREs Data Mining and Knowledge Discovery **8** (2018)

23. Warfield, S.K., Zou, K.H., Wells, W.M.: Simultaneous truth and performance level estimation (STAPLE): an algorithm for the validation of image segmentation. IEEE Trans. Med. Imaging **23**, 903–921 (2004)

24. Kingma, D.P., Ba, J.: Adam: A Method for Stochastic Optimization (2014)

Multi-modal Transformer for Brain Tumor Segmentation

Jihoon Cho[iD] and Jinah Park[(✉)][iD]

Korea Advanced Institute of Science and Technology, Daejeon, South Korea
{zinic,jinahpark}@kaist.ac.kr

Abstract. Segmentation of brain tumors from multiple MRI modalities is necessary for successful disease diagnosis and clinical treatment. In recent years, Transformer-based networks with the self-attention mechanism have been proposed. But they do not show the performance beyond the U-shaped fully convolutional network. In this paper, we apply HFTrans network to the brain tumor segmentation task of BraTS 2022 challenge by focusing on the multi-modalities of MRI with the benefits of Transformer. By applying BraTS-specific modifications of preprocessing, aggressive data augmentation, and postprocessing, our method shows superior results in comparisons between previous best performers. We show that the final result on the BraTS 2022 validation dataset achieves dice scores of 82.94%, 85.48%, and 92.44% and Hausdorff distances of 14.55 mm, 12.96 mm, and 3.77 mm for enhancing tumor, tumor core, and whole tumor, respectively.

Keywords: Transformer · multi-modality · brain tumor segmentation

1 Introduction

Gliomas are the most prevalent type of malignant adult brain tumor. Following the WHO grade system, gliomas are categorized from 1 to 4 based on how aggressively the cell divide. In the case of glioblastoma, which is WHO grade 4 astrocytoma, it has extreme intrinsic heterogeneity in appearance, shape, and histology, so multi-protocol magnetic resonance imaging (MRI) is required to detect the brain tumors accurately. Popularly used modalities of MRI are T1-weighted (T1), post-contrast T1-weighted (T1ce), T2-weighted (T2), and T2 Fluid Attenuated Inversion Recovery (FLAIR). These modalities are utilized to divide the tumor's sub-regions following the annotation protocol. However, the manual segmentation process for the identification of brain tumor sub-regions is labor-intensive and time-consuming work of domain experts. Therefore, automated brain tumor segmentation solutions can contribute to many clinical tasks such as disease diagnosis and treatment planning.

During the last decade, convolutional neural network (CNN) has become the standard method for medical image segmentation. U-Net [16], one of the variants of Fully Convolutional Network (FCN) [11], has made remarkable achievements

S. Bakas et al. (Eds.): BrainLes 2022, LNCS 13769, pp. 138–148, 2023.
https://doi.org/10.1007/978-3-031-33842-7_12

on brain tumor segmentation [9, 12]. However, despite the powerful feature representation capability of CNN, limited receptive fields of CNN-based methods compared to large-sized medical images face the absence of a global context.

Recently in medical image segmentation, many works have proposed the network fused CNN and vision transformer [7] to take advantage of feature representation ability and the global context, and some works have shown great performances in brain tumor segmentation [8, 17]. However, CNN-based methods do not use a transformer still show the best performance in multi-modal brain tumor segmentation until now [9, 12].

In this work, we apply the Hybrid-Fusion Transformer (HFTrans) [6] for multi-parametric MRI brain tumor segmentation. HFTrans has multiple encoders for modality-specific feature embeddings and Transformer layer for integrating the multi-modal characteristics. Therefore, it is possible to fully utilize the multi-modal characteristics. We modify the settings to be suitable for the BraTS challenge including data preprocessing, data augmentation, training scheme, and postprocessing. As a result, evaluation on BraTS 2022 validation dataset [3, 4, 13] shows that remarkable results for 3D brain tumor segmentation.

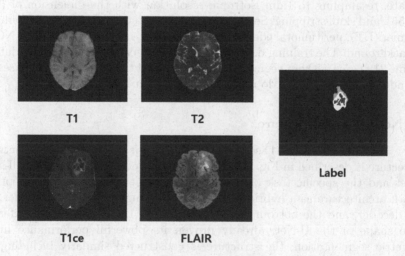

Fig. 1. Four MRI sequences and segmentation label of BraTS 2022 dataset. In the segmentation label, dark grey, grey, and white represent the necrotic tumor core (NCR), peritumoral edematous tissue (ED), and enhancing tumor (ET). (Color figure online)

2   Methods

2.1   Data

The dataset of BraTS 2022 challenge [1, 2] consists of 2,000 brain MRI scans acquired from multiple centers with different equipment (Fig. 1). Each brain MRI scan have four MRI sequences which are T1, T2, T1ce, and FLAIR. MRI

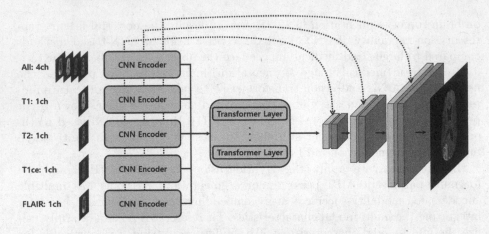

Fig. 2. Overview of the network architecture.

sequences are provided after preprocessing of co-registration to the anatomical template, resampling to 1mm isotropic resolution with the dimension of (240, 240, 155), and skull stripping. Segmentation labels consist of four classes: enhancing tumor (ET), peritumoral edematous tissue (ED), necrotic tumor core (NCR), and background. The training dataset contains 1251 cases, the validation dataset contains 219 cases without segmentation labels, and the remaining 570 cases are kept hidden for testing. We do not use any additional data for training.

2.2   Network Architecture

We use HFTrans [6] as the baseline network for our method, and the network architecture is described in Fig. 2. Considering the medical domain's small-sized dataset and the specific task of brain tumor segmentation, we have kept the network architecture as a hybrid structure consisting of the CNN encoder, the CNN decoder, and the bottom bottleneck layer of the Transformer. Referring to the shape of the U-Net, already proven its powerful performance in 3D volumetric segmentation, the structure is constructed similarly including the skip-connection path from the CNN encoder to the CNN decoder. The bottom bottleneck layers are processed through the self-attention mechanism from the multiple Transformer layers through the patch-embedded 1D sequences with the positional embedding. The most distinctive difference between HFTrans and the other Transformer-based networks [5,17] is that the HFTrans has additional CNN encoders for each modality. Features of each modality are also tokenized for the 3D Transformer layers. Therefore the network can train meaningful features balancing the importance of modalities in spatial space by all of the embedded tokens conducting the self-attention process.

Given the input patch size is 128 ×128 × 128, CNN encoders produce the five feature representations of $C \times 16 \times 16 \times 16$ where the C is the channel size. After $2 \times 2 \times 2$ patch-sized embedding to five representations, 2560 sequences are prepared with the feature dimension of K. Transformer layers emphasize the important weights using the global self-attention mechanism between sequences. In order to generate segmentation results the same size as the original 3D images, we recover the sequence data to the 4D feature map.

In the implementation, we construct the CNN encoders with the four residual CNN blocks consisting of two consecutive CNN layers with instance normalization and leaky ReLU activation function. For the bottom bottle layers, six Transformer layers and $K = 512$ are used. We reduce the channel dimension for saving the computational budget of the CNN decoder. Consequently as $128 \times 16 \times 16 \times 16$ sized 4D feature map can be generated for the decoder. And then progressive up-sampling is conducted with the spatial information merged from all five CNN encoders.

2.3 Data Preprocessing

As a first step, we crop the redundant background region (identified with voxel value zero) for efficient training. All of the images are resized to (192, 224, 160) by searching the crop size that all scans' brain regions can be captured considering the CNN encoder's pooling operation. And then, we normalize each image in the form of a standard normal distribution (with zero mean and one standard deviation) except for the background region.

2.4 Augmentations

Since it is difficult to utilize the whole-sized image as a training input due to the VRAM limitation, patch-based approach is used with the dimension of (128, 128, 128). For the patch selection, we select the patch randomly with the probability of $\frac{2}{3}$, and the tumor-centered patch is selected with the probability of $\frac{1}{3}$ to train the tumor representation efficiently. And then, we apply the on-the-fly augmentation during the training phase to prevent the overfitting problem. Intensity-based augmentation can be applied separately to each modality, but the geometric transformation is applied at once to keep the co-registered spatial space. The following data augmentations are applied sequentially using TorchIO framework [15] (Fig. 3).

1. **Rotation:** With the probability of 0.2, rotate the volume for each x, y, z axis individually with the uniformly sampled value from $[-30°, 30°]$. Volume size does not change and if an empty area occurs, replace the region with the background of zero voxel value.
2. **Scale:** With the probability of 0.2, scale the volume for each x, y, z axis individually with the uniformly sampled value from $[0.7, 1.4]$. Volume size is preserved and when zooming out on the image, fill the occurred region with the background of zero voxel value.
3. **Flip:** With the probability of 0.5 for each x, y, z axis independently, volume is flipped along the axis.

4. **Gaussian Noise:** With the probability of 0.15, add a Gaussian noise sampled from the normal distribution of zero mean and standard deviation of uniformly sampled from [0, 0.1].
5. **Gaussian Blur:** With the probability of 0.1 for each modality, blur the volume using the Gaussian filter having uniformly sampled standard deviation from [0.5, 1.5].
6. **Brightness:** With the probability of 0.15, multiply the random value uniformly sampled from [0.7, 1.3].
7. **Contrast:** With the probability of 0.15, multiply the random value uniformly sampled from [0.65, 1.5], and then clipped to the intensity range of the original image.
8. **Gamma Correction:** With the probability of 0.15, apply the gamma correction with the log of the gamma value uniformly sampled from [−0.35, 0.4].

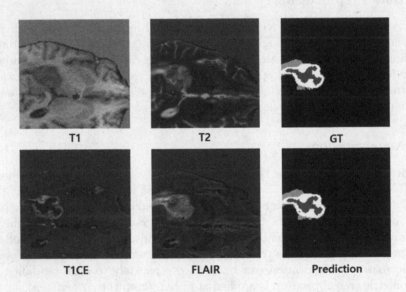

Fig. 3. Visualization of $128 \times 128 \times 128$ training patches after the data augmentation. A huge number of possible patch images make the network prevent overfitting.

2.5   Loss Function and Optimization

The evaluation targets of the BraTS challenge are slightly different from the segmentation labels. Three kinds of sub-regions are considered in the evaluation, 1) the enhancing tumor (ET), 2) the tumor core (TC) consists of enhancing tumor and the necrotic tumor core, and 3) the whole tumor (WT) consists of the enhancing tumor, the necrotic tumor core, and peritumoral edematous tissue. Reflecting these differences, we optimize each sub-region of evaluation separately with dice loss [14]. Additionally, the cross-entropy loss is applied to the brain tumor sub-region of the labels. We have used a stochastic gradient descent optimizer with an initial learning rate of 0.0001 and we have adjusted the learning rate with a polynomial policy with a power of 0.9. We have trained the models during 1000 epochs using four Nvidia RTX 3090 GPUs with batch-size 4.

$$L_{total} = L_{ce} + L_{diceET} + L_{diceTC} + L_{diceWT} \tag{1}$$

2.6 Inference

In inference, we only used the brain regions without redundant background regions for computational efficiency. A prediction has been conducted using the sliding window method. The window size is the same as the patch size during the training phase and the stride is half of the patch size. As for post-processing, we have multiplied the Gaussian importance map, which is weighted to the center using the Gaussian distribution, to the prediction preventing the borderline artifact caused by the sliding window approach [10]. The segmentation results are predicted with the ensemble of the cross-validation training network.

3   Results

3.1   Experiments on BraTS2020 Dataset

We have compared the performance of our method with nnU-Net [10] and Trnas-BTS [17]. For the efficiency of the comparisons, we train the networks with the BraTS 2020 dataset which has 369 training images. Local test results are presented in Table 1. Our proposed method has notable result of 79.43% dice score in TC class and achieves the best performance of 83.73% in the average dice score. The winner of recent BraTS challenges, nnUnet, shows the worst scores in the comparison; but, when training the network with whole-sized images utilizing the FCN's characteristic, nnUnet shows the competitive results with our method.

Table 1. Segmentation results tested on the BraTS 2020 dataset. We trained the networks with the patch of $128 \times 128 \times 128$ dimension except for nnUnet (whole).

Dice Score (%)	ET	TC	WT	Avg.
nnUnet [10]	77.84	78.39	92.09	82.77
nnUnet (whole) [10]	**79.15**	78.74	92.69	83.53
TransBTS [17]	78.64	77.41	**93.11**	83.05
Ours	78.75	**79.43**	93.02	**83.73**

3.2   Experiments on BraTS2022 Dataset

In order to evaluate the performance of our approach using the training dataset only, we have trained the models as five-fold cross-validation on the 2022 BraTS dataset. We randomly split the dataset for each fold. Evaluation results of the cross-validation is shown in Table 2. Due to an increase in the number of training data, the dice scores of the ET and TC were increased by about 10% than the result of BraTS 2020. However, fold 5 shows worse results in ET and TC than other folds. It could potentially harm prediction, so we tested about ensemble on the validation dataset.

Table 2. five-fold cross-validation results of the BraTS 2022 Training dataset.

Dice Score (%)	ET	TC	WT	Avg.
fold 1	89.26	92.73	93.80	91.93
fold 2	89.54	92.67	93.37	91.86
fold 3	91.41	94.17	93.86	93.15
fold 4	87.73	92.10	92.33	90.72
fold 5	84.71	77.58	92.40	84.90
Average	88.53	89.85	93.15	90.51

The validation results for the different configurations are presented in Table 3. As predicted, the dice scores of TC and ET were degraded in fold 5. Additionally, when we applied the test-time augmentation method of flipping on the x, y, z axis for the robustness, results were not improved. Therefore, we only ensemble with the four networks except for fold 5. Finally, we got the 86.95% of average dice score and 10.43 mm of average 95% Hausdorff distance with the Gaussian importance map.

Table 3. Segmentation results tested on BraTS 2022 validation dataset. BL represents our method based on HFTrnas without post-processing, EN is the ensemble of the five-fold cross-validation, and EN* is the ensemble without fold 5. GM is the Gaussian importance map, and TTA is the test-time augmentation with flipping.

Method	Dice Score (%)				HD Distance (mm)			
	ET	TC	WT	Avg.	ET	TC	WT	Avg.
BL	81.98	85.02	92.20	86.40	13.02	10.37	3.89	**9.09**
BL + EN	83.08	84.72	92.40	86.73	14.37	13.04	3.68	10.36
BL + EN*	82.80	85.34	92.36	**86.83**	14.51	12.93	3.70	10.38
BL + EN + GM	82.74	84.85	92.48	86.69	16.08	13.13	3.75	10.99
BL + EN* + GM	82.94	85.48	92.44	**86.95**	14.55	12.96	3.77	**10.43**
BL + EN + GM + TTA	82.30	84.89	92.53	86.57	17.82	14.64	3.72	12.06
BL + EN* + GM + TTA	82.45	85.56	92.49	86.83	16.17	12.92	3.70	10.93

3.3 Qualitative Results

In Fig. 4, visualizations of segmentation results are provided. We choose several cases of best, median, worst, and 25th and 75th percentile cases based on the segmentation accuracy. As you can see, our method predicts the whole tumor region very well even in the worst case. However, in some cases, our method has a problem missing some details of sub-tumor regions.

3.4 Hidden Testset Results

Table 4 presents the results of the hidden testset. The results on datasets of BraTS Testing Cohort and SSAfrican show great performances which are 88.44% and 92.42 of average dice scores and 11.53 mm and 3.12 mm of average 95% Hausdorff distances respectively. However, in the case of pediatric data, poor results are shown due to the different characteristics between the child and adult brains.

Table 4. Segmentation results tested on BraTS 2022 test dataset.

BraTS Testing Cohort	Dice Score (%)			HD Distance (mm)		
	ET	TC	WT	ET	TC	WT
Mean	86.14	86.72	92.47	12.41	16.89	5.30
StdDev	19.83	24.54	9.65	59.69	68.46	23.09
Median	92.55	95.90	95.56	1	1.41	1.73
25th percentile	84.86	90.34	91.07	1	1	1
75th percentile	96.10	97.85	97.51	2	3	4.12
Pediatric Data	Dice Score (%)			HD Distance (mm)		
	ET	TC	WT	ET	TC	WT
Mean	-	33.29	69.71	-	185.59	68.86
StdDev	-	39.94	32.87	-	181.60	136.50
Median	-	0.05	85.01	-	111.85	4.58
25th percentile	-	0	69.98	-	5.69	3.32
75th percentile	-	76.41	90.29	-	373.13	20.45
SSAfrican Data	Dice Score (%)			HD Distance (mm)		
	ET	TC	WT	ET	TC	WT
Mean	88.12	92.94	96.20	3.22	2.89	3.24
StdDev	13.20	7.98	4.59	3.71	2.41	5.97
Median	94.00	95.97	97.27	2.45	2.24	1.41
25th percentile	84.62	92.53	96.18	1	1	1
75th percentile	96.17	97.61	98.25	4.12	3.16	2.83

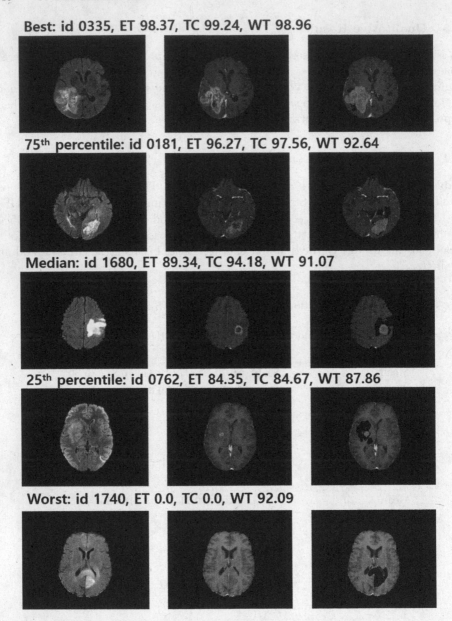

Fig. 4. Qualitative Results of BraTS 2022 validation dataset. The cases of best, worst, median, and 75th and 25th percentile were selected. FLAIR (left), T1ce (middle), and prediction (right) are presented within each row. In the prediction results, purple, yellow, and blue represent the necrotic tumor core (NCR), peritumoral edematous tissue (ED), and enhancing tumor (ET). (Color figure online)

4   Discussion

Depending on the fold of the cross-validation, various results are shown up to 8% of the average dice score. It makes the worse results in combining the five ensemble models on the validation dataset. We guess that the divided five-fold dataset has a bias like a specific tumor type. Therefore, considering the distribution of tumor proportions during the splitting of the dataset will be helpful to improve the performance. Additionally, the longer training time has guaranteed good performance in our training experience. However, the total iteration for the training is limited by the many experiences with the model architecture and hyperparameter tuning. These are limitations of the final model for this challenge. Nonetheless, our work shows competitive results to previous best performers so we have proven the benefit of our method.

Acknowledgements. This research was supported by the Capacity Enhancement Program for Scientific and Cultural Exhibition Services through the National Research Foundation of Korea (NRF) funded by Ministry of Science and ICT (No. NRF-2018X1A3A1069693) and Korea Institute of Energy Technology Evaluation and Planning (KETEP) grant funded by the Korea government (MOTIE) (20201510300280, Development of a remote dismantling training system with force-torque responding virtual nuclear power plant).

References

1. Bakas, S., et al.: Segmentation labels and radiomic features for the pre-operative scans of the TCGA-GBM collection (2017). https://doi.org/10.7937/K9/TCIA.2017.KLXWJJ1Q
2. Bakas, S., et al.: Segmentation labels and radiomic features for the pre-operative scans of the TCGA-LGG collection (2017). https://doi.org/10.7937/K9/TCIA.2017.GJQ7R0EF
3. Bakas, S., et al.: Advancing the cancer genome atlas glioma MRI collections with expert segmentation labels and radiomic features. Sci. Data 4(1), 1–13 (2017)
4. Bakas, S., et al.: Identifying the best machine learning algorithms for brain tumor segmentation, progression assessment, and overall survival prediction in the brats challenge. arXiv preprint arXiv:1811.02629 (2018)
5. Chen, J., et al.: Transunet: transformers make strong encoders for medical image segmentation. arXiv preprint arXiv:2102.04306 (2021)
6. Cho, J., Park, J.: Hybrid-fusion transformer for multisequence MRI. In: Medical Imaging and Computer-Aided Diagnosis. Springer, Cham (2022, in press)
7. Dosovitskiy, A., et al.: An image is worth 16x16 words: transformers for image recognition at scale. arXiv preprint arXiv:2010.11929 (2020)
8. Hatamizadeh, A., Nath, V., Tang, Y., Yang, D., Roth, H., Xu, D.: Swin UNETR: swin transformers for semantic segmentation of brain tumors in MRI images. arXiv preprint arXiv:2201.01266 (2022)
9. Isensee, F., Jäger, P.F., Full, P.M., Vollmuth, P., Maier-Hein, K.H.: nnU-Net for brain tumor segmentation. In: Crimi, A., Bakas, S. (eds.) BrainLes 2020. LNCS, vol. 12659, pp. 118–132. Springer, Cham (2021). https://doi.org/10.1007/978-3-030-72087-2_11

10. Isensee, F., et al.: nnu-net: self-adapting framework for u-net-based medical image segmentation. arXiv preprint arXiv:1809.10486 (2018)
11. Long, J., Shelhamer, E., Darrell, T.: Fully convolutional networks for semantic segmentation. In: Proceedings of the IEEE Conference on Computer Vision and Pattern Recognition, pp. 3431–3440 (2015)
12. Luu, H.M., Park, S.H.: Extending nn-unet for brain tumor segmentation. arXiv preprint arXiv:2112.04653 (2021)
13. Menze, B.H., et al.: The multimodal brain tumor image segmentation benchmark (BRATS). IEEE Trans. Med. Imaging **34**(10), 1993–2024 (2014)
14. Milletari, F., Navab, N., Ahmadi, S.A.: V-net: fully convolutional neural networks for volumetric medical image segmentation. In: 2016 Fourth International Conference on 3D Vision (3DV), pp. 565–571. IEEE (2016)
15. Pérez-García, F., Sparks, R., Ourselin, S.: Torchio: a python library for efficient loading, preprocessing, augmentation and patch-based sampling of medical images in deep learning. Comput. Methods Programs Biomed. 106236 (2021). https://doi.org/10.1016/j.cmpb.2021.106236. https://www.sciencedirect.com/science/article/pii/S0169260721003102
16. Ronneberger, O., Fischer, P., Brox, T.: U-net: convolutional networks for biomedical image segmentation. CoRR abs/1505.04597 (2015). http://arxiv.org/abs/1505.04597
17. Wang, W., Chen, C., Ding, M., Yu, H., Zha, S., Li, J.: TransBTS: multimodal brain tumor segmentation using transformer. In: de Bruijne, M., et al. (eds.) MICCAI 2021. LNCS, vol. 12901, pp. 109–119. Springer, Cham (2021). https://doi.org/10.1007/978-3-030-87193-2_11

An Efficient Cascade of U-Net-Like Convolutional Neural Networks Devoted to Brain Tumor Segmentation

Philippe Bouchet[1], Jean-Baptiste Deloges[1], Hugo Canton-Bacara[1],
Gaëtan Pusel[1], Lucas Pinot[2], Othman Elbaz[2], and Nicolas Boutry[3]( )

[1] EPITA Majeure Santé, Le Kremlin-Bicêtre 94270, France
[2] EPITA Majeure SCIA, Le Kremlin-Bicêtre 94270, France
[3] EPITA Research and Development Laboratory (LRDE),
Le Kremlin-Bicêtre 94270, France
nicolas.boutry@lrde.epita.fr

Abstract. A *glioma* is a fast-growing and aggressive tumor that starts in the glial cells of the brain. They make up about 30% of all brain tumors, and 80% of all malignant brain tumors. Gliomas are considered to be *rare* tumors, affecting less than 10,000 people each year, with a 5-year survival rate of 6%. If intercepted at an early stage, they pose no danger; however, providing an accurate diagnosis has proven to be difficult. In this paper, we propose a cascade approach using state-of-the-art Convolutional Neural Networks, in order to maximize accuracy in tumor detection. Various U-Net-like networks have been implemented and tested in order to select the network best suited for this problem.

Keywords: Neural Networks Cascade · Deep Learning · Brain Tumor Segmentation · U-Net · Res-U-Net · U-Net++ · Attention U-Net · Attention ResU-Net

1 Introduction

The MICCAI BraTS [1] is a challenge that occurs every year since 2012, organized by the Radiological Society of North America, the American Society of Neuroradiology and the Medical Image Computing and Computer Assisted Interventions society (RSNA-ASNR-MICCAI BraTS). The goal of the competition is the evaluation of state-of-the-art methods for the segmentation of intrinsically heterogeneous glioblastoma sub-regions in mpMRI [2] scans using multi-institutional pre-operative baseline multi-parametric magnetic resonance imaging scans [3,4].

As stated in the abstract, intercepting the glioma at an early stage *greatly* increases the patient's survival rate. However, in order to intercept the tumor, it must be accurately diagnosed. Unfortunately, most modern hospitals are not equipped with the technology capable of automatically detecting gliomas [12], thus causing the tumor to grow until it becomes deadly.

S. Bakas et al. (Eds.): BrainLes 2022, LNCS 13769, pp. 149–161, 2023.
https://doi.org/10.1007/978-3-031-33842-7_13

We have been provided with clinically acquired training data, as well as the corresponding segmentation labels of the different glioma sub-regions: Enhancing Tumor (ET), Tumor Core (TC) and the Whole Tumor (WT).

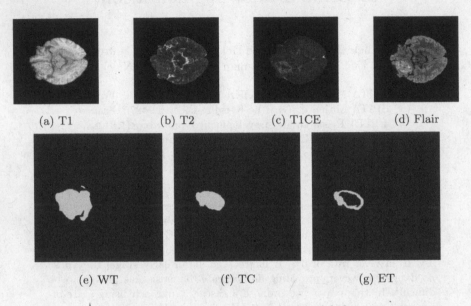

(a) T1   (b) T2   (c) T1CE   (d) Flair

(e) WT   (f) TC   (g) ET

Fig. 1. Modalities and corresponding labels.

As depicted in Fig. 1, the WT describes the complete extent of the tumor. It entails the TC and ET, which is typically depicted by hyper-intense signal in FLAIR. The TC describes the bulk of the tumor. The TC entails the ET, as well as the necrotic parts of the tumor (NCR). The ET is described by areas that show hyper-intensity in T1CE when compared to T1, but also when compared to "healthy" white matter in T1CE. The voxel values for these images are:

- 1: Necrotic Tumor
- 2: Peritumoral edematous/invaded tissue
- 4: Enhancing tumor
- 0: Everything else

Furthermore, by applying the logical bitwise *or* operation on these voxel values, we can find the different tumor regions.

- 1 ∪ 2 ∪ 4: Whole Tumor
- 1 ∪ 4: Tumor Core
- 4: Enhanced Tumor

In this paper, we propose a three-stage cascaded network, implementing a state-of-the-art variation of the U-Net at each stage. Each U-Net model will specialize in segmenting the whole tumor, the tumor core and the enhanced tumor, in that order.

2   State-of-the-Art

2.1   Main Architectures in Biomedical Image Segmentation

Since the apparition of the U-Net [19] in 2016 in the biomedical image segmentation community, it has been established as the gold standard of medical image segmentation ever since. [13] We've seen numerous variations of the model, such as the U-Net++ [21], the ResU-Net [5,6], or the Attention U-Net [14]. Many different state-of-the-art architectures have since been proposed and benchmarked in previous iterations of the BraTS challenge [13]. Concerning these different architectures, let us recall their main advantages compared to the standard U-Net.

2.2   U-Net++

The U-Net++ [20] is a dense network, rendering it capable to extract rather minute details from an image or a volume. Moreover, the network also presents two output methods: a regular single output image, or deep supervision [8], with multiple outputs. Since each output has its own loss, we are able to calculate a weighted sum of the loss, allowing us to have more accurate results, at the cost of slower computation. In contrast, the single output mode is slightly less accurate than the deep supervision mode, however computation time will be much shorter as there is only a single output. It was selected for its versatility.

2.3   Attention ResU-Net

The Attention ResU-Net [11], is a combination of the Attention U-Net [14] and the ResU-Net [5,6], seeking to make use of each of these network's advantages. The ResU-Net is interesting, since it uses residual blocks in order to eliminate gradient related issues, such as the vanishing gradient problem. The Attention U-Net highlights only the relevant activations during training, meaning that the relevant parts of the image get large weights, thus reducing computational resources that are wasted on irrelevant activations of certain weights [14].

2.4   Existing Cascade Networks

Note that we also found several research papers related to cascades of networks used in the context of biomedical image segmentation. Among them, we can cite Wang G. et al. [19] who propose a cascade designed to decompose the multi-class segmentation problem into a sequence of three binary segmentation problems according to the sub region hierarchy. Y. Guo et al. [7] proposed a *Bidirectional Symmetric Cascade Network* (BSCN), such that each layer is supervised by vessel contour labels of specific diameter scale instead of the usual supervised approach which consists of using a ground truth to train different network layers.

3   Methodology

As stated in the opening abstract, this task was carried out using the Python machine learning frameworks *Tensorflow 2.9.1* as well as *numpy* and *nibabel* for handling volumes. We used OVHCloud, as well as the ROMEO supercomputer from the University of Reims Champagne-Ardenne in order to train the models. When we worked on the OVH platform, we had 4 Tesla V100S GPU's in parallel with each 32 Gb of VRAM, and when we worked on ROMEO, we got 4 Tesla P100-SXM2 GPU's with each 16Gb of VRAM. We obtained our benchmark results from testing with 200 patients from the dataset.

3.1   Motivation

Due to the nature of the segmentation problem, we propose a three-stage cascaded model, with variations of state-of-the-art U-Net models at each stage. We seek to train each model of our cascaded ensemble to specialize in the segmentation of different sub-regions of the glioblastoma. Since each sub-region of the brain tumor is contained within its predecessor, we can provide the subsequent models of our cascade with additional information pertaining to the location of the tumor. Moreover, using a three-stage cascaded model allows us to approach the problem with modularity in mind. We are not restricted to using the same model for each stage of our cascade. Instead, we can experiment with different types of U-Net-like models at different stages, for optimal performance.

3.2   Memory Management

In previous years, the MICCAI BraTS challenge provided competitors with a dataset containing the scans of approximately 350 patients. This year we have 1251 patients. The main issue of these data sets is known to be the heterogeneity of the data. Managing and accessing the entirety of the data posed to us an infrastructure problem, especially for regular computers with very little amounts of RAM and VRAM, as we simply cannot load all of the data into one big array.

Much part of our time has been spent designing and setting up the framework in which we would tackle the problem. After having come up with a solution to store all the data in numpy arrays on the disk using the NumPy's *memmap* function, we quickly implemented a framework in order to generate the data and build the models.

3.3   Data Formatting

The medical volumes of this challenge are of dimensions $(240, 240, 155)$, and we decided to combine each modality (T1, T2, T1CE, FLAIR) into a single volume with 4 channels; thus giving us a dimension of $(240, 240, 155, 4)$ for our input data. The ground truth's dimensions remained the same.

Due to this year's limitations in VRAM (limited to 16 GB), running a fully 3-dimensional network has proven to be a difficult and time consuming task. In order to preserve the information pertaining to the shape of the tumor in 3D, we opted for a 2.5D approach, that is, for each modality we fed the network with three horizontal slices of a single patient, instead of the whole 3D volume.

So we compared the 2D and the 2.5D approach for each architecture and each cascade, and found that the 2.5D approach resulted in far more accurate predictions, as more data was being fed into the network at each epoch.

3.4   Normalization

For the normalization step, we proceed in the following manner. Let N be the number of voxels of a given modality x among the T1, T1CE, T2, FLAIR modalities, then the indices i of the voxels of x belonging to $[0, N[$ with $N = 240 \times 240 \times 155$. This leads to:

$$\forall i \in [1, N], \; x_i^{\mathrm{norm}} = \min\left(\max\left(\frac{x_i - \mu}{5\,\sigma}, -1.0\right), 1.0\right) \tag{1}$$

with

$$\mu = \frac{1}{\#(\mathcal{NZ})} \sum_{i \in \mathcal{NZ}} x_i,$$

$$\sigma = \frac{1}{\#(\mathcal{NZ})} \sqrt{\sum_{i \in \mathcal{NZ}} (x_i - \mu)^2}.$$

where the indexes of the non zeros values of the modality x is denoted by $\mathcal{NZ} = \#\{i \; ; \; x_i \neq 0\}$ and $\#$ denotes the cardinality. Note that the operators min and max are used here to ensure that each value of the normalized input x^{norm} lies in $[-1, 1]$.

3.5   Learning Step

We used Keras' built-in *Adam* optimizer, with a constant learning rate of $\alpha_0 = 10^{-4}$. The maximal number of epochs was set at 100 and we used an early stopping based on the validation loss with a patience equal to 5. In order to ensure that we preserved the best network weights, we used the checkpoint callback with the best weights restoration to True.

3.6   Loss Function

For this segmentation task, a voxel can belong to either one of two classes. One label for the tumor, and one for everything else. Knowing this, we can use binary cross-entropy loss at each stage of our cascade to calculate the difference between the network's prediction of the tumor, and the ground truth. We define the binary cross-entropy function BCE:

$$\mathrm{BCE} = -\frac{1}{N}\sum_{i=1}^{N}(y_i\ \log(\hat{y_i}) + (1 - y_i)\ \log(1 - \hat{y_i})) \tag{2}$$

3.7   Evaluation of the Model

Once the model is trained, we can predict an output X, and use the Dice function to check the similarity with the ground truth Y. A value $\epsilon > 0$ is added to avoid a division by zero error, it is set to a very small number as not to modify the accuracy of the Dice function. We recall the Dice formula (up to the added ϵ avoiding divisions by zero):

$$\mathrm{Dice} = \frac{2*|X|\cap|Y|}{|X| + |Y| + \epsilon}, \text{with } \epsilon = 10^{-6}. \tag{3}$$

The closer the Dice coefficient is to 1, the more accurate the prediction is.

4   Our Contributions

The main architectures that won the first places in the BraTS MICCAI challenge in 2020 [1] were all based on U-Net models [9,15,17].

Having noticed this, we decided that it would be interesting to test variations of U-Net networks in order to find the network that is best suited for the task of brain tumor segmentation. Some of these networks, however, have not yet been implemented in Python, so we took it upon ourselves to implement some of these networks. For example, we designed and implemented an algorithm[1] capable of generating a U-Net++ network of size L, as its size can vary.

The main difference between Wang. G *et al.* [19] and our approach is that here we consider at each step the *optimal* network in a set of networks which will be described in Subsect. 4.2.

4.1   Data Analysis

In an effort to understand the data that was provided to us by the MICCAI BraTS challenge, we took it upon ourselves to compute the histogram of the cardinality of non-zero voxels in each patient's volume (we used the FLAIR modality as a reference). For the sake of clarity, we ordered these cardinalities in an increasing manner. We found that there was a sizeable amount of corrupted data, with patients either lacking in voxels, or having an over abundance of voxels in their volumes. We applied this analysis on the entirety of the 1251 patients, as well as the 219 patients in the validation data.

---

[1] https://github.com/sudomane/unetpp/blob/main/unetpp/unetpp.py.

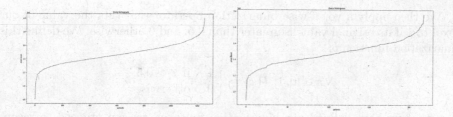

Fig. 2. Brains volumes distributions of training (left) and validation (right) patients

As expected, the distribution of the validation data was the same as the training data, as depicted on Fig. 2. However we were not able to define a threshold corresponding to the minimal size of the brain volume ensuring that data is not "corrupted".

4.2   Proposing a New Cascade of Neural Networks

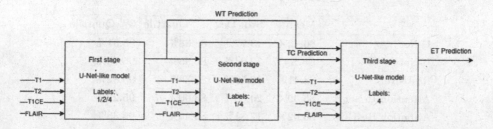

Fig. 3. Flow of data in a cascade model with 3 networks

The idea in this challenge is to build a cascaded model implementing three different U-Net-like networks with sigmoidal outputs (so that each output remains between 0 and 1). Each step of the cascade corresponds to the U-Net-like model with the best accuracy. The accuracy is evaluated with the Dice function in Eq. 3 defined earlier. Ultimately, the cascade will be composed of nothing but the most accurate networks at each step (see Fig. 5 and Fig. 3).

The training procedure is carried out in four steps: one for each network fed with the predictions of the previous ones, and a fourth step to combine the outputs of each networks. Let us define Ξ_k as the function corresponding to the kth network, we obtain the following formulas:

$$\widetilde{WT} = \Xi_1(FLAIR, T1, T1CE, T2),$$
$$\widetilde{TC} = \Xi_2(FLAIR, T1, T1CE, T2, \widetilde{WT}),$$
$$\widetilde{ET} = \Xi_3(FLAIR, T1, T1CE, T2, \widetilde{WT}, \widetilde{TC}).$$

We then apply a voxel-wise binarization operator that sets the value of our voxel to 1 if its original value is greater than 0.5, and 0 otherwise. We define this binarization function b:

$$\forall x \in [0,1], b(x) = \begin{cases} 1 & \text{if } x > 0.5 \\ 0 & \text{otherwise} \end{cases}$$

Now that we have defined our binarization function, we can proceed to reconstruct the 3D volume of our prediction by using the output from each stage of our cascade. Let us establish the formula to reconstruct the prediction volume:

$$4*b(\widetilde{ET})*b(\widetilde{TC})*b(\widetilde{WT})+2*(1-b(\widetilde{TC}))*b(\widetilde{WT})+(1-b(\widetilde{ET}))*b(\widetilde{TC})*b(\widetilde{WT}).$$

5   Results

5.1   Scores on Training Data Set

Table 1. WT Dice results

	Mean	Std. Dev	1st Quartile	3rd Quartile
U-Net	86.42%	13.77%	82.68%	95.51%
U-Net++	**88.54%**	12.04%	86.95%	95.75%
ResU-Net	88.41%	12.59%	87.38%	95.82%
Attention U-Net	83.39%	20.88%	83.00%	95.22%
Attention ResU-Net	86.02%	17.81%	85.46%	95.38%

Table 2. TC Dice results

	Mean	Std. Dev	1st Quartile	3rd Quartile
U-Net	**89.26%**	17.26%	89.97%	97.54%
U-Net++	84.31%	21.35%	84.11%	95.42%
ResU-Net	82.97%	24.20%	81.22%	96.71%
Attention U-Net	81.14%	26.83%	82.42%	96.01%
Attention ResU-Net	85.10%	23.86%	88.13%	97.07%

Table 3. ET Dice results

	Mean	Std. Dev	1st Quartile	3rd Quartile
U-Net	88.19%	20.84%	90.94%	97.44%
U-Net++	80.57%	23.67%	79.12%	93.71%
ResU-Net	89.59%	20.14%	92.39%	98.09%
Attention U-Net	89.62%	20.44%	91.70%	98.36%
Attention ResU-Net	**89.94%**	20.61%	93.00%	98.37%

Note: The U-Net++ model was tested in single output mode.

After having run the predictions on the entirety of the train data set, we collected the information pertaining to the accuracy of the models given to us by the Dice evaluation (see Tables 1, 2, 3).

5.2 Scores on Validation Data

See Table 4.

Table 4. Dice and HD95 of our optimal model.

Dice	WT (Mean)	WT (Std)	TC (Mean)	TC (Std)	ET (Mean)	ET (Std)
	88.68%	12.43%	80.67%	25.07%	75.35%	27.67%
HD95	WT (Mean)	WT (Std)	TC (Mean)	TC (Std)	ET (Mean)	ET (Std)
	11.54	21.23	17.79	56.83	27.79	87.84

6 Discussion

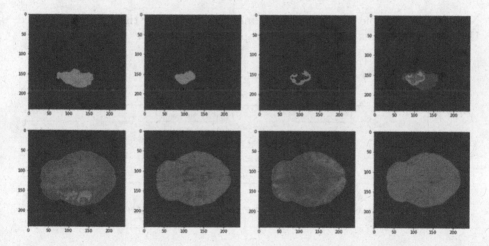

Fig. 4. Prediction on validation data with the complete cascade implementation. In the top row, from left to right: WT prediction, TC prediction, ET prediction, complete prediction.

At the first step (WT), we notice that the network with the best results is the U-Net++, with a mean Dice score of 88.54%. Then at the second step (TC), we notice that the network with the best results is a standard U-Net, with a mean Dice score of 89.26%. Finally, at the third step (ET), we notice that the network with the best results is the Attention ResU-Net, with a mean dice score of 89.94%.

The label for the extended tumor (ET) has proven to be the most difficult to segment, as it is defined with minute detail. However, the Attention ResU-Net performs the best for this label (see Table 3). This can be due to the mechanisms present in the model, such as the use of the attention mechanism, as well as residual blocks which help in eliminating the vanishing gradient problem [11]. Because of its inherent advantages, the Attention ResU-Net seems to be the best suited for the task of segmenting fine detail in MRI scans.

In summary, a cascade model made up of a U-Net++ for the first step, a standard U-Net for the second step, and an Attention ResU-Net for the third step, would provide us with the best results (see Fig. 4).

7   Proposed Solution

Based on the benchmark results, we have chosen the following networks for each region:

– Whole Tumor: U-Net++ [20]
– Tumor Core: U-Net [16]
– Enhanced Tumor: Attention ResU-Net [11]

Now that we are able to determine the final architecture for the optimal cascaded U-Net model, here is a graph of the proposed architecture.

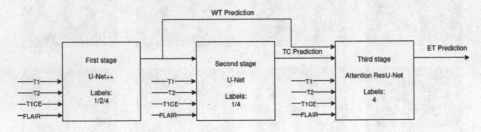

Fig. 5. Optimal cascade with a U-Net++, U-Net and an Attention ResU-Net

8   Final Results

Here are the results on the test data set that MICCAI uses to evaluate the model (Tables 5, 6 and 7).

Table 5. Results on African Data

	Dice ET	Dice TC	Dice WT	Hausdorff ET	Hausdorff TC	Hausdorff WT
Mean	0.8440	0.8943	0.9370	3.324	6.034	4.280
Std	0.1450	0.1148	0.0615	2.911	8.454	6.695
Median	0.9042	0.9286	0.9540	2.911	4	2.236
1st quartile	0.8553	0.8874	0.9368	1.414	1.414	1.414
3rd quartile	0.9283	0.9623	0.9656	3.741	6.034	3.162

Table 6. Testing cohort

	Dice ET	Dice TC	Dice WT	Hausdorff ET	Hausdorff TC	Hausdorff WT
Mean	0.7938	0.8227	0.8803	22.19	21.70	11.69
Std	0.2449	0.2628	0.1357	80.33	71.84	19.56
Median	0.8781	0.9268	0.9250	1.414	3	3.741
1st quartile	0.7912	0.8438	0.8686	1	1.414	2
3rd quartile	0.9316	0.9619	0.9514	3	8.124	8.747

Table 7. Results on Pediatric Data

	Dice TC	Dice WT	Hausdorff TC	Hausdorff WT
Mean	0.2288	0.6657	154.97	30.47
Std	0.3275	0.2725	167.89	51.04
Median	0	0.7592	53.074	14.90
1st quartile	0	0.5662	10.998	5.692
3rd quartile	0.4429	0.8669	373.12	34.79

9 Conclusion

9.1 Future Works

Despite the scores we obtained, we strongly believe in the potential of the three-stage cascade method for the BraTS challenge. Each network of the cascade being able to develop specific features devoted to segmenting a specific sub-region of the glioblastoma. Moreover, each network providing additional information to the subsequent stages in the cascade, causing a guiding effect for each network.

In the future, we would like to implement and test additional features in our three-stage cascaded network. Here are some of the features we would like to test:

- Implement and benchmark the nn-U-Net [10].
- Benchmark with 851 patient instead of 200.
- Improve the overall quality of the training data set by preprocessing data.
- Implement cross-validation.

9.2 Summary

In this paper, we proposed a three-stage cascaded network devoted to brain tumor segmentation. The U-Net-like network employed at each step of the cascade was determined through benchmarking several U-Net variants in order to determine which network performs the best at a certain stage. Moreover, our 2.5D method allows us to optimize the usage of the GPU's VRAM, with minimal performance loss.

Acknowledgements. We would like to thank Guy Fournier, Bastien Verdebout, Kevin Amil and Christina De Azevedo of OVHcloud, for providing us with the infrastructure and resources that have proven to be detrimental to our success. Without their support, we likely would not have succeeded in our task.

We would also like to thank Arnaud Renard and his team for granting us access to the ROMEO Supercomputer of the University of Reims.

Moreover, we would like to thank Philippe Dewost, Christian Chabrerie, and Patrick DeMichel for supporting us throughout the entirety of this project.

References

1. Baid, U., et al.: The RSNA-ASNR-MICCAI BraTS 2021 benchmark on brain tumor segmentation and radiogenomic classification. arXiv.org (2021). https://arxiv.org/abs/2107.02314
2. Bakas, S., et al.: Advancing the cancer genome atlas glioma MRI collections with expert segmentation labels and radiomic features. Nat. Sci. Data **4**, 1–13 (2017). https://doi.org/10.1038/sdata.2017.117
3. Bakas, S., et al.: Segmentation labels and radiomic features for the pre-operative scans of the TCGA-LGG collection (2017). https://doi.org/10.7937/K9/TCIA.2017.GJQ7R0EF
4. Bakas, S., et al.: Segmentation labels and radiomic features for the pre-operative scans of the TCGA-GBM collection (2017). https://doi.org/10.7937/K9/TCIA.2017.KLXWJJ1Q
5. Diakogiannis, F., Waldner, F., Caccetta, P., Wu, C.: Resunet-a: a deep learning framework for semantic segmentation of remotely sensed data. ISPRS J. Photogram. Remote Sens. **16**, 94–114 (2020). https://doi.org/10.1016/j.isprsjprs.2020.01.013
6. Diakogiannis, F.I., Waldner, F., Caccetta, P., Wu, C.: Resunet-a: a deep learning framework for semantic segmentation of remotely sensed data (2020). https://arxiv.org/abs/1904.00592
7. Guo, Y., Peng, Y.: BSCN: bidirectional symmetric cascade network for retinal vessel segmentation. BMC Med. Imaging **20**(1), 1–22 (2020). https://bmcmedimaging.biomedcentral.com/articles/10.1186/s12880-020-0412-7
8. Lee, C.Y., Xie, S., Gallagher, P., Zhang, Z., Tu, Z.: Deeply-supervised nets (2014). https://doi.org/10.48550/ARXIV.1409.5185. https://arxiv.org/abs/1409.5185
9. Luu, H.M., Park, S.H.: Extending nn-UNet for brain tumor segmentation (2021). https://arxiv.org/abs/2112.04653
10. Luu, H.M., Park, S.H.: Extending nn-UNet for brain tumor segmentation. In: Crimi, A., Bakas, S. (eds.) BrainLes 2021. LNCS, vol. 12963, pp. 173–186. Springer, Cham (2022). https://doi.org/10.1007/978-3-031-09002-8_16

11. Maji, D., Sigedar, P., Singh, M.: Attention res-UNet with guided decoder for semantic segmentation of brain tumors. Biomed. Signal Process. Control **71**, 103077 (2022). https://doi.org/10.1016/j.bspc.2021.103077. https://www.sciencedirect.com/science/article/pii/S1746809421006741

12. Wilson, C.B., Prados, M.D.: Surgery for low-grade glioma: rationale for early intervention. https://pubmed.ncbi.nlm.nih.gov/8846605/

13. Menze, B.H., et al.: The multimodal brain tumor image segmentation benchmark (BRATS). IEEE Trans. Med. Imaging **34**(10), 1993–2024 (2015). https://doi.org/10.1109/TMI.2014.2377694

14. Oktay, O., et al.: Attention u-net: learning where to look for the pancreas (2018). https://doi.org/10.48550/ARXIV.1804.03999. https://arxiv.org/abs/1804.03999

15. Peiris, H., Chen, Z., Egan, G., Harandi, M.: Reciprocal adversarial learning for brain tumor segmentation: a solution to brats challenge 2021 segmentation task (2022). https://arxiv.org/abs/2201.03777

16. Ronneberger, O., Fischer, P., Brox, T.: U-net: convolutional networks for biomedical image segmentation (2015). https://arxiv.org/abs/1505.04597

17. Siddiquee, M.M.R., Myronenko, A.: Redundancy reduction in semantic segmentation of 3D brain tumor MRIs (2021). https://arxiv.org/abs/2111.00742

18. Vu, M.H., Nyholm, T., Löfstedt, T.: TuNet: end-to-end hierarchical brain tumor segmentation using cascaded networks. In: Crimi, A., Bakas, S. (eds.) BrainLes 2019. LNCS, vol. 11992, pp. 174–186. Springer, Cham (2020). https://doi.org/10.1007/978-3-030-46640-4_17

19. Wang, G., Li, W., Ourselin, S., Vercauteren, T.: Automatic brain tumor segmentation using cascaded anisotropic convolutional neural networks. In: Crimi, A., Bakas, S., Kuijf, H., Menze, B., Reyes, M. (eds.) BrainLes 2017. LNCS, vol. 10670, pp. 178–190. Springer, Cham (2018). https://doi.org/10.1007/978-3-319-75238-9_16. https://arxiv.org/pdf/1709.00382.pdf

20. Zhou, Z., Siddiquee, M.M.R., Tajbakhsh, N., Liang, J.: UNet++: a nested U-Net architecture for medical image segmentation (2018). https://doi.org/10.48550/ARXIV.1807.10165. https://arxiv.org/abs/1807.10165

21. Zhou, Z., Siddiquee, M.M.R., Tajbakhsh, N., Liang, J.: UNet++: redesigning skip connections to exploit multiscale features in image segmentation (2020). https://arxiv.org/abs/1912.05074

Tuning U-Net for Brain Tumor Segmentation

Michał Futrega(✉), Michał Marcinkiewicz(✉), and Pablo Ribalta(✉)

NVIDIA, Santa Clara, CA 95051, USA
{mfutrega,michalm,pribalta}@nvidia.com

Abstract. We propose a solution for BraTS22 challenge that builds on top of our previous submission—Optimized U-Net method. This year we focused on improving the model architecture and training schedule. The proposed method further improves scores on both our internal cross validation and challenge validation data. The validation mean dice scores are: ET 0.8381, TC 0.8802, WT 0.9292, and mean Hausdorff95: ET 14.460, TC 5.840, WT 3.594.

Keywords: U-Net · Brain Tumor Segmentation · Deep Learning · MRI

1 Introduction

Gliomas are one of the most common kind of brain tumors [1] that affect humans. Their accurate segmentation is a difficult task due to their variable shape represented in multi-modal magnetic resonance imaging (MRI). Manual segmentation of such brain tumors is time-consuming, prone to human error, has to be performed by a trained medical expert. Moreover, the manual process lacks consistency and reproducibility, which is detrimental to the results and can result in incorrect diagnosis and treatment. An automatic solution could potentially solve many of the most persistent issues with the manual work—it could greatly accelerate the segmentation process, pre-selecting scans that require immediate attention for a final evaluation. Also, since most of the automatic solutions are reproducible, an automatic segmentation of given scans would always yield identical results, free from variance and human error.

The rapid progress in development of deep learning (DL) algorithms shows great potential for application of deep neural networks (DNNs) in computer-aided automatic or semi-automatic methods for medical data analysis. The drastic improvements of convolutional neural networks (CNNs) resulted in models being able to approach or surpass the human level performance in plethora of applications, such as image classification [2] or microscope image segmentation [3], among many others. DL-based models are great candidates for brain tumor segmentation, as long as sufficient amount of training data is supplied. The Brain Tumor Segmentation Challenge (BraTS) provides a large, high-quality dataset consisting of multi-modal MRI brain scans with corresponding segmentation masks [4–8].

S. Bakas et al. (Eds.): BrainLes 2022, LNCS 13769, pp. 162–173, 2023.
https://doi.org/10.1007/978-3-031-33842-7_14

Since its publication, U-Net [9] has become one of the most widely used models for medical image segmentation, based on the number of citations. In the recent BraTS editions, U-Net-based models were very successful at the BraTS challenge, usually claiming the top spots. For instance, in 2018, Myronenko *et al.,* modified a U-Net model by adding a variational autoencoder branch for regularization [10]. In 2019, Jiang *et al.,* employed a two-stage U-Net pipeline to segment the substructures of brain tumors from coarse to fine [11]. In 2020, Isensee *et al.,* applied the nnU-Net framework [12] with specific BraTS designed modifications regarding data post-processing, region-based training, data augmentation, and minor modifications to the nnU-Net pipeline [13]. In 2021, our submission based on U-Net (Futrega *et al.* [14]) won the validation phase and took the third place during the test phase.

Those achievements prove that U-Net-based architectures consistently deliver excellent performance on medical segmentation tasks, such as brain tumor segmentation, becoming a de facto a standard baseline model to compare new solution against. Since the U-Net is conceptually a simple network design, consisting almost exclusively of convolutional layers (and optionally normalization layers), it is straightforward to add various modifications that are aligned with new discoveries in Deep Learning and Computer Vision. For instance, a plethora of U-Net variants has been designed, such as: Attention U-Net [15] incorporating attention blocks, Residual U-Net [16] incorporating blocks with residual connections, Dense U-Net [17] exploiting dense connections between layers, Inception U-Net [18] using inception blocks, U-Net++ [19] using multiscale features in its skip-connections, SegResNetVAE [10] joining a variational autoencoder for regularization, or UNETR [20] which treats U-Net as a visual transformer, just to name a few. Also, there were works that focused less on architecture and more on the way the data flows through the model, for example via an addition of deep-supervision [21] or drop-block [22].

In our previous submission [14], we selected an optimal U-Net variant/extension and training schedule for the BraTS21 challenge via ablation studies. We tested U-Net [9], Attention U-Net [15], Residual U-Net [16], SegResNetVAE [10] and UNETR [20] for U-Net variants, and experimented with Deep Supervision [21], Drop-Block [22]. Additionally, we investigated different loss functions (combinations of Cross Entropy, Focal, and Dice), and we optimized our model by increasing the encoder depth, adding one-hot-encoding channel for the foreground voxels to the input data, and increasing the number of convolutional filters.

In this paper, we continue to investigate the possible U-Net modifications to push its performance further. We focused on improving model architecture by modifying the U-Net convolutional block. The new block is having the following structure: instance normalization, 3D convolution, ReLU vs 3D Convolution, instance normalization, leaky ReLU. Furthermore, we increased the number of filters, and prepared a more robust final solution by building the ensemble from the best models trained on 10-fold cross validation and used test time augmentation for evaluation.

2 Method

2.1 Data

The training data for the BraTS challenge [4–8] is the same as in 2021: a set of 1,251 brain MRI scans along with segmentation annotations (masks) of regions of interest—tumor regions. Each data sample encompasses four modalities: native (T1), post-contrast T1-weighted (T1Gd), T2-weighted (T2), and T2 Fluid Attenuated Inversion Recovery (T2-FLAIR). Because the samples were acquired with different clinical protocols and various scanners from multiple data-contributing institutions, the $240 \times 240 \times 155$ voxel 3D volumes were skull-stripped and co-registered to $1\,mm^3$ isotropic resolution. All volumes are provided as NIfTI files [23].

Segmentation masks were annotated manually by one to four experts. All annotations consist of three different tumor classes: the GD-enhancing tumor (ET), the peritumoral edematous (ED), and the necrotic tumor core (NCR). Voxels that are not labeled as part of the tumor can be considered as (fourth) background class.

There were two additional subsets of data: A total of 219 additional validation samples without associated segmentation masks were released. The predictions

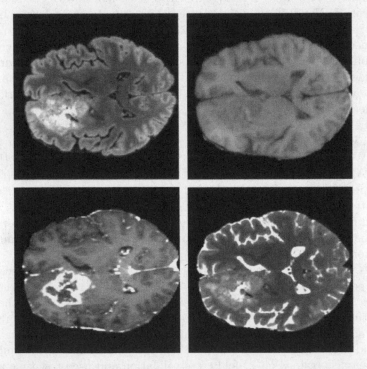

Fig. 1. Example, with ID 00000 from the BraTS21 training dataset. Each panel presents a different modality. From top left to bottom right: FLAIR, T1, T1Gd T2.

on the validations samples were to be evaluated on an online platform. For the test phase, an additional cohort of 530 cases was used by the organizers to run the evaluation on (Fig. 1).

2.2   Data Pre-processing

The goal of data pre-processing is to prepare a dataset for training and inference. In order to facilitate the training process, the pre-processed dataset should have standardized properties, for example, normalized voxel intensity values, removed redundant parts like boundary background voxels or encoded new features. We applied the following pre-processing steps:

1. **Modalities stacking:** For each example, its modalities are given as a separate files. In order to create a single volume per example we stacked all four modalities such that each example has a shape $(4, 240, 240, 155)$ (input tensor is in the (C, H, W, D) layout, where C-channels, H-height, W-width and D-depth)
2. **Background cropping:** To make training the neural network faster, we removed redundant background voxels (with voxel value zero) on the borders of each volume. Those voxels do not provide any meaningful information and can be ignored by the neural network.
3. **Normalizing voxel values:** To standardize the voxel values, all volumes were normalized by first subtracting its mean and then divided by the standard deviation. The background voxels were not normalized so that their value remained at zero.
4. **Foreground one hot encoding:** To distinguish between the background voxels and normalized voxels which have values close to zero, an additional input channel was created with one-hot encoding for foreground voxels and stacked with the input data, making channel dimension equal to 5.

2.3   Data Augmentation

Data augmentation is a technique that alleviates the overfitting problem by artificially extending a dataset during the training phase. To make our method more robust, we used a similar augmentation techniques as in our last paper [14]. The following data augmentations were used during training phase:

1. **Biased crop:** From the input volume, a patch of dimensions $(5, 128, 128, 128)$ was randomly cropped. Additionally, with probability of 0.4 the patch selected via random biased crop is guaranteed that some foreground voxels (with positive class in the ground truth) are present in the cropped region.
2. **Flips:** With probability of 0.5, for each x, y, z axis independently, volume was flipped along that axis.
3. **Gaussian Noise:** With probability of 0.15, random Gaussian noise with mean zero and standard deviation sampled uniformly from $(0, 0.33)$ is sampled for each voxel and added to the input volume.

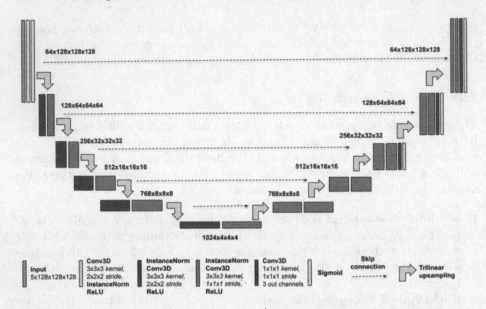

Fig. 2. U-Net architecture. The encoder is transforming the input by reducing its spatial dimensions, and then the decoder is upsampling it back to the original input shape. Additional two output heads are used for deep supervision loss (green bars). (Color figure online)

4. **Gaussian Blur:** With probability of 0.15, Gaussian blurring with standard deviation of the Gaussian Kernel sampled uniformly from $(0.5, 1.5)$ is applied to the input volume.
5. **Brightness:** With probability of 0.15, a random value is sampled uniformly from $(0.7, 1.3)$ and then input volume voxels are multiplied by it.

2.4   Model Architecture

We selected U-Net [9] architecture (shown in the Fig. 2) as our model. U-Net is characterized by a symmetric U-shape, and can be divided into two parts, i.e., encoder and decoder. The first part is the contracting path (encoder) which is transforming the input volume into a smaller spatially but higher dimensional space. The contracting path is followed by a decoder—an expanding path that upsamples the data to the original input shape. Skip connections between corresponding levels in encoder and decoder are added to preserve more information that might be lost by downsampling. The output of a given encoder block is concatenated to the input to the corresponding decoder block.

The encoder has a modular structure consisting of repeating convolution blocks. Encoding starts with processing the input of shape $5 \times 128 \times 128 \times 128$ with two convolutional blocks, each build of 3D convolution with kernel size $3 \times 3 \times 3$ and $1 \times 1 \times 1$ stride, instance normalization and ReLU activation. Then contracting blocks start processing the feature map (output from the input block) with two convolutional blocks that are organized in the following transformation: instance normalization, 3D convolution with $3 \times 3 \times 3$ kernel size, ReLU activation. The difference between the first and second block is the stride used in 3D convolution. The first block (dark blue on the Fig. 2) is using stride $2 \times 2 \times 2$ to reduce the spatial dimensions by a factor of two, while the second one (light blue on the Fig. 2) is using stride $1 \times 1 \times 1$ to further refine the feature map.

After the spatial dimensions of the feature map is transformed to the size of $4 \times 4 \times 4$, decoding part commences. The decoder also has a modular structure, but its goal is to decode a spatially small but high dimensional input representation from the encoder into a spatially large but low dimensional one by expanding the spatial dimensions back to the original one, i.e., $128 \times 128 \times 128$. The convolutional block in the decoder is first upsampling the spatial dimension by trilinear interpolation to match feature map dimension from the equivalent encoder level (see skip connections on the Fig. 2) and concatenates both features along the channel dimension. Then it transforms concatenated feature maps by two repeated blocks of: instance normalization, 3D convolution with $3 \times 3 \times 3$ kernel and $1 \times 1 \times 1$ stride and ReLU activation.

In order to prepare a final prediction from the decoder output, we used a 3D convolution with $1 \times 1 \times 1$ both kernel and stride to make feature map channels equal to 3 and apply a sigmoid activation at the very end. Additionally, we used deep-supervision (Subsect. 2.5) for loss computation on decoder outputs with a lower resolution.

2.5   Loss Function

As the *nnU-Net for Brain Tumor Segmentation* [13] paper states, the classes present in the annotations were converted into three partially overlapping regions: whole tumor (WT) representing classes 1, 2, 4; tumor core (TC) representing classes 1, 4; and enhancing tumor (ET) representing the class 4. The leaderboard score is computed based on those overlapping regions instead of classes present in the labels. We wanted the function that we tried to optimize to reflect as closely as possible the scoring function, therefore we constructed the loss function based on classes used for ranking calculation. We set the output feature map to have three channels (one per class) which at the very end are transformed via the sigmoid activation, generally used for multi-label classification.

Each region was optimized separately with a sum of binary cross-entropy and the Dice loss [24]. For Dice loss, its batched variant was used, i.e., Dice loss was computed over all samples in the batch instead of averaging the Dice loss over each sample separately.

Deep Supervision [21]. Similarly as in our previous submission [14], we added two additional output heads for decoder output shapes $(64, 64, 64)$ and $(32, 32, 32)$ that are used to enable deep supervision—a technique that helps with a better gradient flow by computing loss function on different decoder levels. To compute the deep supervision loss, labels were first downsampled to the corresponding output shape with nearest neighbor interpolation. For labels y_i and predictions p_i for $i = 1, 2, 3$, where $i = 1$ corresponds to the last output head, $i = 2$ is the output head on the penultimate decoder level and $i = 3$ is before the penultimate, the final loss function is computed as follows:

$$\mathcal{L}(y_1, y_2, y_3, p_1, p_2, p_3) = \mathcal{L}(y_1, p_1) + \frac{1}{2}\mathcal{L}(y_2, p_2) + \frac{1}{4}\mathcal{L}(y_3, p_3). \tag{1}$$

2.6   Inference

Because our pre-processing results in cropping out the background voxels around the skull, the input volumes can have arbitrary size, instead of the fixed patch size $(128, 128, 128)$ used during the training phase. Thus, we used a sliding window inference[1], where the window has the same size as the training patch, i.e., $(128, 128, 128)$ and adjacent windows overlap by half the size of a patch. The predictions on the overlapping regions are then averaged with Gaussian importance weighting, such that the weights of the center voxels have higher importance, as in the original nnU-Net paper [12].

One of the known ways to improve robustness of predictions is to apply test time augmentations. During inference, we have created eight versions of the input volume, such that each version corresponds to one of eight possible flips along the x, y, z axis combination. Then we run inference for each version of the input volume and transform the predictions back to the original input volume orientation by applying the same flips to predictions as were used for the input volume. Finally, the probabilities from all predictions were averaged.

The output map from the network consists of three channels with the probabilities for each of three overlapping regions: ET, TC, WT. To find the optimal thresholds, we run grid search to find the optimal cutoff for each class. We found the following strategy as the optimal one: if the WT probability for a given voxel is less than 0.45 then its class is set to 0 (background), otherwise if the probability for TC is less than 0.35 the voxel class is 2 (ED), and finally if the probability for ET is less than 0.375 voxel has class 1 (NCR), or otherwise 4 (ET).

3   Results

3.1   Implementation

Our solution is written in PyTorch [25] and extends NVIDIA's implementation of the nnU-Net with publicly available code on the NVIDIA Deep Learning Examples GitHub repository[2]. Proposed solution is using the NVIDIA NGC PyTorch 22.05 Docker container[3] which allows for the full encapsulation of dependencies, reproducible runs, as well as easy deployment on any system. All training and

---

[1] MONAI sliding window implementation was used.

[2] https://github.com/NVIDIA/DeepLearningExamples/tree/master/PyTorch/Segmentation/nnUNet.

[3] https://ngc.nvidia.com/catalog/containers/nvidia:pytorch.

inference runs were performed with use of Mixed Precision [26], which speeds-up the model and reduces the GPU memory consumption. Experiments were run on NVIDIA DGX A100 (8×A100 80 GB) system.[4]

3.2 Training Schedule

Each experiment was trained for 600 epochs using the AdamW optimizer [27] with three different learning rates: 0.0005, 0.0007, 0.0009 and a weight decay equal to 0.0001. Additionally, during the first 1000 steps, we used a linear warm-up of the learning rate, starting from 0 and increasing it to the target value, and then it was decreased with a cosine annealing scheduler [28]. The weights for 3D convolutions were initialized with Kaiming initialization [29].

3.3 Experiments

For model evaluation, we used 5-fold cross validation and compared the average of the highest Dice score reached on each of the 5-folds. However, for the final submission, we have retrained the best configuration on 10-folds cross valida-tion. The evaluation on the validation set was run after every epoch. For each fold, we have stored the two checkpoints with the highest mean Dice score on the validation set reached during the training phase. Then during the inference phase, we ensembled the predictions from stored checkpoints by averaging the probabilities (Table 1).

Table 1. Averaged Dice scores of ET, TC, WT classes from 5-fold cross validation for Optimized U-Net (Opt U-Net) used for 2021 submission and Tuned U-Net used in 2022 edition.

5-fold CV	Optimized U-Net	Tuned U-Net
Fold 0	0.9118	**0.9148**
Fold 1	0.9141	**0.9150**
Fold 2	0.9176	**0.9217**
Fold 3	0.9268	**0.9274**
Fold 4	0.9076	**0.9105**
Mean Dice	0.9156	**0.9179**

Next, to make our method more robust, we trained it on a 10-fold cross vali-dation. By increasing the number of folds, the model has more data for training and as a result should have better accuracy. After increasing the number of folds, the mean Dice score has moved from 0.9179 to 0.9202 (Fig. 3 and Table 2).

---

[4] https://www.nvidia.com/en-us/data-center/a100.

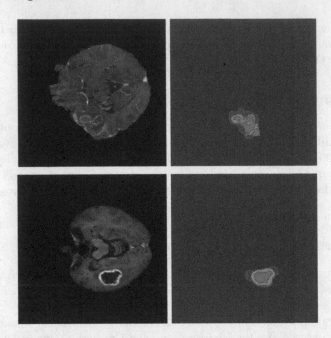

Fig. 3. Predictions from the challenge validation dataset. On the left column input image is visualized while on the right model predictions where the meaning of colors is the following: purple - background, blue - NCR, turquoise - ED, yellow - ET. (Color figure online)

Table 2. Dice scores for ET, TC, WT classes from 10-fold cross validation. Table shows result before (left) post-processing and after (right)

10-fold CV	ET	TC	WT	ETpost	TCpost	WTpost
Fold 0	0.9064	0.9373	0.9454	0.9068	0.9380	0.9455
Fold 1	0.8626	0.9203	0.9352	0.8630	0.9204	0.9358
Fold 2	0.8789	0.9242	0.9396	0.8791	0.9246	0.9397
Fold 3	0.9033	0.9307	0.9271	0.9035	0.9308	0.9268
Fold 4	0.8902	0.9233	0.9405	0.9233	0.9233	0.9427
Fold 5	0.9051	0.9405	0.9394	0.9054	0.9405	0.9394
Fold 6	0.9131	0.9354	0.9355	0.9132	0.9358	0.9352
Fold 7	0.9174	0.9341	0.9452	0.9177	0.9343	0.9456
Fold 8	0.8892	0.9231	0.9324	0.8896	0.9235	0.9325
Fold 9	0.8712	0.9152	0.9434	0.8713	0.9158	0.9433
Mean	0.8937	0.9284	0.9386	0.8940	0.9287	0.9386

Finally, we experimented with a post-processing strategy. It is known from previous BraTS editions that removing small regions with enhanced tumor can be beneficial to the final score. It is so because if there is no enhancing tumor in the label, then the Dice score for zero false positive prediction is 1, and 0 otherwise. The best strategy we found for our 10-fold cross-validation is the following: find ET connected components, for components smaller than 16 voxels with mean probability smaller than 0.9, replace their class to NCR, next if there is overall less than 4 voxels with ET and their mean probability is smaller than 0.9 replace all ET voxels to NCR. Additionally, we have experimented with optimal thresholds for converting probabilities for each of three overlapping regions: ET, TC, WT. To find the optimal thresholds, we run grid search to find the optimal cutoff for each class. We found the following strategy as the optimal one: if the WT probability for a given voxel is less than 0.45 then its class is set to 0 (background), otherwise if the probability for TC is less than 0.35 the voxel class is 2 (ED), and finally if the probability for ET is less than 0.375 voxel has class 1 (NCR), or otherwise 4 (ET).

4   Conclusions

In this work, we further optimized our submission from the previous year. We demonstrated that by modifying the U-Net architecture (using instance normalization before convolution, and more convolutional filters) and training schedule (training with test-time augmentations and increasing cross validation from 5 to 10 folds) we increased our cross validation score from 0.9156 to 0.9204.

References

1. Goodenberger, M.L., Jenkins, R.B.: Genetics of adult glioma. Cancer Genet. **205**(12), 613–621 (2012). https://doi.org/10.1016/j.cancergen.2012.10.009
2. Russakovsky, O., et al.: ImageNet large scale visual recognition challenge. Int. J. Comput. Vis. **115**(3), 211–252 (2015). https://doi.org/10.1007/s11263-015-0816-y
3. Zeng, T., Wu, B., Ji, S.: DeepEM3D: approaching human-level performance on 3D anisotropic EM image segmentation. Bioinformatics **33**(16), 2555–2562 (2017). https://doi.org/10.1093/bioinformatics/btx188
4. Baid, U., et al.: The RSNA-ASNR-MICCAI BraTS 2021 benchmark on brain tumor segmentation and radiogenomic classification (2021)
5. Menze, B.H., Jakab, A., Bauer, S., Kalpathy-Cramer, J., Farahani, K., Kirby, J., et al.: The multimodal brain tumor image segmentation benchmark (BRATS). IEEE Trans. Med. Imaging **34**(10), 1993–2024 (2015). https://doi.org/10.1109/TMI.2014.2377694
6. Bakas, S., Akbari, H., Sotiras, A., Bilello, M., Rozycki, M., Kirby, J., et al.: Advancing the cancer genome atlas glioma MRI collections with expert segmentation labels and radiomic features. Sci. Data **4** (2017). https://doi.org/10.1038/sdata.2017.117
7. Bakas, S., Akbari, H., Sotiras, A., Bilello, M., Rozycki, M., Kirby, J., et al.: Segmentation labels and radiomic features for the pre-operative scans of the TCGA-GBM collection, July 2017. https://doi.org/10.7937/K9/TCIA.2017.KLXWJJ1Q
8. Bakas, S., Akbari, H., Sotiras, A., Bilello, M., Rozycki, M., Kirby, J., et al.: Segmentation labels and radiomic features for the pre-operative scans of the TCGA-GBM collection, July 2017. https://doi.org/10.7937/K9/TCIA.2017.GJQ7R0EF

9. Ronneberger, O., Fischer, P., Brox, T.: U-Net: convolutional networks for biomedical image segmentation. In: Navab, N., Hornegger, J., Wells, W.M., Frangi, A.F. (eds.) MICCAI 2015. LNCS, vol. 9351, pp. 234–241. Springer, Cham (2015). https://doi.org/10.1007/978-3-319-24574-4_28

10. Myronenko, A.: 3D MRI brain tumor segmentation using autoencoder regularization. In: Crimi, A., Bakas, S., Kuijf, H., Keyvan, F., Reyes, M., van Walsum, T. (eds.) BrainLes 2018. LNCS, vol. 11384, pp. 311–320. Springer, Cham (2019). https://doi.org/10.1007/978-3-030-11726-9_28

11. Jiang, Z., Ding, C., Liu, M., Tao, D.: Two-stage cascaded U-Net: 1st place solution to BraTS challenge 2019 segmentation task. In: Crimi, A., Bakas, S. (eds.) BrainLes 2019. LNCS, vol. 11992, pp. 231–241. Springer, Cham (2020). https://doi.org/10.1007/978-3-030-46640-4_22

12. Isensee, F., Jäger, P.F., Kohl, S.A., Petersen, J., Maier-Hein, K.H.: nnU-Net: a self-configuring method for deep learning-based biomedical image segmentation. Nat. Methods **18**(2), 203–211 (2021)

13. Isensee, F., Jäger, P.F., Full, P.M., Vollmuth, P., Maier-Hein, K.H.: nnU-Net for brain tumor segmentation. In: Crimi, A., Bakas, S. (eds.) BrainLes 2020. LNCS, vol. 12659, pp. 118–132. Springer, Cham (2021). https://doi.org/10.1007/978-3-030-72087-2_11

14. Futrega, M., Milesi, A., Marcinkiewicz, M., Ribalta, P.: Optimized U-Net for brain tumor segmentation (2021). https://doi.org/10.48550/ARXIV.2110.03352. https://arxiv.org/abs/2110.03352

15. Oktay, O., et al.: Attention U-Net: learning where to look for the pancreas (2018)

16. He, K., Zhang, X., Ren, S., Sun, J.: Deep residual learning for image recognition (2015)

17. Huang, G., Liu, Z., van der Maaten, L., Weinberger, K.Q.: Densely connected convolutional networks (2016)

18. Szegedy, C., et al.: Deep residual learning for image recognition (2014)

19. Zhou, Z., Rahman Siddiquee, M.M., Tajbakhsh, N., Liang, J.: UNet++: a nested U-Net architecture for medical image segmentation. In: Stoyanov, D., et al. (eds.) DLMIA/ML-CDS -2018. LNCS, vol. 11045, pp. 3–11. Springer, Cham (2018). https://doi.org/10.1007/978-3-030-00889-5_1

20. Hatamizadeh, A., Yang, D., Roth, H., Xu, D.: UNETR: transformers for 3D medical image segmentation (2021)

21. Zhu, Q., Du, B., Turkbey, B., Choyke, P.L., Yan, P.: Deeply-supervised CNN for prostate segmentation (2017)

22. Ghiasi, G., Lin, T.Y., Le, Q.V.: DropBlock: a regularization method for convolutional networks (2018)

23. Cox, R., et al.: A (sort of) new image data format standard: NiFTI-1, vol. 22, January 2004

24. Milletari, F., Navab, N., Ahmadi, S.-A.: V-Net: fully convolutional neural networks for volumetric medical image segmentation. In: International Conference on 3D Vision (3DV) (2016)

25. Paszke, A., et al.: PyTorch: an imperative style, high-performance deep learning library. In: Wallach, H., Larochelle, H., Beygelzimer, A., d' Alché-Buc, F., Fox, E., Garnett, R. (eds.) Advances in Neural Information Processing Systems, vol. 32, pp. 8024–8035. Curran Associates, Inc. (2019). http://papers.neurips.cc/paper/9015-pytorch-an-imperative-style-high-performance-deep-learning-library.pdf

26. Micikevicius, P., et al.: Mixed precision training (2018)

27. Kingma, D.P., Ba, J.: Adam: a method for stochastic optimization (2017)

28. Loshchilov, I., Hutter, F.: SGDR: stochastic gradient descent with warm restarts (2017)
29. He, K., Zhang, X., Ren, S., Sun, J.: Delving deep into rectifiers: surpassing human-level performance on ImageNet classification (2015)
30. Antonelli, M., et al.: The medical segmentation decathlon. Nat. Commun. **13**, 4128 (2022)
31. NVIDIA nnU-Net implementation. https://github.com/NVIDIA/DeepLearning Examples/tree/master/PyTorch/Segmentation/nnUNet. Accessed 30 Sept 2021
32. Dosovitskiy, A., et al.: An image is worth 16×16 words: transformers for image recognition at scale (2021)
33. Vaswani, A., et al.: Attention is all you need (2017)
34. Kingma, D.P., Welling, M.: Auto-encoding variational bayes (2014)
35. Lin, T.-Y., Goyal, P., Girshick, R., He, K., Dollár, P.: Focal loss for dense object detection. In: International Conference on Computer Vision (ICCV) (2017)

Diffraction Block in Extended nn-UNet for Brain Tumor Segmentation

Qingfan Hou[1], Zhuofei Wang[2], Jiao Wang[1], Jian Jiang[1], and Yanjun Peng[1]([⊠])

[1] College of Computer Science and Engineering, Shandong University of Science and Technology, Qingdao, China
pengyanjuncn@163.com
[2] University of Bristol, Bristol, UK

Abstract. Automatic brain tumor segmentation based on 3D mpMRI is highly significant for brain diagnosis, monitoring, and treatment planning. Due to the limitation of manual delineation, automatic and accurate segmentation based on a deep learning network has a tremendous practical necessity. The BraTS2022 challenge provides many data to develop our network. In this work, we proposed a diffraction block based on the Fraunhofer single-slit diffraction principle, which emphasizes the effect of associated features and suppresses isolated features. We added the diffraction block to nn-UNet, which took first place in the BraTS 2020 competition. We also improved nn-UNet by referring to the solution proposed by the 2021 winner, including using a larger network and replacing the batch with a group normalization. In the final unseen test data, our method is ranked first for Pediatric population data and third for BraTS continuous evaluation data.

Keywords: Brain Tumor Segmentation · nn-UNet · Diffraction Block

1 Introduction

Brain segmentation is of great significance in the diagnosis, treatment, aid surgery, and post-treatment planning of tumors [1]. Due to the highly variable appearance, shape, and position of gliomas in the brain, the segmentation of gliomas and their subregions through multi-parametric magnetic resonance imaging (mpMRI) scans is one of the most critical tasks in biomedical imaging areas. The high proliferation rate and mortality rate of glioblastoma multiforme (GBM) make the accuracy and efficiency of segmentation vital. However, manual segmentation using mpMRI scans is a time-consuming, complex task that relies heavily on the experience of specialists. Specialists must have sufficient anatomical knowledge and be skilled in using software tools to mark the boundaries and regions of tumor tissues. In manual segmentation, specialists can only segment tumor regions slice by slice and only use a single image modality simultaneously. Hence, the manual segmentation results are more variable than the ground truth results. Therefore, there are better choices than manual segmentation in mpMRI, while a fully automatic segmentation method can integrate multimodal information to provide the best segmentation results.

The Brain Tumor Segmentation Challenge (BraTS) [2–6] provides a wealth of well-annotated and publicly available data for model development and a suitable platform for comparing models. The BraTS 2022 offers 1,251 labeled training data and 219 unlabeled validation data. All BraTS mpMRI scans describe Native T1-weighted image, post-contrast T1-weighted (T1Gd), T2-weighted, and T2 Fluid Attenuated Inversion Recovery (T2-FLAIR) volumes, all $240 \times 240 \times 155$ in size. An example image set is presented in Fig. 1. All imaging datasets were annotated manually according to the same annotation protocol. Annotations include the GD-enhancing tumor (ET--label 4), the peritumoral edematous/invaded tissue (ED--label 2), and the necrotic tumor core (NCR--label 1). The unlabeled validation data required participants to upload the segmentation masks to the platform for evaluation, allowing multiple submissions to facilitate improvements in the segmentation performance of the model. The segmentation targets are three regions: whole tumor (WT), tumor core (TC), and enhancing tumor (ET).

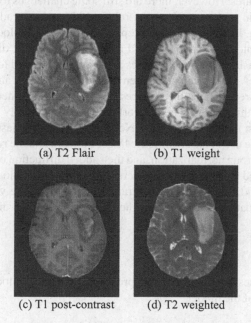

(a) T2 Flair   (b) T1 weight

(c) T1 post-contrast   (d) T2 weighted

Fig. 1. Example of image modalities in the BraTS 2022 dataset

In recent years, the successful entries in BraTS have been entirely based on the U-Net [7], the network with skip-connection based on an encoder-decoder structure. Myronenko [8] used 3D U-Net with large asymmetric encoders and added variation autoencoders (VAE) branches at the end of the sampling path to standardize the shared encoders. Jiang et al. [9] proposed a two-stage cascade U-Net. The first stage used U-Net variants to train rough prediction, and in the second stage, rough prediction and the original graph of the previous stage are used as inputs for training to refine prediction. Both extend the encoder-decoder structure. Isensee et al. [10] took nn-UNet [11] as the baseline in the 2020 Challenge and optimized it specifically for BraTS. Luu et al. [12]

Extended nn-UNet by using a more extensive network, replacing batch normalization with group normalization, and using axial attention in decoders. With a larger dataset and many attempts, we can see that the segmentation accuracy of the winners is getting higher every year.

We also studied different deep-learning methods for automatic brain tumor segmentation tasks. The ARU-GD (Attention Res-UNet with Guided Decoder) proposed by Dhiraj et al. [13] uses a hybrid network framework and proposes a new guided decoder that trains each decoder layer using an individual loss function and output in each decoder layer. Sun et al. [14] proposed a multi-pathway architecture method based on 3D FCN (fully convolutional network), in which 3D dilated convolution is adopted in multi-pathway architecture to extract different receptive fields of feature from multi-modal MRI images more effectively. Wang et al. [15] proposed a dynamic focal dice loss function, which could be dynamically adjusted according to the training performance of each class during training, and pay more attention to smaller tumor sub-regions with more complex structures. However, there are still some challenges to be addressed in the segmentation of brain tumors, such as the relationship between adjacent features that needs more attention. Based on this, we propose the diffraction block.

The diffraction block is based on the Fraunhofer single-slit diffraction principle, which aims to emphasize associated features and suppress isolated features. The diffraction block establishes relationships between high-value features and features within a specific range, then recalibrates the features based on the obtained relationships. We expect that through this process, the network enhances the ability to use the relationships concerning first modifying the nn-UNet with reference to last year's champion's scheme, including the use of an asymmetric larger network and the replacement of batch normalization with group normalization, and then added diffraction blocks to the adapted nn-UNet and adjusted the specific parameters of the diffraction blocks for the network. The 5-fold cross-validation results on the training dataset and the validation set results from the online evaluation platform show the effectiveness of the diffraction block.

2 Method

This section discusses the details of our proposed diffraction block and the network architecture details of the model.

2.1 Diffraction Block

A diffraction block is a computational unit abstracted from the Fraunhofer single-slit diffraction. The structure of the diffraction block is depicted in Fig. 2.

By calculating the influence radius R of the input X, the intensity of the influence of each eigenvalue on the surrounding is determined. Finally, the influence matrix F_a of each point under the influence of surrounding pixels is obtained.

process of discrimination

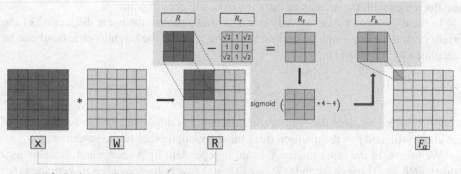

Calculate influence radius R

Fig. 2. Diffraction block

In Fraunhofer single-slit diffraction, when the slit width of the diffraction plane is no more significant than the wavelength of the light beam, the light beam passing through the slit in the diffraction plane will show a distinct diffraction pattern on the screen. The diffraction pattern has a bright central band followed by an alternative dark, and a bright band on both sides is obtained. Figure 3 shows the variation of the intensity distribution with the distance of Fraunhofer single-slit diffraction.

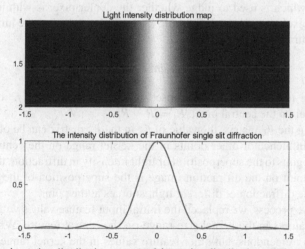

Fig. 3. The light intensity distribution map and intensity distribution of Fraunhofer single-slit diffraction

The light intensity of the bright central band reaches its maximum value at the center and decreases with the increasing distance from the central point.

In the diffraction block, we only consider and simulate the beam diffraction of the bright central band in single-slit diffraction. The width of the bright central band can be calculated by formula (1).

$$\Delta x = 2f \frac{\lambda}{a} \tag{1}$$

where Δx is the width of the bright central brand, λ is the wavelength, a is the width of the single-slit, and f is the distance from the diffraction plane to the screen.

We take x_i in the input matrix X as an independent light source and its value as a wavelength λ. . Through formula (2), we calculate the influence radius of x_i in the input matrix X on the surrounding x_i:

$$R = d \frac{X}{W} \tag{2}$$

where R is the matrix of influence radius r_i of x_i, X is input, d is constant, and W is the training parameter of diffraction block. By training W, the network automatically adjusts the range of influence of each feature in input X.

In Fig. 2, we can see that in the process of discrimination, we calculate the distance matrix R_r between pixels (assuming that the pixel distance between the center pixel and pixels in the 4-connected region is 1), then subtract the influence radius matrix R to obtain the matrix R_t, which is used to judge whether the center pixel is within the influence range of other pixels in the kernel. Formula (3) is used to calculate the influence of each pixel on the central pixel.

$$F_k = sigmoid\,(R_t \times 4 - 4) \tag{3}$$

where F_k is the influence matrix composed of the influence value f_{ki} of other pixels within the kernel on the central pixel, $R_t = R - R_r$.

By summing the F_k matrix, the value of f_{ai} in the F_a matrix can be obtained, which represents the influence of other points in the kernel range on the central point. This process is analogous to the superposition of light intensity in diffraction; that is, the light intensity of a point on the diffraction image is the superposition of the light intensity generated by the diffraction of different light sources at the point.

By the above process, we replaced the initial input feature values with the influence values of all features in the kernel size range on the central feature. When the central feature value is tremendous, but other feature values in the kernel range are small, the influence value becomes smaller than the input value. The influence value becomes larger when other large feature values are in the range. We expect that this explicit approach allows the network to emphasize associated features and suppress isolated features, focusing more on the relationships between features.

2.2 Model

In this section, the details of our model will be described, starting from the nn-UNet baseline, which won first place in BraTS 2020, and the modifications to this baseline will be explained.

Baseline nn-UNet. In the BraTS 2020 Challenge, Isensee et al. proposed the nn-UNet, which selected 3D U-Net with an encoder-decoder structure connected through skip-connection as the core network structure. In this network, mpMRI volumes, concatenated as four channels, were taken as input. The patch size is $128 \times 128 \times 128$ with a batch size of 2. The encoder carries out five downsamplings, performed with strided convolutions, and the size of the feature map size in its bottleneck is $4 \times 4 \times 4$. The initial number of convolution kernels is set to 32, which is doubled with each downsampling, and the maximum number is 320. The number of convolution kernels in the decoder is as same as the encoder, and upsampling is implemented as convolution transposed. After each convolution, the network uses leaky ReLUs [16] with slope 0.01 as the activation function, and instance normalization [17] is used for feature map normalization. The softmax nonlinearity at the network's last layer is replaced by sigmoid activation, treating each voxel as a multiclass classification problem. Besides the two lowest layers in the decoder, a sigmoid is added for output to achieve depth supervision and improve gradient propagation. The optimization objective of the training is the sum of Dice [18, 19] and a binary cross-entropy loss that optimizes each of the regions independently. The Loss operates in the following three areas: GD-enhancing tumor (ET), tumor core (TC) including the edematous/invaded tissue (NCR) and GD-enhancing tumor (ET), and whole tumor (WT) consisting of all three classes (ET + ED + NCR).

Larget Network, Group Normalization, and Diffraction Block. The diffraction block was added to the nn-UNet baseline. Diffraction blocks were used at all decoder layers except the two lowest layers and the final output layer. The first change we made to nn-UNet involved asymmetrically expanding the network by doubling the number of filters in the encoder while maintaining the same number in the decoder. Myronenko [8] used this asymmetrically large encoder, and Luu et al. [12] also used this approach in extended nn-UNet. As the amount of training data has increased significantly over previous years, increasing the size of the network will help it to be able to model a larger variety of data. The maximum number of filters was also increased from 320 to 512. The second modification replaces all batch normalization with group normalization [20]. Even with mixed-precision training, 3D convolutional networks require much GPU memory, limiting the batch size used during training. In low batch size regimes, group normalization has been found to perform better than batch normalization, and prior competition winners have also elected to use it [8, 9]. The modified network structure is shown in Fig. 4.

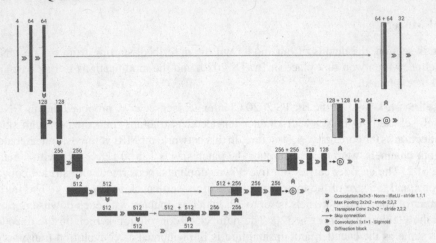

Fig. 4. Structure of lager nn-UNet with asymmetric scaling on the encoder.

2.3   Training Details

The training process for the entire model followed nn-UNet training steps and referenced the BraTS 2021 champion's methodology. Each attempted network was trained with five-fold cross-validation, following the data augmentation parameters used by nn-UNet in BraTS 2020 during training, including but not limited to rotation and scaling with a probability of 0.3 and a scale range of (0.65, 1.6), the use of elastic deformation with a probability of 0.3, additional brightness augmentation with a probability of 0.3, and increase the aggressiveness of the Gamma augmentation. Aggressive data augmentation improves the generalization and robustness of the model. The optimization objectives of the training are the sum of dice loss and a binary cross-entropy loss. The proposed network was trained on a batch size of 1 for 1000 epochs, each consisting of 250 mini batches at each training. We used a stochastic gradient descent optimization with a Nesterov momentum of 0.9, and the initial learning rate was 0.01. The learning rate gradually decreased according to formula (4).

$$lr = 0.01 \times (1 - \frac{epoch}{1000})^{0.9} \tag{4}$$

All experiments were conducted with Pytorch 1.8 on NVIDIA RTX 2080ti GPU with 11 GB VRAM. The following models were developed:

- **BL**: baseline nn-UNet, batch normalization with a batch size of 2
- **BL + L**: baseline with large U-Net, batch size of 2, train on all training samples
- **BL + L + GN**: nn-UNet with larger U-Net, group normalization, batch size of 1
- **BL + L + GN + DB**: nn-UNet with larger U-Net, group normalization, diffraction block, batch size of 1

3 Result

3.1 Quantitative Results

We train each configuration as five-fold cross-validation on the training cases (no external data is used). Table 1 shows the dice scores for the three tumor sub-regions of the four models from the cross-validation. The model BL + L increasing the size of the U-Net yields a slight improvement. The model BL + L + GN combines large U-Net and group normalization to improve the performance of the tumor core and the whole tumor while significantly increasing GPU memory usage. Combining large U-Net, group normalization, and diffraction blocks slightly improves performance for all three regions compared to BL.

Table 1. Training set results (n = 1251). Dice metrics of the networks on 5-fold cross-validation. ET: enhancing tumor, TC: tumor core, WT: whole tumor.

Model	ET	TC	WT	Average
BL	88.27	92.06	93.68	91.34
BL + L	**88.72**	**92.93**	93.86	**91.83**
BL + L + GN	88.24	92.36	93.78	91.46
BL + L + GN + DB	88.37	92.82	**93.93**	91.71

Table 2 shows the aggregated Dice scores and 95% Hausdorff distances (HD95) calculated by the online evaluation platform. The model with the changes made has improved segmentation results in all three subregions compared to the baseline. Among them, the BL + L + GN + DB model significantly improved in the ET and TC regions compared with BL + L + GN, and the results are very similar in the WT.

Table 2. The online evaluation platform calculated dice scores and 95% Hausdorff distances (HD95). ET: enhancing tumor, TC: tumor core, WT: whole tumor.

Model	Dice				HD95			
	ET	TC	WT	Average	ET	TC	WT	Average
BL	83.63	87.00	92.56	87.73	22.47	12.30	3.61	12.79
BL + L + GN	84.64	87.83	**92.75**	88.41	20.73	6.83	**3.48**	10.35
BL + L + GN + DB	**85.22**	**88.64**	92.71	**88.86**	**15.63**	**5.85**	3.53	**8.34**

3.2 Qualitative Results

Figure 5 provides a qualitative overview of the performance of the model BL + L + GN + DB segmentation. It shows our three generated results on the validation set. We have selected the best, median, and worst predictions based on the Dice score (average of the three validation regions). As can be seen from Fig. 5, the whole tumor segmentation is of high quality. The segmentation of the tumor core and enhanced tumor of the worst example reveals that the network failed to segment the enhanced tumor and the tumor core.

BraTS2021_00153
ET:98.68, TC: 99.34, WT: 99.07

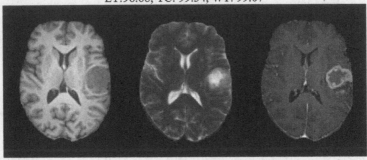

BraTS2021_01704
ET: 84.52, TC: 95.24, WT: 97.50

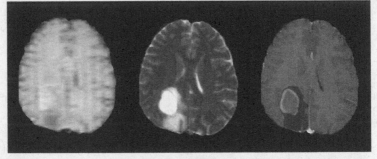

BraTS2021_01784
ET: 0, TC: 3.12, WT: 93.06

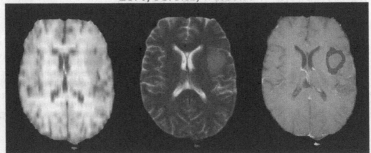

Fig. 5. Qualitative validation set results. Within each row, the raw T1 image is shown to the left, the T2 image in the middle, and the overlay with the generated segmentation on the T1ce image is shown on the right. Blue: necrotic tumor core, yellow: GD-enhancing tumor, purple: edematous tissues.

3.3   Test Set Results

Table 3. Quantitative results for the pediatric population of diffuse intrinsic pontine glioma (DIPG) test set.

	Dice		HD95	
	TC	WT	TC	WT
Mean	33.37	81.78	158.044	6.487
StdDev	37.86	16.17	176.26	6.760
Median	5.89	88.04	32.16	4.182
25th percentile	0	81.83	5.608	3
75th percentile	73.26	90.56	373.128	6.555

Table 3 provides quantitative results for the DIPG of the test set from challenge organizers. Our submission took first place in the BraTS 2022 competition.

Table 4. Quantitative results for BraTS 2021 Challenge test data.

	Dice			HD95		
	ET	TC	WT	ET	TC	WT
Mean	87.31	87.98	92.84	11.674	15.281	4.702
StdDev	18.00	23.36	9.28	57.642	65.004	17.240
Median	93.08	96.16	95.80	1	1.414	1.414
25th percentile	85.61	91.70	91.84	1	1	1
75th percentile	96.23	97.94	97.68	2	3	3.742

Table 4 provides quantitative results for BraTS 2021 Challenge test data from challenge organizers. Our submission took third place in the BraTS 2022 competition.

Table 5. Quantitative results for SSA adult patient populations of brain diffuse glioma (Africa-BraTS) of test data.

	Dice			HD95		
	ET	TC	WT	ET	TC	WT
Mean	90.89	94.91	97.03	2.468	2.097	3.314
StdDev	11.35	7.91	2.87	2.687	2.013	6.216
Median	95.12	97.36	97.82	1	1.414	1
25th percentile	90.32	95.81	96.66	1	1	1
75th percentile	96.82	98.43	98.38	2.468	2.013	1.732

Table 5 provides quantitative results for Africa-BraTS of test data from challenge organizers.

4   Discussion

In BraTS 2022 competition, we propose a diffraction block based on Fraunhofer single-slit diffraction principle. The diffraction block establishes the relationship between high-value and other features, emphasizes associated features, and suppresses isolated features. We also made some modifications on nn-UNet, including using a larger network and group normalization instead of batch normalization. Finally, we added diffraction blocks to the adjusted nn-UNet. The results demonstrate that the diffraction block and the adjustment of the nn-UNet improve the segmentation performance.

The 3D input of the mpMRI data is more conducive to producing a good segmentation network because it contains more contextual and local information among the nearby slices. However, the memory capacity required is also huge. In particular, when we propose a complex operator, although most of the operators can be obtained by combining the basic tensor operations and some advanced functions in Pytorch, such combinations tend to result in low GPU computation efficiency and long computation time. To solve this problem, we have implemented diffraction blocks using a mixture of C++ and CUDA programming. Compared with the direct implementation of diffraction blocks using Pytorch, the GPU data loading is fast enough, the computational resources are hardly idle, and the GPU utilization can reach 99.84%.

After analyzing the results from the online platform, we found that the primary source of error is the tumor core region and the enhanced tumor region. The post-processing approach is the source of error for the enhanced tumor regions, as Isensee et al. [10] on this part. In short, they argue that removing small sporadic enhancing tumor regions in post-processing can improve the ranking. In the poorer segmentation results, the source of error in the tumor core region seems to come from the fact that there is no clear boundary between the tumor core and the enhancing tumor region, causing the network to incorrectly classify the enhancing tumor region into the tumor core region.

Acknowledgements. We want to acknowledge Fabian Isensee for developing the nn-UNet framework and sharing the models from the 2020 competition and Huan Minh Luu for modifying the nn-UNet and communicating the models from last year's competition.

This paper is the results of the research project funded by the National Natural Science Foundation of China (61976126) and Shandong Natural Science Foundation (ZR2019MF003).

References

1. Rajput, S., Raval, M.S.: A review on end-to-end methods for brain tumor segmentation and overall survival prediction. arXiv preprint arXiv:2006.01632 (2020)
2. Baid, U., et al.: The RSNA-ASNR-MICCAI BraTS 2021 Benchmark on Brain Tumor Segmentation and Radiogenomic Classification. arXiv:2107.02314 (2021)
3. Menze, B.H., Jakab, A., Bauer, S., Kalpathy-Cramer, J., Farahani, K., Kirby, J., et al.: The multimodal brain tumor image segmentation benchmark (BRATS). IEEE Trans. Med. Imaging **34**(10), 1993–2024 (2015). https://doi.org/10.1109/TMI.2014.2377694
4. Bakas, S., Akbari, H., Sotiras, A., Bilello, M., Rozycki, M., Kirby, J.S., et al.: Advancing the cancer genome atlas glioma MRI collections with expert segmentation labels and radiomic features. Nat. Sci. Data **4**, 170117 (2017). https://doi.org/10.1038/sdata.2017.117

5. Bakas, S., et al.: Segmentation labels and radiomic features for the pre-operative scans of the TCGA-GBM collection. The Cancer Imaging Archive (2017). https://doi.org/10.7937/K9/TCIA.2017.KLXWJJ1Q

6. Bakas, S., et al.: Segmentation labels and radiomic features for the pre-operative scans of the TCGA-LGG collection. The Cancer Imaging Archive (2017). https://doi.org/10.7937/K9/TCIA.2017.GJQ7R0EF

7. Ronneberger, O., Fischer, P., Brox, T.: U-Net: convolutional networks for biomedical image segmentation. In: Navab, N., Hornegger, J., Wells, W.M., Frangi, A.F. (eds.) MICCAI 2015. LNCS, vol. 9351, pp. 234–241. Springer, Cham (2015). https://doi.org/10.1007/978-3-319-24574-4_28

8. Myronenko, A.: 3D MRI brain tumor segmentation using autoencoder regularization. In: Crimi, A., Bakas, S., Kuijf, H., Keyvan, F., Reyes, M., van Walsum, T. (eds.) BrainLes 2018. LNCS, vol. 11384, pp. 311–320. Springer, Cham (2019). https://doi.org/10.1007/978-3-030-11726-9_28

9. Jiang, Z., Ding, C., Liu, M., Tao, D.: Two-stage cascaded U-Net: 1st place solution to BraTS challenge 2019 segmentation task. In: Crimi, A., Bakas, S. (eds.) BrainLes 2019. LNCS, vol. 11992, pp. 231–241. Springer, Cham (2020). https://doi.org/10.1007/978-3-030-46640-4_22

10. Isensee, F., Jäger, P.F., Full, P.M., Vollmuth, P., Maier-Hein, K.H.: nnU-net for brain tumor segmentation. In: Crimi, A., Bakas, S. (eds.) BrainLes 2020. LNCS, vol. 12659, pp. 118–132. Springer, Cham (2021). https://doi.org/10.1007/978-3-030-72087-2_11

11. Isensee, F., Jaeger, P.F., Kohl, S.A., Petersen, J., Maier-Hein, K.H.: nnU-Net: a self-configuring method for deep learning-based biomedical image segmentation. Nat. Methods 18(2), 203–211 (2021)

12. Luu, H.M., Park, S.H.: Extending nn-UNet for brain tumor segmentation. arXiv preprint arXiv:2112.04653 (2021)

13. Maji, D., Sigedar, P., Singh, M.: Attention res-UNet with guided decoder for semantic segmentation of brain tumors. Biomed. Signal Process. Control 71, 103077 (2022)

14. Sun, J., Peng, Y., Guo, Y., Li, D.: Segmentation of the multimodal brain tumor image used the multi-pathway architecture method based on 3D FCN. Neurocomputing 423, 34–45 (2021)

15. Wang, P., Chung, A.C.: Relax and focus on brain tumor segmentation. Med. Image Anal. 75, 102259 (2022)

16. Maas, A.L., Hannun, A.Y., Andrew, Y.N.: Rectifier nonlinearities improve neural network acoustic models. Proc. ICML 30(1), 3 (2013)

17. Ulyanov, D., Vedaldi, A., Lempitsky, V.: Instance normalization: the missing ingredient for fast stylization. arXiv preprint arXiv:1607.08022 (2016)

18. Milletari, F., Navab, N., Ahmadi, S.A.: V-net: Fully convolutional neural networks for volumetric medical image segmentation. In: International Conference on 3D Vision (3DV), pp. 565–571. IEEE (2016)

19. Drozdzal, M., Vorontsov, E., Chartrand, G., Kadoury, S., Pal, C.: The importance of skip connections in biomedical image segmentation. Carneiro, G., et al. (eds.) Deep Learning and Data Labeling for Medical Applications, vol. 10008, pp. 179–187. Springer International Publishing Cham (2016). https://doi.org/10.1007/978-3-319-46976-8_19

20. Wu, Y., He, K.: Group normalization. In: Ferrari, V., Hebert, M., Sminchisescu, C., Weiss, Y. (eds.) ECCV 2018. LNCS, vol. 11217, pp. 3–19. Springer, Cham (2018). https://doi.org/10.1007/978-3-030-01261-8_1

Infusing Domain Knowledge into nnU-Nets for Segmenting Brain Tumors in MRI

Krzysztof Kotowski[1], Szymon Adamski[1], Bartosz Machura[1], Lukasz Zarudzki[3], and Jakub Nalepa[1,2(✉)]

[1] Graylight Imaging, Gliwice, Poland
kotowski.polsl@gmail.com,
{sadamski,bmachura,jnalepa}@graylight-imaging.com
[2] Silesian University of Technology, Gliwice, Poland
jnalepa@ieee.org
[3] Maria Sklodowska-Curie Memorial Cancer Center and Institute of Oncology, Gliwice, Poland

Abstract. Accurate and reproducible segmentation of brain tumors from multi-modal magnetic resonance (MR) scans is a pivotal step in clinical practice. In this BraTS Continuous Evaluation initiative, we exploit a 3D nnU-Net for this task which was ranked at the 6th place (out of 1600 participants) in the BraTS'21 Challenge. We benefit from an ensemble of deep models enhanced with the expert knowledge of a senior radiologist captured in a form of several post-processing routines. The experimental study showed that infusing the domain knowledge into the deep models can enhance their performance, and we obtained the average Dice score of 0.81977 (enhancing tumor), 0.87837 (tumor core), and 0.92723 (whole tumor) over the validation set. For the test data, we had the average Dice score of 0.86317, 0.87987, and 0.92838 for the enhancing tumor, tumor core and whole tumor. Our approach was also validated over the hold-out testing data which encompassed the BraTS 2021 Challenge test set, as well as new data from out-of-sample sources including independent pediatric population of diffuse intrinsic pontine glioma patients, together with an independent multi-institutional dataset covering under-represented Sub-Saharian African adult patient population of brain diffuse glioma. Our technique was ranked 2nd and 3rd over the pediatric and Sub-Saharian African populations, respectively, proving its high generalization capabilities.

Keywords: Brain Tumor · Segmentation · Deep Learning · U-Net · Expert Knowledge

1 Introduction

Brain tumor segmentation from multi-modal MR scans is an important step in oncology care. Accurate delineation of tumorous tissue is pivotal for further diagnosis, prognosis and treatment, and it can directly affect the treatment pathway.

S. Bakas et al. (Eds.): BrainLes 2022, LNCS 13769, pp. 186–194, 2023.
https://doi.org/10.1007/978-3-031-33842-7_16

Hence, ensuring the reproducibility, robustness, e.g., against different scanners, and quality of an automated segmentation process are critical to design personalized patient care. The state-of-the-art brain tumor segmentation algorithms are commonly divided into the *atlas-based, unsupervised, supervised,* and *hybrid* techniques. In the *atlas-based* algorithms, manually segmented atlases are used to segment the unseen scans [19]. *Unsupervised* approaches elaborate intrinsic characteristics of the *unlabeled* data [7,12,20]. Once the labeled data is available, we can use the *supervised* techniques [9,22,23]. Deep learning models span across various networks architectures [16] and include ensembles of deep nets [13], U-Net architectures [11,18], encoder-decoder approaches [6], and more [8,17].

We use a 3D nnU-Net architecture (Sect. 3) operating over multi-modal MR scans [10], in which brain tumors are segmented into the enhancing tumor (ET), peritumoral edema (ED), and necrotic core (NCR). We utilize five-fold ensembling with stratification based on the distribution of NCR, ET, and ED, together with the post-processing routines that capture the expert knowledge of a senior radiologist. The experiments performed over the BraTS'21 training, validation, and test datasets showed that our architecture delivers accurate multi-class segmentation, and that infusing the expert knowledge into the deep models may significantly improve their abilities nnU-Nets (Sect. 4).

2   Data

The 2021 release of the Brain Tumor Segmentation (BraTS) set [1–4,15] includes MRI training data of 1251 patients with gliomas. Each study was contoured by one to four experienced and trained readers. The data captures four co-registered MRI modalities, being the native pre-contrast (T1), post-contrast T1-weighted (T1Gd), T2-weighted (T2), and T2 Fluid Attenuated Inversion Recovery (T2-FLAIR) sequences. All pixels are labeled, and the following labels are considered: healthy tissue, Gd-enhancing tumor (ET), peritumoral edema/invaded tissue (ED) and the necrotic tumor core (NCR) [5].

The data was acquired with different protocols and scanners at multiple institutions. The studies were interpolated to the same shape ($240 \times 240 \times 155$, hence there are 155 images of 240×240 size, with voxel size of $1\,mm^3$), and they were skull-stripped. Finally, there are 219 patients in the validation set V (see examples in Fig. 1), for which the manual annotations are not provided.

3   Methods

We built upon the nnU-Net framework [10], which automatically configures itself, including preprocessing, basic post-processing, architecture and training configurations. We train the network over the BraTS'21 training data with the averaged (across all target classes) cross-entropy and soft Dice as the loss function. A patch size of $128 \times 128 \times 128$ with a batch size of 2 was selected.

In our recent BraTS paper [14], we investigated 15 combinations of an array of post-processing routines that capture the expert knowledge, and showed that

| T1 | T1Gd | T2 | T2-FLAIR |

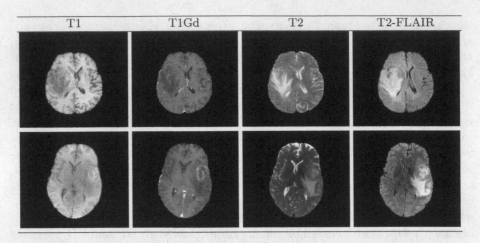

Fig. 1. Example scans of two patients (separate rows) included in the validation set.

utilizing the FillTC method allows us to statistically significantly improve the results for Dice obtained for TC and WT ($p < 0.005$) (Table 1).

Table 1. The post-processing approach utilized to infuse the expert knowledge into the nnU-Net segmentation framework.

Method's short name	Algorithm	Expert knowledge
FillTC	Any voxels surrounded by TC in 2D in any slice on any plane are iteratively relabeled to NCR. The planes are filled in the following order: axial, coronal, sagittal	Edema cannot be surrounded by necrosis only. Necrosis cannot have "holes" (tissue not labeled by model to any class) inside it. If enhancing tumor is "closed" (ring-shaped) in 2D everything inside it which is not enhancing has to be necrosis. Large tumors usually do not contain "holes" of healthy tissue

4   Experiments

4.1   Experimental Setup

The DNN models were implemented using `Python3` with `Keras` and `PyTorch`. The experiments were run on a high-performance computer equipped with an NVIDIA Tesla V100 GPU (32 GB) and 6 Intel Xeon E5-2680 (2.50 GHz) CPUs.

4.2   Training Process

The metric for training was a sum of the Dice score and cross-entropy. Training was performed on ET, ED, and NCR classes, with the maximum number of epochs set to 500. The optimizer was the stochastic gradient descent with the Nesterov momentum with the initial learning rate of 10^{-2}. The learning rate is decayed gradually to a value close to zero in the last epoch [10].

The training set was split into five non-overlapping stratified folds (each base model is trained over four folds, and one fold is used for validation during the training process; see Table 2). We stratify the dataset at the patient level with respect to the distribution of the size of the NCR, ED, and ET examples. The fold sizes were equal to 251, 253, 250, 248, and 249 patients.

Table 2. Characteristics of the folds (average volume of the corresponding tumor subregion is reported in cm^3) used for training our model.

	WT vol.	NCR vol.	ED vol.	ET vol.
Fold 1	95.16	14.21	59.85	21.10
Fold 2	96.63	15.38	60.42	20.82
Fold 3	93.97	13.77	57.74	22.47
Fold 4	97.18	14.65	60.72	21.82
Fold 5	96.80	13.43	62.36	21.00

4.3   Experimental Results

In this section, we present the results obtained over the BraTS'21 validation and test sets (as returned by the Synapse portal)[1]. The quantitative results are gathered in Table 3—they confirm that our approach delivers accurate segmentation of all regions of interest. Also, our model allowed us to take the 6th place in the BraTS'21 Challenge (across 1600 participants from all over the globe). In Fig. 2, we can appreciate the example of an MRI scan from the validation set which was segmented without and with infusing the expert knowledge into the algorithm (for this patient, we observed the largest improvement in TC Dice). Although there are cases for which the segmentation quality (as quantified by Dice) was around 0.50 (ET), 0.67 (TC) and 0.79 (WT), the qualitative analysis reveals that they are still sensible (Fig. 3). Such cases could be further investigated manually, within a semi-automated clinical process—hence, quantifying the confidence of the segmentation returned by the deep model is of high practical importance, and it constitutes our current research efforts.

In Table 4, we gather the results obtained over the unseen hold-out testing data. It encompassed the BraTS 2021 Challenge test data, as well as new data from out-of-sample sources including independent pediatric population of diffuse

---

[1] Our team name is `Graylight Imaging`.

Table 3. Segmentation performance quantified by Dice, sensitivity, specificity, and Hausdorff (95%) distance over the BraTS'21 **validation** and **test** sets obtained using our approach (as returned by the validation server). The scores (average μ, standard deviation s, median m, and the 25 and 75 quantile) are presented for the whole tumor (WT), tumor core (TC), and enhancing tumor (ET).

	Dice ET	Dice TC	Dice WT	Haus. ET	Haus. TC	Haus. WT	Sens. ET	Sens. TC	Sens. WT	Spec. ET	Spec. TC	Spec. WT
Validation set												
μ	0.8198	0.8784	0.9272	17.8533	7.5973	3.6368	0.8222	0.8594	0.9289	0.9998	0.9998	0.9994
s	0.2462	0.1787	0.0735	73.6816	36.0452	5.7308	0.2601	0.1991	0.0788	0.0004	0.0003	0.0008
m	0.8979	0.9412	0.9457	1.4142	1.7321	2.0826	0.9148	0.9370	0.9557	0.9999	0.9999	0.9996
25q	0.8242	0.8784	0.9032	1.0000	1.0000	1.4142	0.8304	0.8513	0.9122	0.9998	0.9998	0.9992
75q	0.9520	0.9687	0.9689	2.4495	3.8708	3.6212	0.9664	0.9736	0.9787	1.0000	1.0000	0.9999
Test set												
μ	0.8632	0.8799	0.9284	13.0853	15.8731	4.7724	0.8761	0.8892	0.9292	0.9998	0.9997	0.9995
s	0.2038	0.2342	0.0899	61.4577	66.6866	17.0157	0.2147	0.2190	0.0946	0.0003	0.0008	0.0008
m	0.9351	0.9635	0.9573	1.0000	1.4142	1.7321	0.9523	0.9693	0.9584	0.9999	0.9999	0.9998
25q	0.8516	0.9175	0.91300	1.0000	1.0000	1.0000	0.8875	0.9095	0.9176	0.9997	0.9998	0.9995
75q	0.9660	0.9822	0.9777	2.0000	3.0000	4.0000	0.9788	0.9876	0.9812	1.0000	1.0000	0.9999

Without injecting expert knowledge   **With** injecting the expert knowledge

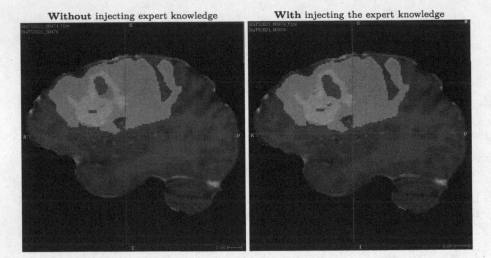

Fig. 2. The prediction for a patient with ID: 474 from the BraTS'21 validation data for which the largest improvement of TC Dice was achieved after infusing the expert knowledge into the post-processing routine (green—ED, yellow—ET, red—NCR). (Color figure online)

intrinsic pontine glioma patients (Pediatric population), together with an independent multi-institutional dataset covering under-represented Sub-Saharian African adult patient population of brain diffuse glioma. We can appreciate that our technique can indeed generalize well over the unseen test data—it was ranked 2nd over the pediatric population, and 3rd over the Sub-Saharian African adult patient population, across all participating teams.

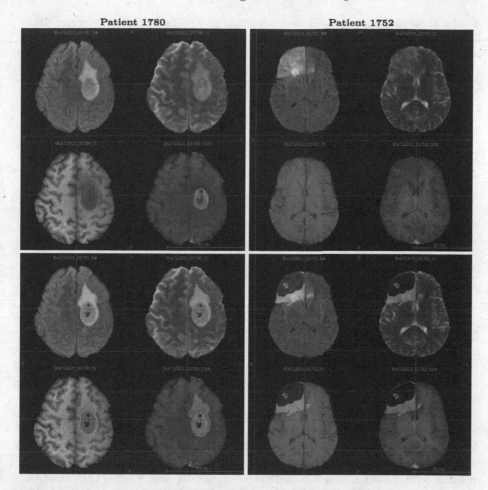

Fig. 3. Examples of high- and low-quality contouring (patients with ID: 1780 and 1752, respectively) from the validation set (green—ED, yellow—ET, red—NCR). The Dice values amounted to 0.98990 (ET), 0.99232 (TC), and 0.98318 (WT) for patient 1780, and to 0.49577 (ET), 0.67378 (TC), and 0.78600 (WT) for patient 1752. (Color figure online)

Table 4. Segmentation performance quantified by Dice, sensitivity, specificity, Hausdorff (95%) distance and precision over the BraTS 2021 testing cohort, pediatric test population and Sub-Saharan African test population obtained using our approach (as returned by the validation server). The scores (average μ, standard deviation s, median m, and the 25 and 75 quantile) are presented for the whole tumor (WT), tumor core (TC), and enhancing tumor (ET).

	Dice ET	Dice TC	Dice WT	Haus. ET	Haus. TC	Haus. WT	Sens. ET	Sens. TC	Sens. WT	Spec. ET	Spec. TC	Spec. WT	Prec. ET	Prec. TC	Prec. WT
BraTS testing cohort															
μ	0.8578	0.8767	0.9275	13.7210	15.8530	4.7301	0.8739	0.8922	0.9304	0.9998	0.9997	0.9995	0.8590	0.8898	0.9374
s	0.2052	0.2348	0.0905	63.2727	66.6884	17.0133	0.2177	0.2166	0.0958	0.0003	0.0009	0.0008	0.1949	0.2286	0.0957
m	0.9271	0.9607	0.9568	1.0000	1.4142	1.7321	0.9522	0.9707	0.9611	0.9999	0.9999	0.9997	0.9226	0.9658	0.9704
25q	0.8499	0.9123	0.9130	1.0000	1.0000	1.0000	0.8850	0.9127	0.9176	0.9997	0.9998	0.9994	0.8437	0.9245	0.9316
75q	0.9612	0.9795	0.9765	2.0000	3.0000	4.0000	0.9785	0.9882	0.9819	1.0000	1.0000	0.9999	0.9622	0.9834	0.9860
Pediatric test population															
μ		0.2968	0.8075		181.0460	7.9224		0.3517	0.7662		0.9992	0.9997		0.3192	0.9240
s		0.3702	0.2045		180.1919	10.6302		0.4222	0.2267		0.0010	0.0004		0.3527	0.0616
m		0.0019	0.8695		74.7178	4.4155		0.0011	0.8269		0.9997	0.9998		0.0907	0.9282
25q		0.0000	0.8095		6.7082	3.2935		0.0000	0.7240		0.9986	0.9996		0.0000	0.8844
75q		0.6883	0.9038		373.1287	7.3286		0.8673	0.8933		0.9999	0.9999		0.6598	0.9714
Sub-Saharan African (SSA) population															
μ	0.9076	0.9487	0.9698	2.2225	1.8814	3.2766	0.8793	0.9430	0.9639	0.9998	0.9998	0.9996	0.9549	0.9626	0.9771
s	0.1116	0.0763	0.0237	2.5241	1.5352	6.8043	0.1605	0.0832	0.0334	0.0002	0.0002	0.0005	0.0356	0.0866	0.0327
m	0.9536	0.9761	0.9756	1.0000	1.0000	1.0000	0.9469	0.9628	0.9688	0.9999	0.9999	0.9998	0.9667	0.9836	0.9872
25q	0.9086	0.9565	0.9650	1.0000	1.0000	1.0000	0.8810	0.9415	0.9522	0.9997	0.9998	0.9996	0.9439	0.9718	0.9712
75q	0.9660	0.9828	0.9829	2.4495	2.0000	2.2361	0.9680	0.9811	0.9840	0.9999	0.9999	0.9999	0.9749	0.9890	0.9941

5   Conclusion

In this paper, we utilized an ensemble of five nnU-Net models with our custom stratification based on the distribution of NCR, ET, and ED volumes for accurate brain tumor segmentation. To further improve the segmentation capabilities of the nnU-Nets, we infused the expert knowledge into the framework through introducing a post-processing routine. It significantly improves TC and WT Dice, without deteriorating any other metric. Additionally, it is robust to specific cases with missing classes in ground truth, because it extends the TC volume with additional voxels instead of removing any voxels. Our algorithm allowed us to take the 6th place in the BraTS'21 Challenge over the hidden test data (out of 1600 participants). Additionally, the approach was validated over the hold-out test data, including the BraTS 2021 Challenge test data, independent pediatric population of diffuse intrinsic pontine glioma patients, and an independent multi-institutional dataset covering under-represented Sub-Saharan African adult patient population of brain diffuse glioma. Our technique was ranked 2nd and 3rd over the Pediatric and Sub-Saharan African adult populations, respectively, proving its high generalization capabilities.

The research undertaken in this paper constitutes an interesting departure point for further efforts. We currently focus on improving the segmentation quality of ET and TC by creating specialized models that could deal better with the aforementioned specific cases. Also, we believe that exploiting the expert knowledge which could be captured as various forms of pre- and post-processing routines (and also as the elements of the deep learning model's training strategies) could help us improve the segmentation quality even further, not only in brain tumor segmentation tasks, but also in other medical image analysis tasks.

However, following a rigorous validation procedure—as in BraTS—is of utmost practical importance [21], in order to objectively assess such improvements.

Acknowledgments. JN was supported by the Silesian University of Technology funds through the grant for maintaining and developing research potential. This work was supported by the Polish National Centre for Research and Development grant: POIR.01.01.01-00-0092/20 (*Methods and algorithms for automatic coronary artery calcium scoring on cardiac computed tomography scans*).

This paper is in memory of Dr. Grzegorz Nalepa, an extraordinary scientist and pediatric hematologist/oncologist at Riley Hospital for Children, Indianapolis, USA, who helped countless patients and their families through some of the most challenging moments of their lives.

References

1. Baid, U., et al: The RSNA-ASNR-MICCAI BraTS 2021 benchmark on brain tumor segmentation and radiogenomic classification (2021)
2. Bakas, S., et al.: Advancing the cancer genome atlas glioma MRI collections with expert segmentation labels and radiomic features. Nat. Sci. Data **4**, 1–13 (2017). https://doi.org/10.1038/sdata.2017.117
3. Bakas, S., et al.: Segmentation labels and radiomic features for the pre-operative scans of the TCGA-GBM collection. The Cancer Imaging Archive (2017). https://doi.org/10.7937/K9/TCIA.2017.KLXWJJ1Q
4. Bakas, S., et al.: Segmentation labels and radiomic features for the pre-operative scans of the TCGA-LGG collection. The Cancer Imaging Archive (2017). https://doi.org/10.7937/K9/TCIA.2017.GJQ7R0EF
5. Bakas, S., et al.: Identifying the best machine learning algorithms for brain tumor segmentation, progression assessment, and overall survival prediction in the BRATS challenge. CoRR abs/1811.02629 (2018). http://arxiv.org/abs/1811.02629
6. Bontempi, D., Benini, S., Signoroni, A., Svanera, M., Muckli, L.: CEREBRUM: a fast and fully-volumetric convolutional encoder-decoder for weakly-supervised segmentation of brain structures from out-of-the-scanner MRI. Med. Image Anal. **62**, 101688 (2020)
7. Chander, A., Chatterjee, A., Siarry, P.: A new social and momentum component adaptive PSO algorithm for image segmentation. Expert Syst. Appl. **38**(5), 4998–5004 (2011)
8. Estienne, T., et al.: Deep learning-based concurrent brain registration and tumor segmentation. Front. Comput. Neurosci. **14**, 17 (2020)
9. Geremia, E., Clatz, O., Menze, B.H., Konukoglu, E., Criminisi, A., Ayache, N.: Spatial decision forests for MS lesion segmentation in multi-channel magnetic resonance images. Neuroimage **57**(2), 378–390 (2011)
10. Isensee, F., Jaeger, P., Kohl, S., Petersen, J., Maier-Hein, K.: nnU-Net: a self-configuring method for deep learning-based biomedical image segmentation. Nat. Methods **18**, 1–9 (2021). https://doi.org/10.1038/s41592-020-01008-z
11. Isensee, F., Kickingereder, P., Wick, W., Bendszus, M., Maier-Hein, K.H.: No new-net. In: Crimi, A., Bakas, S., Kuijf, H., Keyvan, F., Reyes, M., van Walsum, T. (eds.) BrainLes 2018. LNCS, vol. 11384, pp. 234–244. Springer, Cham (2019). https://doi.org/10.1007/978-3-030-11726-9_21

12. Ji, S., Wei, B., Yu, Z., Yang, G., Yin, Y.: A new multistage medical segmentation method based on superpixel and fuzzy clustering. Comput. Math. Methods Med. **2014**, 747549:1–747549:13 (2014)

13. Kamnitsas, K., et al.: Ensembles of multiple models and architectures for robust brain tumour segmentation. In: Crimi, A., Bakas, S., Kuijf, H., Menze, B., Reyes, M. (eds.) BrainLes 2017. LNCS, vol. 10670, pp. 450–462. Springer, Cham (2018). https://doi.org/10.1007/978-3-319-75238-9_38

14. Kotowski, K., Adamski, S., Machura, B., Zarudzki, L., Nalepa, J.: Coupling nnU-Nets with expert knowledge for accurate brain tumor segmentation from MRI. In: Crimi, A., Bakas, S. (eds.) BrainLes 2021. LNCS, vol. 12963, pp. 197–209. Springer, Cham (2022). https://doi.org/10.1007/978-3-031-09002-8_18

15. Menze, B.H., et al.: The multimodal brain tumor image segmentation benchmark (BRATS). IEEE Trans. Med. Imaging **34**(10), 1993–2024 (2015)

16. Myronenko, A.: 3D MRI brain tumor segmentation using autoencoder regularization. In: Crimi, A., Bakas, S., Kuijf, H., Keyvan, F., Reyes, M., van Walsum, T. (eds.) BrainLes 2018. LNCS, vol. 11384, pp. 311–320. Springer, Cham (2019). https://doi.org/10.1007/978-3-030-11726-9_28

17. Nalepa, J., Marcinkiewicz, M., Kawulok, M.: Data augmentation for brain-tumor segmentation: a review. Front. Comput. Neurosci. **13**, 83 (2019)

18. Nalepa, J., et al.: Fully-automated deep learning-powered system for DCE-MRI analysis of brain tumors. Artif. Intell. Med. **102**, 101769 (2020)

19. Pipitone, J., et al.: Multi-atlas segmentation of the whole hippocampus and subfields using multiple automatically generated templates. Neuroimage **101**, 494–512 (2014)

20. Simi, V., Joseph, J.: Segmentation of glioblastoma multiforme from MR images - a comprehensive review. Egypt. J. Radiol. Nucl. Med. **46**(4), 1105–1110 (2015)

21. Wijata, A.M., Nalepa, J.: Unbiased validation of the algorithms for automatic needle localization in ultrasound-guided breast biopsies. In: 2022 IEEE International Conference on Image Processing (ICIP), pp. 3571–3575 (2022). https://doi.org/10.1109/ICIP46576.2022.9897449

22. Wu, W., Chen, A.Y.C., Zhao, L., Corso, J.J.: Brain tumor detection and segmentation in a CRF (conditional random fields) framework with pixel-pairwise affinity and superpixel-level features. Int. J. Comput. Assist. Radiol. Surg. **9**(2), 241–253 (2014). https://doi.org/10.1007/s11548-013-0922-7

23. Zikic, D., et al.: Decision forests for tissue-specific segmentation of high-grade gliomas in multi-channel MR. In: Ayache, N., Delingette, H., Golland, P., Mori, K. (eds.) MICCAI 2012. LNCS, vol. 7512, pp. 369–376. Springer, Heidelberg (2012). https://doi.org/10.1007/978-3-642-33454-2_46

Multi-modal Brain Tumour Segmentation Using Transformer with Optimal Patch Size

Ramtin Mojtahedi[1][iD], Mohammad Hamghalam[1,2][iD],
and Amber L. Simpson[1,3(✉)][iD]

[1] School of Computing, Queen's University, Kingston, ON, Canada
amber.simpson@queensu.ca
[2] Department of Electrical Engineering, Qazvin Branch, Islamic Azad University,
Qazvin, Iran
[3] Department of Biomedical and Molecular Sciences, Queen's University,
Kingston, ON, Canada

Abstract. Early diagnosis and grading of gliomas are crucial for determining therapy and the prognosis of brain cancer. For this purpose, magnetic resonance (MR) studies of brain tumours are widely used in the therapy process. Due to the overlap between the intensity distributions of healthy, enhanced, non-enhancing, and edematous areas, automated segmentation of tumours is a complicated task. Convolutional neural networks (CNNs) have been utilized as the dominant deep learning method for segmentation tasks. However, they suffer from the inability to capture and learn long-range dependencies and global features due to their limited kernels. Vision transformers (ViTs) were introduced recently to tackle these limitations. Although ViTs are capable of capturing long-range features, their segmentation performance falls as the variety of tumour sizes increases. In this matter, ViT's patch size plays a significant role in the learning process of a network, and finding an optimal patch size is a challenging and time-consuming task. In this paper, we propose a framework to find the optimal ViT patch size for the brain tumour segmentation task, particularly for segmenting smaller tumours. We validated our proposed framework on the BraTS'21 dataset. Our proposed framework, could improve the segmentation dice performance for 0.97%, 1.14%, and 2.05% for enhancing tumour, tumour core, and whole tumour, respectively, in comparison with default ViT (ViT-base). This research lays the groundwork for future research on the semantic segmentation of tumour segmentation and detection using vision transformer-based networks for optimal outcomes. The implementation source code is available at: https://github.com/Ramtin-Mojtahedi/BRATS_OVTPS.

Keywords: MRI Segmentation · Vision Transformer · Brain Tumour

1 Introduction

Primary brain tumours are referred to as gliomas and are divided into several categories based on the cells believed to have originated them. These include

S. Bakas et al. (Eds.): BrainLes 2022, LNCS 13769, pp. 195–204, 2023.
https://doi.org/10.1007/978-3-031-33842-7_17

oligodendrogliomas, ependymomas, mixed gliomas, and astrocytic tumours (astrocytoma, anaplastic astrocytoma, and glioblastoma) [1]. The proper delineation and segmentation of brain tumours is a crucial step in determining their volume, shape, borders, and other features; hence, automated tumour segmentation is now the subject of extensive study to speed up the MRI analysis and enable doctors to accurately plan therapy [2–5]. In the BraTS'21 challenge, the enhancing tumour (ET), tumour core (TC), and whole tumour (WT) are the sub-regions that are taken into consideration for assessment. Areas in T1Gd that exhibit hyper-intensity both when compared to healthy white matter in T1Gd and to T1 when compared to T1 explain the ET. The TC defines the majority of the tumour, which is usually what is removed. The ET and the necrotic (NCR) areas of the tumour are included in the TC. When compared to T1, NCR often shows up as hypo-intense in T1-Gd. The TC and the peritumoural edematous or invading tissue, which is often represented by a hyper-intense signal in FLAIR, are included in the WT, which reflects the whole extent of the illness [6].

In recent years, meachine learning (ML) methods have been utilized in brain tumour diagnosis where convolutional neural networks (CNNs) and vision transformers (ViTs) are the two main segmentation methods that have been widely used on this matter [7]. CNN-based networks have been introduced ahead of ViTs and have shown promised performance on a variety of medical image segmentation tasks since the introduction of the ground-breaking U-shaped encoder-decoder topology, known as U-Net [8,9]. The U-Net is a highly supervised encoder-decoder network in which dense, layered skip connections bridge the encoder and decoder components of the network. There are many degrees of freedom involved with adapting the U-Net to new issues in terms of the network's architecture, pre-processing, training, and assessment. These hyperparameters are interconnected and significantly affect the outcome. Later, Zhang et al. introduced RESUNET, which is a backboned U-Net structure equipped with residual blocks. Utilizing residual blocks allows the development of a deeper network without having to worry about vanishing or exploding gradient issues. It also makes network training simple. Rich skip connections in the RESUNET also facilitate better information flow across layers, which facilitates better gradient flow during training (backpropagation) [10]. Another powerful CNN-based network was introduced by Zhou et al., known as UNet++. The proposed design is basically a deeply supervised encoder-decoder network where the encoder and decoder sub-networks are linked by a number of layered, dense skip connections. The semantic gap between the feature maps of the encoder and decoder sub-networks is intended to be closed by the newly developed skip connections [9]. To overcome these restrictions by manual setting up Un-Net-based networks, Isensee et al. [11] developed the nnU-Net architecture. Their proposed network is a deep learning-based segmentation technique that adapts automatically to every new segmentation task, including preprocessing, network design, training, and post-processing. The main design decisions in this process are modelled as a set of fixed parameters, interdependent rules, and empirical choices.

The above-mentioned fully convolutional networks are efficient. However, they perform poorly when learning global features and long-range spatial dependencies as a result of their limited kernel size and receptive fields [12]. ViT was introduced by Dosovitsky et al. and utilized in the computer vision tasks inspired by their high performance in the language domain. ViTs are able to resolve CNN's localized learning with their capability in learning long-range dependencies, and self-attention mechanism [13]. ViT-based models provide meaningful results while using less processing power throughout the training phase as compared to cutting-edge convolutional networks. As one of the most effective transformer-based networks, Hatamizadeh et al. [14] developed UNEt TRansformers (UNETR). In their proposed network a transformer is used as the encoder in a U-Net-based architecture to learn sequence representations of the input volumes. In order to predict the segmentation outputs, the extracted features from the transformer encoder are combined with the CNN-based decoder using skip connections. Their proposed network employs an isotropic network architecture with fixed-size feature resolutions and an unchangeable embedding size while achieving state-of-the-art performance in 3D volumetric segmentation. On the other hand, UNETR is unable to perform computations at various resolutions or provide context at various sizes. Although their suggested network would be successful at segmenting large objects, it can't show the same level of performance without using an optimal patch size when segmenting small objects, such as tiny tumours.

Accordingly, the primary objective of this study was to propose a framework to find an optimal patch size for ViTs to improve their performance, particularly in segmenting small brain tumours. Particularly, we designed a framework backed by the UNETR architecture to achieve higher segmentation performance based on the average tumour volumes. We validated our proposed framework on the glioma sub-regions available in BraTS'21 dataset, as shown in Fig. 1.

2   Method

2.1   ViT Structure

The input image is divided into equal-sized patches in the ViT transformer architecture, and a sequence of linear embeddings of these patches is passed to the vanilla transformer. These image patches are processed and work similarly to the tokens used in natural language processing (NLP). Using a 1D series of input embeddings, the transformer's function [14]. The 3D input images are also translated to 1D embedding vectors. The 3D input images are also translated to 1D embedding vectors. The 3D medical images are presented in the framework being used with an input size of (X, Y, Z). In addition, the transformer patches are represented as P. In this way, the size of the flattened uniform sequences being constructed $U = (X, Y, Z)/(P \times P \times P)$ using nonoverlapping patches that are shown with $y_v \in R^{U \times P^3}$.

To preserve the spatial details of the recovered patches, the projected patch embeddings are supplemented by 1D learnable positional embeddings

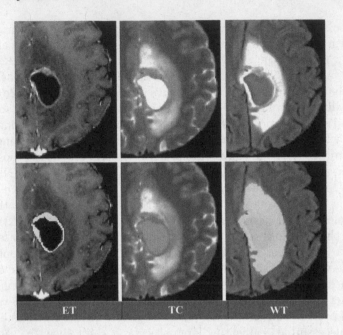

Fig. 1. Glioma sub-regions, including Enhancing Tumour (ET), Tumour Core (TC), and Whole Tumour (WT).

($\mathbf{E}_{pos} \in R^{U \times T}$) with T dimensional embedding size. The details of the transformer's multi-headed self-attention (MSA) and multilayer perceptron (MLP) blocks can be found in [15].

2.2   Model Pipeline

The backbone framework that we used for our experiments, UNETR, uses a contracting-expanding pattern with a stack of transformers, ViT, as the encoder, and skips connections to the decoder. As discussed in [8], Its decoder extracts different representations of the input images, with the size of the image divided by the patch size multiplied by the transformer's embedding size. In addition, a deconvolutional layer was added to the transformer's final layer to convert the feature map and double its resolution. The enlarged feature map is then concatenated with the feature map from the previous transformer output and fed into three successive $3 \times 3 \times 3$ convolutional layers, followed by a deconvolutional layer to upsample the output. This procedure is continued for all consecutive layers until the original input resolution is reached. At this point, the final output is fed into a $1 \times 1 \times 1$ convolutional layer with a SoftMax activation function to predict segmented objects.

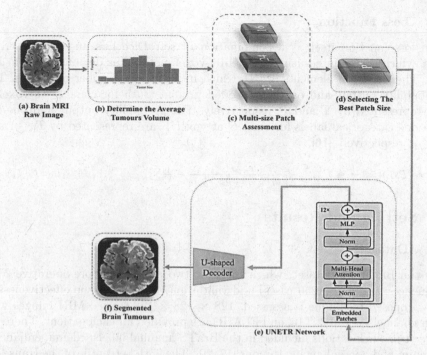

Fig. 2. The model pipeline for the suggested framework is shown. The framework receives the raw 3MRI images of the brain in step (a). The average volume is then calculated in step (b). The three determined patch sizes $P \in [16, 24, 32]$ and the evaluation of the averaged tumour volume led to the selection of the optimal patch size in steps (c, d). To achieve segmented tumours in step (e), we train the model and segment it on our backboned UNETR network (f).

Choosing an effective patch size is critical due to its impact on the features' receptive field and spatial information. As discussed, selecting an optimal patch size $(P*)$ impacts the extracted features, which are reshaped into a tensor with the size of $\frac{X}{P*} \times \frac{Y}{P*} \times \frac{Z}{P*} \times E$, where E is the transformer's embedding size. This significantly impacts on the performance of the network on segmenting brain tumours.

The suggested framework looks for the ideal patch size for the segmentation task. As shown in Fig. 2, the average tumour volume is first calculated using the supplied input. Then, based on an experimentally discovered non-linear connection between the average tumour volume size and the performance, the best patch size is chosen. This guarantees that the model operates at its peak level when segmenting brain tumours. Patch size were selected based on our available computational resources and the resolutions introduced in [13].

2.3   Loss Function

The loss function itself is a combination of soft Dice loss and cross-entropy loss, which is computed using a voxel-by-voxel method, as demonstrated in Eq. (1). The employed elements are D, which indicates the number of classes. The probability output and one-hot encoded ground truth for class C at voxel V are represented by T and P, respectively. The probability output and one-hot encoded categorical labels for class C at voxel V are represented by $T_{K,M}$, and $P_{K,M}$, respectively [16].

$$Loss(P,T) = 1 - \frac{2}{C} \sum_{M=1}^{C} \frac{\Sigma_{K=1}^{V} P_{K,M} T_{K,M}}{\Sigma_{K=1}^{V} P_{K,M}^2 + \Sigma_{K=1}^{V} T_{K,M}^2} - \frac{1}{V} \sum_{K=1}^{V} \sum_{M=1}^{C} P_{K,M} log(T_{K,M}) \quad (1)$$

3   Setting and Results

3.1   Datasets

On the BraTS'21 dataset, which includes two datasets of pre-operative MRI sequences: training (1250 cases) and validation (219 cases), the effectiveness of the proposed technique is assessed. 128 × 128 × 128 resized MRI images with four channels (T1, T2, T1c, and FLAIR) are provided for each patient. There are three tumour locations included in the BraTS' manual labels: edema, enhancing tumour, and non-enhancing tumour [17–20]. The 95th percentile of the Hausdorff Distance (HD95) and the Dice Similarity Coefficient (DSC) are metrics to assess the segmentation performance in BraTS'21.

3.2   Setup and Experimental Results

Table 1 illustrates the parameters and pre-processing techniques we employed to conduct the experiments. The parameters used for the ViT network were selected based on the ViT-Base discussed in [13]. We also ran the experiments with various input image sizes and discovered that cropping the input images to the size of 128 × 128 × 128 generates the best results compatible with our computational resources. For all experiments, the training and validation split ratio considered as 80:20.

The model's performance results were achieved for the training dataset based on 1-fold cross validation for the training data. The dice similarity coefficient (DSC) and loss function, which were defined in Eq. (1), were used to judge how well the model worked for tumour segmentation. The results for the training data are shown in Table 2.

Table 3 shows the results for the validation dataset based on the given submission to Synapse. The results are provided for the metrics of dice: Hausdorff distance 95 (HD95), precision, sensitivity, and specificity.

As shown in Table 2 and Table 3, the best performance results focusing on the average training and validation results of the smaller tumours were achieved for the patch size of 24. The average volume size of tumours in the training dataset is 14814.9 mm^3 for the TC, 60262.8 mm^3 for the WT, and 22028.4 mm^3 for the

Table 1. Specifications of the utilized parameters and pre-processing techniques.

Parameter	Description of the Value/Method
Input Image Size [X × Y × Z]	[240 × 240 × 155]
Optimizer	Adam
[Learning Rate, Weight_Decay]	[0.0001, 1e−5]
Spacing Transformation [mm³]	1 × 1 × 1
Other Transformations	Random Flip, Normalizing Intensity, Intensity Shifting, Background Removal
ViT Layers	12
ViT Hidden Size	768
ViT MLP Size	3072
ViT Heads	12
ViT Number of Parameters	86 M
Batch Size	1
Computational Resource	NVIDIA A100 – 40 GB
Training Epochs	20
Evaluation	Every 2 Epochs
Validation/Training Split Ratio	1-Fold Cross-validation

Table 2. Segmentation results for the training dataset.

Patch Size	Dice TC [%]	Dice WT [%]	Dice ET [%]	Ave. Dice [%]	Loss Value	Training Time [Min.]
16	71.96	79.16	77.32	76.14	0.38	186.26
24	**73.8**	**80.45**	**79.23**	**77.83**	**0.37**	**266.6**
32	73.37	80.49	79.47	77.91	0.36	334.70

Table 3. Segmentation results for the validation dataset.

Patch Size	Dice [%]			Sensitivity [%]			Specificity [%]			HD95		
	ET	WT	TC	ET	WT	TC	ET	WT	TC	ET	WT	TC
16	67.62	79.34	67.77	68.69	80.96	68.83	99.96	99.84	99.93	51.32	41.03	34.96
24	**68.59**	**80.48**	**69.82**	67.58	**79.02**	**71.03**	**99.97**	79.02	**99.93**	**44.08**	**34.72**	**26.88**
32	68.84	80.45	69.52	70.57	82.67	72.5	99.96	9.84	99.92	47.46	38.8	31.69

ET, with an average of 32368.7 mm³ and an average of 18421.65 mm³ for the smaller tumours of the TC and ET, respectively. Empirically and with respect to the mentioned average volume sizes, the relationship between optimal patch size (P^*) and the averaged volume size of the tumours is attained as Eq. (2), where P is the patch size, V is the voxel spacing (1 mm³), and S is the averaged volume size of tumours for brain tumours. Finding the patch with the squared difference of a voxel's cube root and the average volume size of tumours results in the optimal patch.

$$P^* = \operatorname*{Argmin}_{S \in [16,24,32]} (|\sqrt[3]{S \times V} - P|) \tag{2}$$

The achieved results are aligned with the proposed framework, as the patch size of 24 minimizes the proposed formula introduced in Eq. (2) by focusing on smaller tumours as the most challenging part of the segmentation tasks and corroborating the proposed framework. An example of the predicted results is shown in Fig. 3.

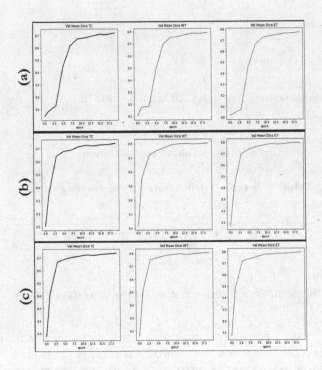

Fig. 3. Comparing Dice scores for three patch sizes experimented for three nested tumours of TC, WT, and ET, including (a) with patch size of 16, (b) with patch size of 24, and (c) with patch size of 32.

4   Discussion and Conclusion

This paper proposed a framework backboned by the UNETR network to find an optimal patch size for semantic segmentation of brain glioma tumors. Our proposed framework detects the optimal patch size for the vanilla vision transformer based on the average volume size of the three subtypes of tumours, ET, WT, and TC. Among the experimented patch sizes and using the proposed framework in

Eq. (1), the patch size of 24 ($P^* = 24$) achieved the best results focusing on the smaller tumours of ET and WT, which are more difficult to be segmented compared to the larger tumours of WT, when we assess it compared to the average of tumours with respect to the achieved average results both on the training, as shown in Fig. 3, and validation results. To elaborate, Our proposed framework with the achieved optimal patch size of 24, could improve the segmentation dice performance for 0.97%, 1.14%, and 2.05% for enhancing tumour, tumour core, and whole tumour, respectively, in comparison with default ViT (ViT-base) with patch size of 16. Through assessing the overall results, WT achieves the best Dice performance, which is aligned with our expectations due to its larger surface compared to ET and TC. The same patterns were observed for other metrics in Hausdorff distance, specificity, and sensitivity. The findings of this research could be used as a backbone for the development of multi-patch vision transformer-based networks and finding optimal patch sizes for vision transformers.

References

1. Banu, Z.: Glioblastoma multiforme: a review of its pathogenesis and treatment. Int. Res. J. Pharm. **9**, 7–12 (2019)
2. Ribalta Lorenzo, P., et al.: Segmenting brain tumors from FLAIR MRI using fully convolutional neural networks. Comput. Methods Programs Biomed. **176**, 135–148 (2019)
3. Soleymanifard, M., Hamghalam, M.: Multi-stage glioma segmentation for tumour grade classification based on multiscale fuzzy C-means. Multimedia Tools Appl. **81**, 8451–8470 (2022)
4. Hamghalam, M., Lei, B., Wang, T.: Brain tumor synthetic segmentation in 3D multimodal MRI scans. In: Crimi, A., Bakas, S. (eds.) BrainLes 2019. LNCS, vol. 11992, pp. 153–162. Springer, Cham (2020). https://doi.org/10.1007/978-3-030-46640-4_15
5. Hamghalam, M., Lei, B., Wang, T.: Convolutional 3D to 2D patch conversion for pixel-wise glioma segmentation in MRI scans. In: Crimi, A., Bakas, S. (eds.) BrainLes 2019. LNCS, vol. 11992, pp. 3–12. Springer, Cham (2020). https://doi.org/10.1007/978-3-030-46640-4_1
6. Menze, B.H., Jakab, A., Bauer, S., Kalpathy-Cramer, J., Farahani, K., Kirby, J., et al.: The multimodal brain tumor image segmentation benchmark (BRATS). IEEE Trans. Med. Imaging **34**(10), 1993–2024 (2015). https://doi.org/10.1109/TMI.2014.2377694
7. Akinyelu, A.A., Zaccagna, F., Grist, J.T., Castelli, M., Rundo, L.: Brain tumor diagnosis using machine learning, convolutional neural networks, capsule neural networks and vision transformers, applied to MRI: a survey. J. Imaging **8**, 205 (2022)
8. Ronneberger, O., Fischer, P., Brox, T.: U-Net: convolutional networks for biomedical image segmentation. In: Navab, N., Hornegger, J., Wells, W.M., Frangi, A.F. (eds.) MICCAI 2015. LNCS, vol. 9351, pp. 234–241. Springer, Cham (2015). https://doi.org/10.1007/978-3-319-24574-4_28

9. Zhou, Z., Rahman Siddiquee, M.M., Tajbakhsh, N., Liang, J.: UNet++: a nested U-Net architecture for medical image segmentation. In: Stoyanov, D., et al. (eds.) DLMIA/ML-CDS -2018. LNCS, vol. 11045, pp. 3–11. Springer, Cham (2018). https://doi.org/10.1007/978-3-030-00889-5_1

10. Zhang, Z., Liu, Q., Wang, Y.: Road extraction by deep residual U-Net. IEEE Geosci. Remote Sens. Lett. **15**, 749–753 (2018)

11. Isensee, F., Jaeger, P.F., Kohl, S.A., Petersen, J., Maier-Hein, K.H.: nnU-Net: a self-configuring method for deep learning-based biomedical image segmentation. Nat. Methods **18**, 203–211 (2020)

12. Hu, H., Zhang, Z., Xie, Z., Lin, S.: Local relation networks for image recognition. In: 2019 IEEE/CVF International Conference on Computer Vision (ICCV) (2019)

13. Dosovitskiy, A., et al.: An image is worth 16×16 words: transformers for image recognition at scale. In: ICLR 2021 (2021)

14. Hatamizadeh, A., et al.: UNETR: transformers for 3D medical image segmentation. In: 2022 IEEE/CVF Winter Conference on Applications of Computer Vision (WACV) (2022)

15. Mojtahedi, R., Hamghalam, M., Do, R.K.G., Simpson, A.L.: Towards optimal patch size in vision transformers for tumor segmentation. In: Li, X., Lv, J., Huo, Y., Dong, B., Leahy, R.M., Li, Q. (eds.) MMMI 2022. LNCS, vol. 13594, pp. 110–120. Springer, Cham (2022). https://doi.org/10.1007/978-3-031-18814-5_11

16. Milletari, F., Navab, N., Ahmadi, S.-A.: V-net: fully convolutional neural networks for volumetric medical image segmentation. In: 2016 Fourth International Conference on 3D Vision (3DV) (2016)

17. Baid, U., et al.: The RSNA-ASNR-MICCAI BraTS 2021 benchmark on brain tumor segmentation and radiogenomic classification. arXiv:2107.02314 (2021)

18. Bakas, S., Akbari, H., Sotiras, A., Bilello, M., Rozycki, M., Kirby, J.S., et al.: Advancing the cancer genome atlas glioma MRI collections with expert segmentation labels and radiomic features. Nat. Sci. Data **4**, 170117 (2017). https://doi.org/10.1038/sdata.2017.117

19. Bakas, S., Akbari, H., Sotiras, A., Bilello, M., Rozycki, M., Kirby, J., et al.: Segmentation labels and radiomic features for the pre-operative scans of the TCGA-GBM collection. The Cancer Imaging Archive (2017). https://doi.org/10.7937/K9/TCIA.2017.KLXWJJ1Q

20. Bakas, S., Akbari, H., Sotiras, A., Bilello, M., Rozycki, M., Kirby, J., et al.: Segmentation labels and radiomic features for the pre-operative scans of the TCGA-LGG collection. The Cancer Imaging Archive (2017). https://doi.org/10.7937/K9/TCIA.2017.GJQ7R0EF

Brain Tumor Segmentation Using Neural Ordinary Differential Equations with UNet-Context Encoding Network

M. S. Sadique⬤, M. M. Rahman⬤, W. Farzana⬤, A. Temtam⬤,
and K. M. Iftekharuddin^(✉)⬤

Old Dominion University, Norfolk, VA 23529, USA
{msadi002,mrahm006,wfarz001,atemt001,kiftekha}@odu.edu
https://sites.wp.odu.edu/VisionLab/

Abstract. Glioblastoma Multiforme (GBM) are the most aggressive brain tumor types and because of their heterogeneity in shape and appearance, their segmentation becomes a challenging task. Automated brain tumor segmentation using Magnetic Resonance Imaging (MRI) plays a key role in disease diagnosis, surgical planning, and brain tumor tracking. Medical image segmentation using deep learning-based U-Net architectures are the state-of-the-art. Despite their improved performance, these architectures require optimization for each segmentation task. Introducing a continuous depth learning with context encoding in deep CNN models for semantic segmentation enable 3D image analysis quantifications in many applications. In this work, we propose Neural Ordinary Differential Equations (NODE) with 3D UNet-Context Encoding (UNCE), a continuous depth deep learning network for improved brain tumor segmentation. We showed that these NODEs can be implemented within the U-Net framework to improve segmentation performance. This year we participated for the Brain Tumor Segmentation (BraTS) continuous evaluation and our model was trained using the same MRI image sets of RSNA-ASNR-MICCAI Brain Tumor Segmentation (BraTS) Challenge 2021. Our model is evaluated on unseen hold-out data included i) the BraTS 2021 Challenge test data, ii) SSA adult patient populations of brain diffuse glioma (Africa-BraTS), and iii) from another independent pediatric population of diffuse intrinsic pontine glioma (DIPG) patients. The mean DSC for the BraTS test dataset are: 0.797797 (ET), 0.825647 (TC) and 0.894891 (WT) respectively. For the Africa-BraTS dataset the performance of our model improves which indicating the generalizability of our model to new, out-of-sample populations for adult brain tumor cases.

Keywords: Glioblastoma · Brain Tumor Segmentation · Neural Ordinary Differential Equations · Deep neural network · U-Net

S. Bakas et al. (Eds.): BrainLes 2022, LNCS 13769, pp. 205–215, 2023.
https://doi.org/10.1007/978-3-031-33842-7_18

1   Introduction

High-grade gliomas with grade III and IV according to World Health Organization (WHO) are the most aggressive and severe malignant brain tumors of the central nervous system (CNS) in adults, with extreme intrinsic heterogeneity in appearance, shape, and histology [1]. Patients diagnosed with the most aggressive type of brain tumor have a median survival time of two years or less [2]. The precise and robust segmentation of brain tumors and the prediction of the patient's overall survival are the basis for subsequent clinical steps and supportive for improving the treatment possibilities of the disease [3]. Conventional segmentation models based on clinical information and handcrafted features from multi-modal (MRI) neuroimaging are time-consuming, may be inaccurate due to human error, and also require anatomical knowledge. The manual extraction of handcrafted features is based on the prior knowledge of disease and can also be limited to the existing imaging techniques. This often limits the ability to take full advantage of all rich information embedded in the multi-modal (MRI) neuroimages for the brain tumor segmentation [4,5].

Automatic brain tumor segmentation is a difficult task. Compared to the classical hand-crafted feature extraction methods, deep learning models can learn a hierarchy of features that could represent the rich embedded information as hierarchical abstraction at many different levels [6–9]. In addition, the robustness in performance remains an open and difficult challenge in deep learning based models. Recent studies have shown that deep learning tools for brain tumor segmentation have been developed and achieved a better performance compared to classical models [3,10–13]. The current state-of-the-art for the medical image segmentation models are deep learning-based networks that follow U-Net architecture [14]. These models have made it feasible to build large-scale trainable models with a large number of receptive field at high computational cost of millions of parameters. To achieve reasonable performance, these models often require adding layers to increase the receptive field which comes at the cost of more parameters, computation, and memory requirements. It is a very challenging task to optimize deep learning models for every segmentation task. Therefore, proper regularization and hyper-parameter tuning are required for developing an efficient deep learning network.

In the previous BraTS challenge we implemented context encoding [15] with deep CNN models which have shown promise for semantic segmentation of brain tumors due to improved representative feature learning. We propose to use a continuous depth deep learning model called Neural Ordinary Differential Equations (NODEs) [16,17] within UNet-Context Encoding (UNCE) [18] framework for automatic brain tumor segmentation. We implemented this technique on the BraTS 2022 challenge datasets. Our model performance indicates that these NODEs can be used within U-Net framework to improve the segmentation results.

2   Method

2.1   Datasets

For training and validation data for the BraTS 2022 challenge, we use the same datasets provided by the RSNA-ASNR-MICCAI Brain Tumor Segmentation (BraTS) Challenge 2021 dataset obtained from multiple different institutions under standard clinical conditions [1]. In the BraTS Challenge 2022 Task, a total of 1251 cases with voxel-level annotations of different tumor sub-tissues: necrotic (NC), peritumoral edema (ED), and enhancing tumor (ET) are presented.

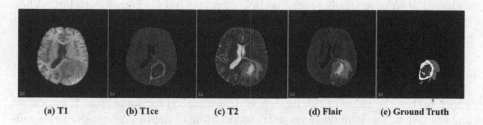

| (a) T1 | (b) T1ce | (c) T2 | (d) Flair | (e) Ground Truth |

Fig. 1. Examples of four different MRI modalities: (a) T1, (b) T2, (c) T1ce, (d) FLAIR of a training sample with Ground Truth.

For online evaluation in the validation phase, there are 219 cases provided without any associated ground truth. Ground truth annotations of every tumor sub-region for brain tumor segmentation were approved by expert neuroradiologists [19–22]. Each patient case has four MRI modalities: T1-weighted (T1), T1-weighted contrast enhancement (T1ce), T2-weighted (T2), and T2-weighted fluid-attenuated inversion recovery (T2- FLAIR). All modality sequences are co-registered, skull-stripped, denoised, and bias-corrected [23]. Figure 1 shows an example from training cases of four MRI modalities (T1, T1ce, T2 and FLAIR).

2.2   UNCE-NODE Network

Neural-ODEs: Approximation of the derivative of any differentiable function using neural network provides more flexibility in the data modeling process. Residual neural networks appear to follow the modeling pattern of an ODE: namely that the continuous relationship is modeled at the level of the derivative. This is the main idea of neural ODEs: a chain of residual blocks in a neural network is basically a solution of the ODE with the Euler method. Euler's method is a discretization of the continuous relationship between the input and output domains of the data. Neural networks are also discretization of this continuous relationship, only the discretization is through hidden states in a latent space. Residual neural networks create a pathway through this latent space by allowing states to depend directly on each other, just like the updates in Euler's method.

Considering a neural network where the hidden states all have the same dimension. Each hidden state depends on a neural layer, $\mathbf{f}$, which itself depends on parameters θ_t, where t is the layer depth. Then

$$h_{t+1} = f(h_t, \theta_t) \tag{1}$$

If we have residual network, then this looks

$$h_{t+1} = h_t + f(h_t, \theta_t) \tag{2}$$

where $t \in \{0...T\}, h_t \in \mathbb{R}^d$, and f a differentiable function. In ResNets, $\mathbf{f}$ consists of several convolutional layers. The update with residual $f(h_t)$ can be seen as a $\Delta t = 1$ step of an Euler discretization of a continuous transformation. When we let $\Delta t \rightarrow 0$ we take more, smaller steps using more layers, which in the limit becomes an ordinary differential equation (ODE), specified by a neural network:

$$\lim_{\Delta t \rightarrow 0} = \frac{h_{t+\Delta t} - h_t}{\Delta t} = \frac{\delta h_t}{\delta t} = f(h(t), t, \theta) \tag{3}$$

where $h(t)$ is the value of the hidden state evaluated for some time t, which we understand as a continuous parametrization of layer depth. We consider the continuous limit of each discrete layer in the network. Instead of a discrete number of layers between the input and output domains, we allow the progression of the hidden states to become continuous.

A neural network is a differentiable function, so we can train it with gradient-based optimization routines. Ordinary Differential Equations (ODE) can be solved using standard ODE solvers such as Runge-Kutta [24, 25]. Since the model is a learnable ODE, we use an ODE solver to evolve the input to an output in the forward pass and calculate a loss. In particular, for weight updating during back propagation, we need a gradient of loss function by the input and the dynamics parameters. Unfortunately, during the forward pass an ODE solver might require hundreds of function evaluations, which may lead to exploding memory requirements. The mathematical trick to retrieve the gradient of the Neural ODE loss with respect to the network parameters by solving another ODE backwards in time, sidestepping the need to store intermediate function evaluations, is called adjoint sensitivity method (for more details see Algorithm 1 in Chen et al., 2018 [17]).

The advantages and motivation to use NODE networks for semantic segmentation are: They are memory efficient given intermediate computations (e.g. activation maps), so we don't need to store all the parameters and gradients while back propagating. Adaptive computation: we can balance speed and accuracy with the discretization scheme, moreover, having it different while training and inference. Parameter efficiency: the parameters of nearby "layers" are automatically tied together.

In this work, we have implemented a continuous depth deep neural network within an UNCE network framework that integrates multiple volumetric MRI processing tasks. Inspired by the work of context encoding networks [13], the UNCE architecture is substantially augmented for brain tumor segmentation.

Two models (a) UNCE deep learning-baseline and (b) UNCE deep learning with NODE for tumor segmentation are trained using the BraTS 2021 challenge datasets. The overall pipeline for the brain tumor segmentation using UNCE-NODE is shown in Fig. 2. The UNCE captures global texture features using a semantic loss to provide regularization in training. The architecture consists of encoding, context encoding, and decoding modules. The encoding module extracts high-dimensional features of the input. The context encoding module produces updated features and a semantic loss to regularize the model by ensuring all segmentation classes are represented. The decoding module reconstructs the feature maps to produce segmentation masks as output. UNCE-Neural ODEs present a new architecture with much potential for reducing parameter and memory costs, improving the performance. Figure 2 below shows the architecture of the 3D UNCE-baseline and UNCE-NODE models and its different components. The U-Net architecture consists of a contracting and an expanding path that aims to build a bottleneck in its innermost part through a combination of convolution, instance norm, and softmax operations. After this bottleneck, the image is reconstructed by combining convolutions and upsampling.

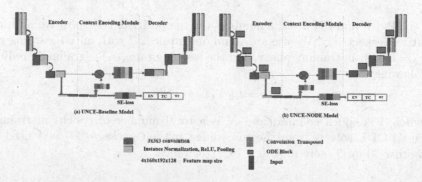

Fig. 2. The Brain Tumor Segmentation pipeline. (a) UNCE-Baseline and (b) UNCE-NODE are fully automatic, end-to-end deep learning pipelines that segment brain tumor sub-regions from 3D MRI across different modalities.

Implementation: To justify the heterogeneity of the medical field, all images are resampled to the same target spacing. The MRI scans provided for the competition are co-registered, skull-stripped, denoised and bias corrected. Since the dataset was collected from different institutions and MRI scanners, the intensities show substantial variations across examples. Consequently, we perform normalization of all examples to have zero mean and unit standard deviation. The dimension of each training sample is $240 \times 240 \times 155$. The size of the images is reduced by cropping to a size of $192 \times 160 \times 128$ to manage computational memory and cost. To generate additional training images, we augment data by adding uniform white noise with limited amplitude. A critical feature of the proposed UNCE is the context encoding module, which computes scaling factors related to the representation of all classes. These factors are learned simultaneously in the training phase via the semantic loss error regularization, defined by L_{se}. The scaling factors capture global information of all classes, essentially learning to mitigate the training bias that may arise due to imbalanced class representation in data. To calculate the Semantic Error loss (SE-loss), we construct another fully connected layer with a sigmoid activation function upon the encoding layer, to predict object classification in the image [13]. Accordingly, the final loss function consists of 2 terms:

$$L = L_{dice} + L_{se} \tag{4}$$

where L_{dice} is a Dice calculated by the difference between prediction and ground truth, and L_{se} is the sematic loss. Dice loss is computed as:

$$L_{dice} = 1 - DSC \tag{5}$$

where DSC is dice similarity coefficient [26]. The DSC is defined as,

$$DSC = \frac{2TP}{FP + 2TP + FN} \tag{6}$$

where TP, FP and FN are the numbers of true positive, false positive and false negative, respectively. We use an Adam optimizer [27] with initial learning rate of $lr_0 = 0.0001$ in training phase, and the learning rate (lr_i) is gradually reduced by following:

$$lr_i = lr_0 \star (1 - \frac{i}{N})^{0.9} \tag{7}$$

where i is epoch counter, and N is a total number of epochs in training. We used ODE solvers from the torchdiffeq python package [17] and used the fifth-order "dopri5" solver, with a 10^{-3} tolerance.

Table 1. Network configurations for UNCE for the BraTS 2022 Challenge Dataset

Parameters	UNCE-Baseline	UNCE-NODE
Target spacing (mm):	$1 \times 1 \times 1$	$1 \times 1 \times 1$
Median image shape: at target spacing	$240 \times 240 \times 155$	$240 \times 240 \times 155$
Patch size:	$192 \times 160 \times 128$	$192 \times 160 \times 128$
Batch size:	2	2
Downsampling strides:	[2, 2, 2]	[2, 2, 2]
Convolution kernel sizes:	[3, 3, 3]	[3, 3, 3]
ODE Block:	No	Yes

Table 1 represents the variants of UNCE network configuration for the Brain Tumor Segmentation (BraTS) 2022 challenge. In the following sections, we summarized the detailed information for the implementation of UNCE network.

We implement the context-aware deep learning network in PyTorch and train the network on an NVIDIA V100 HPC platform using the BraTS training dataset (1251 cases). To train the network, we randomly split the dataset with 80% of data for training and the remaining 20% of the data for validating the trained model. All configurations of UNCE are trained for 300 epochs and the best performing versions based on the validation set are retained for testing. Effective training of the network is observed by the monotonically decreasing loss and the corresponding increase in training dice score. Images are predicted by using the best performing version of the trained model. Once the network is fully trained, the performance of the network is evaluated using the BraTS 2022 validation dataset (219 cases) utilizing the online submission process made available by the challenge organizers. Figure 3 presents an example segmented tumor and the corresponding ground truth of T2 images.

3 Results

The 1251 cases for the brain tumor segmentation task are used for training each configuration of UNCE models. We used the best performing UNCE models using the training dataset provided by the Brain Tumor Segmentation (BraTS) Challenge 2022 organizer to predict the validation cohort.

Table 2. Online Evaluation on Validation dataset(219 cases)

Model	Statistical parameter	Dice Score			Hausdorff95		
		ET	TC	WT	ET	TC	WT
UNCE-Baseline	Mean	0.7810	0.8244	0.9095	15.2337	12.6095	4.5294
	std	0.2389	0.2431	0.0846	65.2718	50.1448	7.6226
	Median	0.8590	0.9255	0.9382	2.2360	2.2360	2.8284
	25quantile	0.7844	0.8300	0.8939	1.4142	1.4142	1.7320
	75quantile	0.9055	0.9554	0.9534	3.09331	5.9154	4.2426
UNCE-NODE	Mean	0.8008	0.8500	0.9108	19.6636	6.9889	4.2722
	std	0.2253	0.2006	0.0748	77.3861	26.3836	5.9913
	Median	0.8644	0.9283	0.9328	2	2.2360	2.4494
	25quantile	0.7983	0.8506	0.8920	1.4142	1.4142	1.7320
	75quantile	0.9091	0.9571	0.9520	3	5	4.3155

We generated the segmented mask from different variants of UNCE configurations and submitted for the online evaluation using the validation datasets. The online evaluation results with DSC and HD95 are reported in Table 2. The dice scores of the UNCE-NODE model are 0.8008, 0.8500, and 0.9108 for enhancing tumor (ET), tumor core (TC), and whole tumor (WT), respectively. The Hausdorff95 distances of the same model are 19.66 for ET, 6.98 for TC, and 4.27 for

Table 3. Online Evaluation on Testing dataset

Test Dataset	Dice Score			Hausdorff95		
	ET	TC	WT	ET	TC	WT
BraTS 2021	0.797797	0.825647	0.894891	23.70354	20.33859	6.05848
Africa-BraTS	0.817089	0.904995	0.944727	4.685421	3.460575	4.27374
DIPG	–	0.365294	0.835283	–	145.4344	9.215518

WT. The evaluation results show a further improvement of dice scores compared to the UNCE-baseline model.

In the testing phase, the unseen hold-out testing data included the BraTS 2021 Challenge test data, as well as new data from out-of-sample sources including i) an independent multi-institutional dataset covering underrepresented SSA adult patient populations of brain diffuse glioma (Africa-BraTS), and ii) from another independent pediatric population of diffuse intrinsic pontine glioma (DIPG) patients. According to the requirement of the challenge, we prepared a docker image of our model and our submitted docker image has been segmented all the unseen hold-out test examples. We have submitted our final model to evaluate the segmentation of the test dataset. The performance of mean dice score coef-ficient (DSC), and Hausdorff distance are shown in Table 3. The online evaluation shows that the average DSC of WT, ET and TC in the testing phase is closer to that of in the validation phase for the BraTS testing cohort. For the Africa-BraTS dataset the performance of our model improves. However, the dice score of the tumor core (TC) is very low for the DIPG dataset, which we believe there is domain shift in the data distribution between the source (BraTS) and target dataset (DIPG).

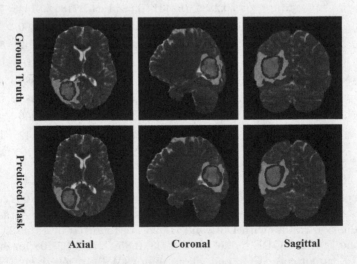

Fig. 3. T2 image overlaid with ground truth and predicted mask. From left to right: axial, coronal, and sagittal view respectively

Figure 3 shows the T2 MRI image overlaid with ground truth in the first row and predicted segmentation mask in the second row respectively for the same case.

4 Discussion

This manuscript explains the application of NODE within the UNCE framework in the Multi-Modality Brain Tumor Segmentation (BraTS) Challenge 2022. The UNCE-NODE model is evaluated on the unseen hold-out testing data included the BraTS 2021 Challenge test data, as well as new data from out-of-sample sources including i) Africa-BraTS, and ii) DIPG patients. For the Africa-BraTS dataset the performance of our model improves which indicating the generalizability of our model to new, out-of-sample populations for adult brain tumor cases. However, the dice score of the tumor core (TC) is very low for the DIPG dataset, which we believe there is domain shift in the data distribution between the source (BraTS) and target dataset (DIPG). It would be interesting, if we could apply domain adaptation with transfer learning approach to perform domain-invariant segmentation. Transfer learning and domain adaptation are both approaches that aim to improve the generalizability of models to a target domain that differs from the source domain on which the model was trained. In future work, we plan to investigate the generalizability of this approach to other age groups and data acquisition pipelines. We hope that this approach may be used to yield automated, objective assessments of age or domain varying patterns in other applications.

Acknowledgements. This work was partially funded through NIH/NIBIB grant under award number R01EB020683. The authors would like to acknowledge partial support of this work by the National Science Foundation Grant No. 1828593.

References

1. Baid, U., et al.: The RSNA-ASNR-MICCAI BraTS 2021 benchmark on brain tumor segmentation and radiogenomic classification. arXiv:2107.02314 (2021)
2. Ostrom, Q.T., Gittleman, H., Truitt, G., Boscia, A., Kruchko, C., Barnholtz-Sloan, J.S.: CBTRUS statistical report: primary brain and other central nervous system tumors diagnosed in the United States in 2011–2015. Neuro-Oncol. **20**(suppl-4), iv1–iv86 (2018)
3. Pereira, S., Pinto, A., Alves, V., Silva, C.A.: Brain tumor segmentation using convolutional neural networks in MRI images. IEEE Trans. Med. Imaging **35**(5), 1240–1251 (2016)
4. Pei, L., Vidyaratne, L., Monibor Rahman, M., Shboul, Z.A., Iftekharuddin, K.M.: Multimodal brain tumor segmentation and survival prediction using hybrid machine learning. In: Crimi, A., Bakas, S. (eds.) BrainLes 2019. LNCS, vol. 11993, pp. 73–81. Springer, Cham (2020). https://doi.org/10.1007/978-3-030-46643-5_7

5. Pei, L., et al.: Deep learning with context encoding for semantic brain tumor segmentation and patient survival prediction. In: Proceedings Volume 11314, Medical Imaging 2020: Computer-Aided Diagnosis; 113140H (2020). https://doi.org/10.1117/12.2550693

6. Mustaqeem, A., Javed, A., Fatima, T.: An efficient brain tumor detection algorithm using watershed & thresholding-based segmentation. Int. J. Image Graph. Sig. Process. 4(10), 34 (2012)

7. Pei, L., Vidyaratne, L., Hsu, W.-W., Rahman, M.M., Iftekharuddin, K.M.: Brain tumor classification using 3D convolutional neural network. In: Crimi, A., Bakas, S. (eds.) BrainLes 2019. LNCS, vol. 11993, pp. 335–342. Springer, Cham (2020). https://doi.org/10.1007/978-3-030-46643-5_33

8. Prastawa, M., Bullitt, E., Ho, S., Gerig, G.: A brain tumor segmentation framework based on outlier detection. Med. Image Anal. 8(3), 275–283 (2004)

9. Ho, S., Bullitt, E., Gerig, G.: Level-set evolution with region competition: automatic 3-D segmentation of brain tumors, p. 10532. Citeseer (2002)

10. Isensee, F., Jaeger, P.F., Kohl, S.A.A., Petersen, J., Maier-Hein, K.H.: nnU-Net: a self-configuring method for deep learning-based biomedical image segmentation. Nat. Methods 18(2), 203–211 (2021). Epub 7 Dec 2020. PMID: 33288961. https://doi.org/10.1038/s41592-020-01008-z

11. Isensee, F., Jäger, P.F., Kohl, S.A., Petersen, J., Maier-Hein, K.H.: Automated design of deep learning methods for biomedical image segmentation. arXiv preprint arXiv:1904.08128, 17 April 2019

12. Myronenko, A.: 3D MRI brain tumor segmentation using autoencoder regularization. In: Crimi, A., Bakas, S., Kuijf, H., Keyvan, F., Reyes, M., van Walsum, T. (eds.) BrainLes 2018. LNCS, vol. 11384, pp. 311–320. Springer, Cham (2019). https://doi.org/10.1007/978-3-030-11726-9_28

13. Pei, L., Vidyaratne, L., Rahman, M.M., et al.: Context aware deep learning for brain tumor segmentation, subtype classification, and survival prediction using radiology images. Sci. Rep. 10, 19726 (2020). https://doi.org/10.1038/s41598-020-74419-9

14. Ronneberger, O., Fischer, P., Brox, T.: U-Net: convolutional networks for biomedical image segmentation. In: Navab, N., Hornegger, J., Wells, W.M., Frangi, A.F. (eds.) MICCAI 2015. LNCS, vol. 9351, pp. 234–241. Springer, Cham (2015). https://doi.org/10.1007/978-3-319-24574-4_28

15. Zhang, H., et al.: Context encoding for semantic segmentation. In: Proceedings of the IEEE Conference on Computer Vision and Pattern Recognition, pp. 7151–7160 (2018)

16. Pinckaers, H., Litjens, G.: Neural ordinary differential equations for semantic segmentation of individual colon glands. arXiv preprint arXiv:1910.10470 (2019)

17. Chen, R.T.Q., et al.: Neural ordinary differential equations. In: Advances in Neural Information Processing Systems, vol. 31 (2018)

18. Rahman, M.M., Sadique, M.S., Temtam, A.G., Farzana, W., Vidyaratne, L., Iftekharuddin, K.M.: Brain tumor segmentation using UNet-context encoding network. In: Crimi, A., Bakas, S. (eds.) BrainLes 2021. LNCS, vol. 12962, pp. 463–472. Springer, Cham (2022). https://doi.org/10.1007/978-3-031-08999-2_40

19. Menze, B.H., et al.: The multimodal brain tumor image segmentation benchmark (BRATS). IEEE Trans. Med. Imaging 34(10), 1993–2024 (2014)

20. Bakas, S., Akbari, H., Sotiras, A., Bilello, M., Rozycki, M., Kirby, J.S., et al.: Advancing the cancer genome atlas glioma MRI collections with expert segmentation labels and radiomic features. Nat. Sci. Data 4, 170117 (2017). https://doi.org/10.1038/sdata.2017.117

21. Bakas, S., Akbari, H., Sotiras, A., Bilello, M., Rozycki, M., Kirby, J., et al.: Segmentation labels and radiomic features for the pre-operative scans of the TCGA-GBM collection. The Cancer Imaging Archive (2017). https://doi.org/10.7937/K9/TCIA.2017.KLXWJJ1Q

22. Bakas, S., Akbari, H., Sotiras, A., Bilello, M., Rozycki, M., Kirby, J., et al.: Segmentation labels and radiomic features for the pre-operative scans of the TCGA-LGG collection. The Cancer Imaging Archive (2017). https://doi.org/10.7937/K9/TCIA.2017.GJQ7R0EF

23. Liu, D., et al.: Imaging-genomics in glioblastoma: combining molecular and imaging signatures. Front. Oncol. **11**, 2666 (2021). https://www.frontiersin.org/article/10.3389/fonc.2021.699265

24. Runge, C.: Ueber die numerische Auflösung von Differentialgleichungen. Math. Ann. **46**, 167–178 (1895)

25. Kutta, W.: Beitrag zur näherungsweisen Integration totaler Differentialgleichungen. Zeitschrift für Mathematik und Physik **46**, 435–453 (1901)

26. Dice, L.R.: Measures of the amount of ecologic association between species. Ecology **26**(3), 297–302 (1945)

27. Kingma, D.P., Ba, J.: Adam: a method for stochastic optimization. In: International Conference on Learning Representations (ICLR) (2015)

An UNet-Based Brain Tumor Segmentation Framework via Optimal Mass Transportation Pre-processing

Jia-Wei Liao[1], Tsung-Ming Huang[2]($\boxtimes$)(iD), Tiexiang Li[3,4]($\boxtimes$), Wen-Wei Lin[5], Han Wang[3], and Shing-Tung Yau[6]

[1] Department of Computer Science and Information Engineering, National Taiwan University, Taipei 106, Taiwan
[2] Department of Mathematics, National Taiwan Normal University, Taipei 116, Taiwan
min@ntnu.edu.tw
[3] Nanjing Center for Applied Mathematics, Nanjing 211135, People's Republic of China
txli@seu.edu.cn
[4] School of Mathematics and Shing-Tung Yau Center, Southeast University, Nanjing 210096, People's Republic of China
[5] Department of Applied Mathematics, National Yang Ming Chiao Tung University, Hsinchu 300, Taiwan
[6] Department of Mathematics, Harvard University, Cambridge, USA

Abstract. This article aims to build a framework for MRI images of brain tumor segmentation using the deep learning method. For this purpose, we develop a novel 2-Phase UNet-based OMT framework to increase the ratio of brain tumors using optimal mass transportation (OMT). Moreover, due to the scarcity of training data, we change the density function by different parameters to increase the data diversity. For the post-processing, we propose an adaptive ensemble procedure by solving the eigenvectors of the Dice similarity matrix and choosing the result with the highest aggregation probability as the predicted label. The Dice scores of the whole tumor (WT), tumor core (TC), and enhanced tumor (ET) regions for online validation computed by Seg-ResUNet were 0.9214, 0.8823, and 0.8411, respectively. Compared with random crop pre-processing, OMT is far superior.

Keywords: Brain Tumor Segmentation · UNet · Optimal Mass Transportation · Density function · 2-Phase OMT framework

1 Introduction

For all kinds of complex problems in the natural sciences, engineering and biology, finance, medical imaging, and social sciences, statistical thinking is the most intuitive and direct. It is effective to explore new areas. However, the success of

S. Bakas et al. (Eds.): BrainLes 2022, LNCS 13769, pp. 216–228, 2023.
https://doi.org/10.1007/978-3-031-33842-7_19

statistical methods mainly relies on whether the distribution and representativeness of the sample data of the problem can fully reflect the overall trend of the solution to the complex problem. Generally speaking, if the sample data of the problem are biased, highly repeatable, under-represented, not normally or uniformly distributed, or the individual data are defective and destroy the collective performance, or it is difficult to collect sufficient samplings, scientists tend to resort to mathematical modeling for the underlying complex problems in order to avoid these issues.

The intuitive idea is to find numerical solutions directly to complex problems in irregular manifolds. If the numerical methods are feasible, they can directly turn into an effective software package. Conversely, if solving the complex problem directly on irregular manifolds is technically challenging, it is better to reduce the original problem to the one in the regular domain. That is, the irregular manifold should be parametrized by a regular domain. For parametrization, the regular 3D parametric domain can be a ball, an ellipsoid, a cube, or a cuboid. Moreover, in recent years, on 2D manifolds, there are conformal, quasi-conformal, or area-preserving parametrizations on discs or spheres [1], while on 3D manifolds, there are spherical, ellipsoidal, or cuboidal volume- or mass-preserving parametrizations [2]. Then we can find the optimal mass transportation (OMT) map that satisfies the minimal deformation on the set of volume- or mass-preserving mappings, which can be formulated as the classical optimal transport problem [3]. Once a mass-preserving optimal transportation mapping has been found between a 3D irregular manifold and a sphere or cube, a complex mathematical model on the irregular manifold domain can be converted into a mathematical model on a regular domain. If the model problem can be solved in the regular domain, then the numerical solution in the desired 3D irregular manifold can be obtained by using the inverse transform of the mass-preserving optimal transportation map.

The main task of this paper is to use the OMT theory combined with deep learning methods to segment brain tumors accurately for medical brain images. 2D and 3D medical images usually have high resolution. But due to the limitation of hardware equipment, most people use 2D images as input data, which may lead to discontinuities along the vertical direction and sawtooth or fault phenomenon as a result of simple stacking. Therefore, it is best to consider the 3D image as a whole to preserve global information. Specifically, we transform the irregular 3D parenchymal brain image into a $128 \times 128 \times 128$ cube by the OMT map and use the characteristics of OMT to design the appropriate density function to enlarge the possible tumor region. Furthermore, we can conveniently make data augmentations for the UNet architecture through the distribution of different density functions, effectively performing accurate segmentation for brain tumors.

The main contributions of this paper are twofold.

(1) The advantage of the OMT map between the brain image and the 128^3 cube can control the density of the possible tumor region and its surroundings so that the tumor region can be properly enlarged in the cube, which is very beneficial for the UNet in identifying and predicting labels. Furthermore, we

can make effective data augmentation through different density control to increase the robustness of the model. The mechanism of the mass-preserving one-to-one OMT map that we propose is unique, compared with other methods which use eight to eighteen 128^3 cubes to hold a brain image for the UNet prediction. Our method can completely skip the procedure of splicing the predictions after dividing them into blocks.

(2) The main motivation of this paper is to participate in the Brain Tumor Segmentation BraTS Challenge organized by the international medical organization MICCAI. The BraTS 2021 database [4–8] contains 1,251 brain image training sets and 219 validation sets. We compare various UNets, namely, Residual UNet [9], SegResNet [10], SwinUNETR [11], HarDNet-FCN [12,13], and find that SegResNet outperforms the others. Therefore, we adopt SegResNet and the combination of Dice loss and focal loss as the segmentation loss function. Moreover, the optimization algorithm for the SegResNet employed in our work is the popular stochastic gradient descent method with Adam acceleration, and with cosine decay learning rate. For the post-processing, we propose an adaptive ensemble procedure by solving the eigenvectors of the Dice similarity matrix and choosing the result with the highest aggregation probability as the predicted label. In particular, in the BraTS2021 Challenge, we have obtained Dice scores 0.9214, 0.8823, and 0.8411 for the online validation of the whole tumor (WT), the tumor core (TC) and the enhanced tumor (ET), respectively, which are highly competitive with the results of state-of-the-art methods [10–12] (see Table 2).

2   Methods

2.1   2-Phase UNet-Based Algorithm with Optimal Mass Transportation

A novel 2-Phase UNet-based algorithm combined with optimal mass transport (2P-UNetB-OMT) for the detection and segmentation of 3D brain tumors has been proposed in [14]. The 2P-UNetB-OMT algorithm with a density function transforms an irregular 3D brain image from magnetic resonance imaging (MRI) into a cube while preserving the local mass ratios between two domains and minimizing transport cost and distortion.

In Phase I, according to the normalized contrast-enhanced histogram equalization grayscale values of the FLAIR modality of a brain image, the associated density function $\rho_\gamma^1(v)$ at each vertex v belonging to the brain is defined as

$$\rho_\gamma^1(v) = \exp(\gamma \cdot \mathrm{HE}(I(v))), \tag{1}$$

where I is the FLAIR grayscale, HE is the contrast-enhanced histogram equalization that maps the grayscale to $[0,1]$, and $\gamma > 0$ is the hyper-parameter. Then, we compute OMT maps with density $\rho_\gamma^1(v)$ from 3D brain images to cubes ($128 \times 128 \times 128$ tensors), and the UNet-based model with these input tensors is used to train a model, called Model 1, to accurately detect the possible WT region.

In Phase II, the possible tumor regions of WT are expanded by m voxels with morphology dilation, denoted by $\mathbb{T}$ contained in mesh $\mathcal{M}$. Define a step-like function $\rho_\gamma^2(v)$ as

$$\rho_\gamma^2(v) = \begin{cases} \exp(\gamma \cdot \mathrm{HE}(I(v))), & \text{if } v \in \mathbb{T}, \\ 1.0, & \text{if } v \notin \mathbb{T}, \end{cases} \quad (2)$$

where γ is a real number between 1 and 2. Then, a new smooth density function $\widetilde{\rho}_\gamma^2(v)$ using the image filtering technique, i.e., by convolving $\rho_\gamma^2(v)$ in (2) with a $m \times m \times m$ blur box tensor, is constructed as follows:

$$\widetilde{\rho}_\gamma^2(v) = \rho_\gamma^2(v) \otimes \frac{\mathbb{1}_{m \times m \times m}}{m^3}. \quad (3)$$

The new OMT maps from 3D brain images to $128 \times 128 \times 128$ tensors can be constructed using density $\widetilde{\rho}_\gamma^2(v)$. The UNet-based model with new OMT tensors is applied to train a new model, called Model 2, to predict the WT, TC, and ET, respectively. The flow chart of the 2P-UNetB-OMT framework is shown in Fig. 1

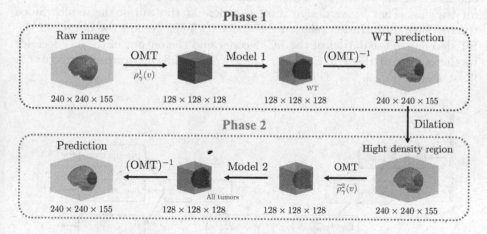

Fig. 1. A flow chart of 2P-UNetB-OMT framework.

2.2 Data Pre-processing

One of the advantages of the OMT maps is that we can transform a brain image into many different tensors by using various parameters γ. Based on the expanded WT region in Phase I, we compute OMT maps with smooth density functions $\widetilde{\rho}_\gamma^2(v)$ with $\gamma = 1.0, 1.5, 1.75,$ and 2.0 in (3) for n brain samples to obtain $4n$ augmented brain tensors to increase data diversity. To avoid over-fitting and enhance the robustness of a model, we apply the following data augmentation techniques to these $4n$ tensors, from which we choose n tensors to train the model:

- **Randomly flipping:** With probability 0.25, we flip the image left and right.
- **Randomly rotating:** With probability 0.25, we rotate the image counter-clockwise by 90°.
- **Randomly adjusting brightness:** With probability 0.1, we set the bright value range from 0.9 to 1.1 and modify the grayscale. Then we truncate the bright value to [0, 1] if necessary.
- **Randomly adding noise:** With probability 0.1, we add the Gaussian noise with a standard deviation of 0.01 to the grayscale image.
- **Normalized image:** We rescale the grayscale range to [0, 1] using Min-Max normalization.

2.3   Model Architecture

To predict the regions of WT, TC, and ET at the same time instead of one by one in Phase II, we develop a multi-head mechanism in the UNet-based model for training. That is, we design three decoders at the end of the model. Since tumors have an inclusion relation $ET \subseteq TC \subseteq WT$, we add the output of the ET decoder to the output of the TC decoder and the output of the TC decoder to the output of the WT decoder. The corresponding network architecture is illustrated in Fig. 2.

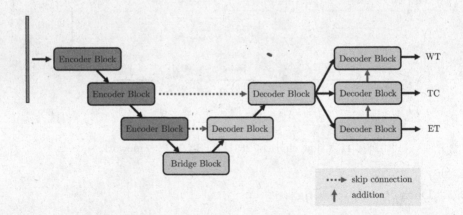

Fig. 2. Architecture of the multi-head mechanism.

The multi-head mechanism can be applied to Residual UNet, SegResNet, SwinUNETR, and HarDNet-FCN, which are the common UNet-based models. SegResNet uses residual blocks and includes normalization layers, ReLU layers, and convolution layers, each layer being used twice. The most significant difference with Residual UNet is that it uses trilinear interpolation as upsampling, which reduces the number of parameters to avoid over-fitting.

2.4 Loss Function

The segmentation task can be seen as pixel-wise classification. The most popular loss function in classification tasks is cross-entropy. However, if the cross-entropy is chosen for the segmentation task, it will suffer from a foreground and background imbalance problem; that is, the loss is small when the objective region is small. To deal with this issue, we adopt the combination of dice loss and focal loss as the segmentation loss. Let $P, G \in \mathbb{R}^{n \times m \times p \times q}$ be the prediction and ground truth, which are used as the following.

Dice Loss. The dice loss is based on the Dice similarity coefficient. Since we want the loss to be as small as possible, we define it as one minus the dice similarity coefficient, which ranges from 0 to 1. In addition, the prediction is a probability distribution. In the case of high-probability predictions and a label of one, the loss becomes small. Specifically, the Dice loss function is expressed as follows:

$$\mathcal{L}_{Dice}(P, G) = 1 - \frac{2 \sum_{i,j,k,c} P_{i,j,k,c} G_{i,j,k,c}}{\sum_{i,j,k,c} P_{i,j,k,c} + \sum_{i,j,k,c} G_{i,j,k,c}} \tag{4}$$

Focal Loss. The focal loss was proposed by Kaiming's team in 2017 [15]. Their team adjusts the cross-entropy by adding a coefficient that addresses the foreground and background imbalance problem. The focal loss is defined as

$$\mathcal{L}_{FL}(P, G) = - \sum_{i,j,k} \alpha \left(1 - P_{i,j,k,C}\right)^{\gamma} \log P_{i,j,k,C}, \tag{5}$$

where C is the category of $G_{i,j,k}$ and $\alpha, \gamma \geq 0$ are hyperparameters.

2.5 Optimization

The most important task in deep learning is updating parameters. Adam [16] is a stochastic optimization method that combines the advantage of Momentum and RMSprop, which is one of the most effective optimization algorithms for training. In addition, it incorporates the bias-correction mechanism.

To further improve results and make the model converge to the global minimum, we use the learning rate schedule. At the beginning of training, the warm-up method sets a lower learning rate to train some epochs. It is known that the deep learning model is very sensitive to the initial weights. So, if we choose a high learning rate, it may bring instability to the resulting model. The warm-up method can guarantee the gradual stabilization of the model at the beginning.

On the other hand, it accelerates the convergence of the model. Here, we adopt the following learning rate γ_t with the cosine decay and warm-up mechanism:

$$\gamma_t = \begin{cases} \frac{\gamma_{max}}{T_{warm}}t, & \text{if } t \leq T_{warm} \\ \gamma_{min} + \frac{1}{2}(\gamma_{max} - \gamma_{min})\left(1 + \cos\left(\frac{t-T_{warm}}{T-T_{warm}}\pi\right)\right), & \text{if } t > T_{warm} \end{cases}, \quad (6)$$

where γ_{max} is the maximum learning rate, γ_{min} is the minimum learning rate, t is the current iteration, T_{warm} is the warm up iteration and T is the total iteration.

2.6   The Adaptive Ensemble Method

In this subsection, we introduce a novel ensemble method that can adapt the weight of aggregation by solving the eigenvector of the Dice similarity matrix.

The irregular 3D brain samples of the validation (testing) set are transformed into tensors using the OMT map with density function $\widetilde{\rho}_{1.5}^2(v)$ in the expanded WT region in Phase I. For each $128 \times 128 \times 128$ brain tensor ($\mathcal{R}_1$), we further build $(M-1)$ $128 \times 128 \times 128$ tensors ($\mathcal{R}_2, \ldots, \mathcal{R}_M$) with data augmentation techniques in Sect. 2.2. For a given model trained at epoch k, let $P_{i,k}$, for $i = 1, 2, \ldots, M$, be the prediction of the brain image from the tensor $\mathcal{R}_i$. For convenience, we reorder the elements of the set $\{P_{1,k_1}, \ldots, P_{M,k_1}, \ldots, P_{1,k_m}, \ldots, P_{M,k_m}\}$ into $\{P_1, \ldots, P_N\}$. Our goal is to aggregate $\{P_i \mid i = 1, \ldots, N\}$. In what follows, we propose a method that automatically detects outliers and gives a higher weight to the important prediction.

First, we compute the Dice similarity coefficient of $\{P_i \mid i = 1, \ldots, N\}$ pairwise, that is, $Dice(P_i, P_j)$ for $i, j = 1, \ldots, N$, and form the adjacency matrix $D \equiv [Dice(P_i, P_j)]$. Next, we calculate the normalized eigenvector $\mathbf{v} = (v_1, \cdots, v_N)^\top$ of D corresponding to the largest eigenvalue $\rho(D)$ as shown in Fig. 3. Notice that the vector component is between 0 and 1, and the sum of all components is 1. Then we define the final prediction $\widehat{P}$ as

$$\widehat{P} = \sum_{i=1}^{N} v_i P_i.$$

3   Results

BraTS 2021 Continuous Challenge database [4–8] contains 2,040 brain images with 1,251 training images and 219 unlabeled brain image samples for validation. The others are unreleased brain image samples for testing. For the 1,251 brain image samples, we randomly choose 1,000 samples for training and 251 for cross-validation.

Residual UNet, SegResNet, and SwinUNETR are implemented in PyTorch and the Medical Open Network for AI (MONAI) [17], and HarDNet-FCN is downloaded from the open source GitHub. The parameters of experiment models

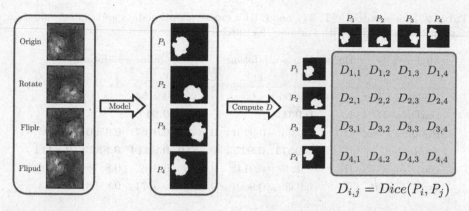

Fig. 3. Adaptive Ensemble Processing: Assume there are four predictions $\{P_1, P_2, P_3, P_4\}$ of the brain image. Let $D = [D_{ij}] \in \mathbb{R}^{4 \times 4}$ with $D_{ij} = Dice(P_i, P_j)$ and $\mathbf{v} = [v_i]$ with $\|\mathbf{v}\|_1 = 1$ be the eigenvector of D corresponding to the spectral radius $\rho(D)$. The ensembling prediction $\widehat{P}$ is taken as $\widehat{P} = \sum_{i=1}^{4} v_i P_i$.

are shown in Table 1. We set the batch size to 12 and train the model with 1,000 epochs. All trainings are performed on a server equipped with two NVIDIA Tesla A100 PCIe 40 GB GPUs.

Table 1. Parameters of our experiment models

Model	Initial Filters	Width	Depth	Activation	Norm	Dropout
Residual UNet	32	2	4	PReLU	Instance	0.25
HarDNet-FCN	32	1	4	Mish	Instance	0.1
SegResNet	32	2	3	ReLU	Instance	0.25
SwinUNETR	32	1	4	LeakyReLU	Instance	0

In Phase I, the OMT maps with the density function $\rho_1^1(v)$ in (1) are used to construct $1,251 + 219$ brain tensors. We use Residual UNet and HarDNet-FCN for training 1,000 brain tensors and inference of 251 cross-validation samples and 219 online validation samples. The WT dice scores for cross-validation and online validation are 0.9306 and 0.9154, respectively, for Residual UNet model as well as 0.9315 and 0.9174, respectively, for the HarDNet-FCN model. The results show that the Dice score for HarDNet-FCN model is better than that for Residual UNet model. Therefore, we use HarDNet-FCN model to expand the WT region.

In Phase II, we compute OMT maps with the smooth density functions $\widetilde{\rho}_\gamma^2(v)$, $\gamma = 1.0, 1.5, 1.75$, and 2.0 in (3) for 1,000 brain samples to obtain 4,000 augmented brain cubes. The data pre-processing technique in Sect. 2.2 is used to randomly generate 1,000 training samples from 4,000 augmented brain cubes.

Table 2. Dice scores of WT, TC, and ET for cross-validation data and online validation data in Phase I and II with various UNet architectures.

Model	Phase	Cross-validation			Online validation		
		WT	TC	ET	WT	TC	ET
Residual UNet	I	0.9306	–	–	0.9154	–	–
HarDNet-FCN	I	**0.9315**	–	–	**0.9174**	–	–
Residual UNet	II	0.9307	0.9101	0.8602	0.9167	0.8560	0.8293
SegResNet	II	**0.9371**	**0.9152**	**0.8819**	**0.9214**	**0.8823**	**0.8411**
HarDNet-FCN	II	0.9349	0.9145	0.8554	0.9187	0.8676	0.7776
SwinUNETR	II	0.9330	0.9091	0.8686	0.9171	0.8568	0.8283

Residual UNet, SegResNet, HarDNet-FCN, and SwinUNETR are used to train these 1,000 training samples. Furthermore, for cross-validation and online validation, we compute OMT maps for 251 and 219 brain samples, respectively, with the density function $\widetilde{\rho}_{1.5}^2(v)$ in the expanded WT region by Phase I. The adaptive ensemble in Sect. 2.6 at epoch k_1, k_2, k_3, i.e., $N = 18$, is used to predict WT, TC, and ET of brain images. We show the Dice scores of 251 cross-validations and 219 online validations with the adaptive ensemble in Table 2. Figure 4 visualizes statistics about the Dice scores of the 219 online validation data for SegResNet, HarDNet-FCN, and SwinUNETR in Phase II. The results in Table 2 and Fig. 4 show that SegResNet produces the best Dice scores for WT, TC, and ET.

Figure 5 plots the Dice scores of the training set (blue line) and the cross-validation set (brown line) for WT, TC, and ET, respectively, every 10 epochs by SegResNet. We see that the Dice scores for WT and TC of the cross-validation set do not increase after 600 epochs. However, the Dice score of ET is still increasing. To obtain a better Dice score of ET, we train SegResNet with 1,000 epochs even though WT and TC seem to be overfitted. Then we select the three best models for WT, TC, and ET, respectively, from 1,000 epochs to perform the adaptive ensemble and get the final Dice scores of WT, TC, and ET as shown in Table 2.

Table 3. Dice score of the cross-validation data and online validation data for random crop and 2P-OMT.

Model	Pre-processing	Cross-validation			Online validation		
		WT	TC	ET	WT	TC	ET
Residual UNet	Random Crop	0.9305	0.9101	0.8610	0.9172	0.8586	0.8090
Residual UNet	2P-OMT	**0.9321**	**0.9146**	**0.8683**	**0.9201**	**0.8667**	**0.8290**
SegResNet	Random Crop	0.9340	0.9082	0.8650	0.9194	0.8542	0.8242
SegResNet	2P-OMT	**0.9371**	**0.9157**	**0.8819**	**0.9214**	**0.8823**	**0.8411**

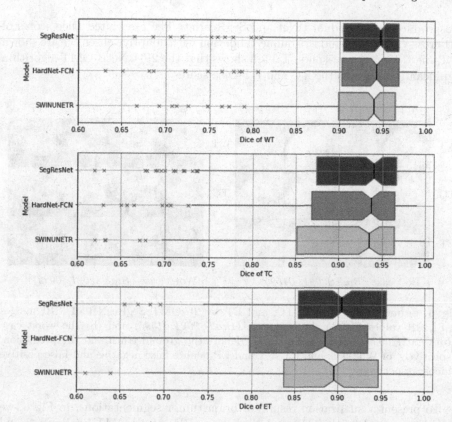

Fig. 4. Statistics about Dice scores above 0.6 of 219 online validation data for Seg-ResNet, HarDNet-FCN, and SwinUNETR in Phase II. SegResNet has the best performance.

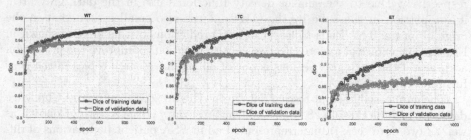

Fig. 5. Dice curves of WT, TC, and ET for the training and validation data by using SegResNet. (Color figure online)

MOANAI package provides random crop pre-processing for the raw brain images. We take twice random crop pre-processing for each brain image to obtain 2000 128 × 128 × 128 training tensors. The data preprocessing technique in Sect. 2.2 is used to randomly augment these training data. The training models are produced by Residual UNet and SegResNet. The associated Dice scores of 251 cross-validations and 219 online validation with adaptive ensemble are shown in Table 3. The comparison in Table 3 shows that the 2P-UNetB-OMT algorithm significantly improves the TC and ET Dice scores.

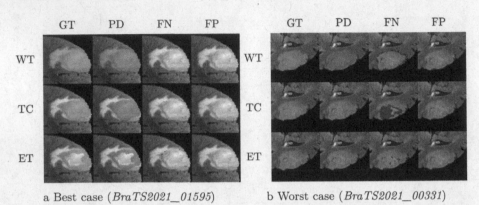

a Best case (*BraTS2021_01595*)   b Worst case (*BraTS2021_00331*)

Fig. 6. Segmentation of WT, TC, and ET by 2P-OMT SegResNet of MRI images in FLAIR values for (a) the best case (*BraTS2021_01595*) and (b) the worst case (*BraTS2021_00331*). Here, GT and PD denote the ground truth and the prediction, respectively, of WT, TC, and ET. FN and FP denote false negative and false positive regions, respectively.

To present visualization results of brain tumor segmentations, in Fig. 6, we show the ground truth (GT) and prediction (PD) of 2P-OMT SegResNet, and the corresponding false negative (FN) and false positive (FP) regions for (a) the best case (*BraTS2021_01595*) and (b) the worst case (*BraTS2021_00331*), respectively. Due to the smaller density function value in the dark gray area, its proportion in the cube by the OMT map is also smaller than that in the original image. This leads to less accurate predictions of this area as shown in Fig. 6b. The choice of a more effective density function to improve the prediction accuracy of the dark gray regions is one of our main research topics in the near future.

The unreleased holdout testing data in the BraTS 2021 Continuous Challenge database include the BraTS 2021 Challenge test data (BraTSTestingCohort), as well as two data sets: i) underrepresented adult SSA patient populations of diffuse glioma in the brain (SSAfricanData) and ii) pediatric population of patients with diffuse intrinsic pontine glioma (PediatricData). The feedback Dice scores of the WT, TC, and ET for BraTSTestingCohort, SSAfricanData, and Pediatric-Data by using 2P-OMT SegResNet present in Table 4. From these results, we see that we perform well on BraTSTestingCohort and SSAfricanData, indicating that our algorithm has an excellent effect on the segmentation of adult diffuse gliomas. However, children's gliomas (PediatricData) are quite different from adults. It is unreasonable to use certain tumor data to verify the segmentation of another tumor and to expect high accuracy.

Table 4. Dice score of unreleased brain image samples for testing data by using 2P-OMT SegResNet.

	BraTSTestingCohort			SSAfricanData			PediatricData	
	WT	TC	ET	WT	TC	ET	WT	TC
mean	0.9106	0.8543	0.8424	0.9327	0.9253	0.8216	0.6892	0.2855
sd	0.0990	0.2496	0.2090	0.0657	0.0660	0.1830	0.2574	0.3574
median	0.9408	0.9508	0.9091	0.9417	0.9486	0.9134	0.7913	0.0680
25 quantile	0.9005	0.8934	0.8432	0.9287	0.9282	0.7952	0.5999	0
75 quantile	0.9615	0.9716	0.9480	0.9563	0.9590	0.9255	0.8758	0.6435

4 Discussion

In this paper, we propose an UNet-based brain tumor segmentation framework via OMT-based pre-processing. Compared to the previous method, this approach has two advantages. The first is that the OMT map transforms an object from an irregular domain to a regular domain with minimal deformation. It can reduce the computational cost of the models and keep the global information of the original image. The second is that it facilitates density control, so data augmentation can be made using different densities. On the one hand, it can enlarge the tumor proportion, which helps the model detect the model. On the other hand, it can increase data diversity, which enhances the model generalization ability.

This framework has a 2-Phase process. In Phase I, we use the OMT map to transform the brain into a cube and predict the WT by HarDNet-FCN. Then we expand the 4 pixels by morphology dilation. It can cover 99.9% TC and ET. In Phase II, we define the density function to enlarge the region proportion generated from Phase I. Finally, we use SegResNet to predict the WT, TC, and ET. For post-processing, we propose an adaptive ensemble method to aggregate the predictions. The Dice scores of 219 online validation data with TC, and ET are 0.8823, and 0.8411, respectively, which significantly improve those obtained by random crop pre-processing. The Dice score of WT is 0.9214 which slightly improves that obtained by random crop pre-processing. How to improve the Dice score of WT in Phase II will be our research direction in the future.

Acknowledgments. This work was partially supported by the Ministry of Science and Technology (MoST), the National Center for Theoretical Sciences, and Big Data Computing Center of Southeast University. W.-W. Lin and T.M. Huang were partially supported by MoST 110-2115-M-A49-004- and MoST 110-2115-M-003-012-MY3, respectively. T. Li was supported in part by the National Natural Science Foundation of China (NSFC) 11971105.

References

1. Yueh, M., Lin, W.-W., Wu, C.-T., Yau, S.: A novel stretch energy minimization algorithm for equiareal parameterizations. J. Sci. Comput. **78**, 1353–1386 (2019). https://doi.org/10.1007/s10915-018-0822-7
2. Yueh, M.-H., Li, T., Lin, W.-W., Yau, S.-T.: A novel algorithm for volume-preserving parameterizations of 3-manifolds. SIAM J. Imaging Sci. **12**, 1071–1098 (2019)
3. Yueh, M.-H., Huang, T.-M., Li, T., Lin, W.-W., Yau, S.-T.: Projected gradient method combined with homotopy techniques for volume-measure-preserving optimal mass transportation problems. J. Sci. Comput. **88**, 64 (2021). https://doi.org/10.1007/s10915-021-01583-z
4. Bakas, S., et al.: Advancing the cancer genome atlas glioma MRI collections with expert segmentation labels and radiomic features. Sci. Data **4**, 170117 (2017)
5. Menze, B.H., et al.: The multimodal brain tumor image segmentation benchmark (BRATS). IEEE Trans. Med. Imaging **34**, 1993–2024 (2015)
6. Baid, U., et al.: The RSNA-ASNR-MICCAI BraTS 2021 benchmark on brain tumor segmentation and radiogenomic classification. Preprint at https://arxiv.org/abs/2107.02314 (2021)
7. Bakas, S., et al.: Segmentation labels and radiomic features for the pre-operative scans of the TCGA-GBM collection. The Cancer Imaging Archive (2017). https://doi.org/10.7937/K9/TCIA.2017.KLXWJJ1Q
8. Bakas, S., et al.: Segmentation labels and radiomic features for the pre-operative scans of the TCGA-LGG collection. The Cancer Imaging Archive (2017). https://doi.org/10.7937/K9/TCIA.2017.GJQ7R0EF
9. Xiao, X., Lian, S., Luo, Z., Li, S.: Weighted Res-UNet for high-quality retina vessel segmentation. In: 2018 9th International Conference on Information Technology in Medicine and Education (ITME), pp. 327–331 (2018)
10. Myronenko, A.: 3D MRI brain tumor segmentation using autoencoder regularization. In: Crimi, A., Bakas, S., Kuijf, H., Keyvan, F., Reyes, M., van Walsum, T. (eds.) BrainLes 2018. LNCS, vol. 11384, pp. 311–320. Springer, Cham (2019). https://doi.org/10.1007/978-3-030-11726-9_28
11. Hatamizadeh, A., et al.: Swin UNETR: Swin transformers for semantic segmentation of brain tumors in MRI images (2022). https://arxiv.org/abs/2201.01266
12. Chao, P., Kao, C.-Y., Ruan, Y., Huang, C.-H., Lin, Y.-L.: HarDNet: a low memory traffic network. In: 2019 IEEE/CVF International Conference on Computer Vision (ICCV), pp. 3551–3560 (2019)
13. Long, J., Shelhamer, E., Darrell, T.: Fully convolutional networks for semantic segmentation (2014). https://arxiv.org/abs/1411.4038
14. Lin, W., et al.: A novel 2-phase residual U-net algorithm combined with optimal mass transportation for 3D brain tumor detection and segmentation. Sci. Rep. **12**, 6452 (2022)
15. Lin, T.-Y., Goyal, P., Girshick, R., He, K., Dollár, P.: Focal loss for dense object detection. In: 2017 IEEE International Conference on Computer Vision (ICCV), pp. 2999–3007 (2017)
16. Kingma, D.P., Ba, J.: Adam: a method for stochastic optimization. In: ICLR (Poster) (2015). http://arxiv.org/abs/1412.6980
17. The MONAI Consortium. Project MONAI (2020). https://doi.org/10.5281/zenodo.4323059

BraTS-Reg

Robust Image Registration with Absent Correspondences in Pre-operative and Follow-Up Brain MRI Scans of Diffuse Glioma Patients

Tony C. W. Mok[✉] and Albert C. S. Chung

The Hong Kong University of Science and Technology, Hong Kong, China
{cwmokab,achung}@cse.ust.hk

Abstract. Registration of pre-operative and follow-up brain MRI scans is challenging due to the large variation of tissue appearance and missing correspondences in tumour recurrence regions caused by tumour mass effect. Although recent deep learning-based deformable registration methods have achieved remarkable success in various medical applications, most of them are not capable of registering images with pathologies. In this paper, we propose a 3-step registration pipeline for pre-operative and follow-up brain MRI scans that consists of 1) a multi-level affine registration, 2) a conditional deep Laplacian pyramid image registration network (cLapIRN) with forward-backward consistency constraint, and 3) a non-linear instance optimization method. We apply the method to the Brain Tumor Sequence Registration (BraTS-Reg) Challenge. Our method achieves accurate and robust registration of brain MRI scans with pathologies, which achieves a median absolute error of 1.64 mm and 88% of successful registration rate in the validation set of BraTS-Reg challenge. Our method ranks 1st place in the 2022 MICCAI BraTS-Reg challenge.

Keywords: Absent correspondences · Patient-specific registration · Deformable registration

1 Introduction

Registration of pre-operative and follow-up images is crucial in evaluating the effectiveness of treatment for patients suffering from diffuse glioma. However, this registration problem is challenging due to the missing correspondences and mass effect caused by resected tissue. While many recent deep learning-based deformable registration algorithms [2,3,9,10,13–15,21] are available, only a few learning-based methods [5] address the missing correspondences problem. In this paper, we propose a 3-step registration pipeline for pre-operative and follow-up brain MRI scans that consists of 1) a multi-level affine pre-alignment, 2) a conditional deep Laplacian pyramid image registration network (cLapIRN) with forward-backward consistency constraint [16–18], and 3) a non-linear instance optimization with inverse consistency. We validate the method using the pre-operative and follow-up images brain MRI scans in the Brain Tumor Sequence Registration Challenge (BraTS-Reg) challenge [1].

© The Author(s), under exclusive license to Springer Nature Switzerland AG 2023
S. Bakas et al. (Eds.): BrainLes 2022, LNCS 13769, pp. 231–240, 2023.
https://doi.org/10.1007/978-3-031-33842-7_20

2   Related Work

Accurate registration of pre-operative and post-recurrence brain MRI scans is crucial to the treatment plan and diagnosis of intracranial tumors, especially brain gliomas [7,20]. To better interpret the location and extent of the tumor and its biological activity after resection, the dense correspondences between pre-operative and follow-up structural brain MRI scans of the patient first need to be established. However, deformable registration between the pre-operative and follow-up scans, including post-resection and post-recurrence, is challenging due to possible large deformations and absent correspondences caused by tumor's mass effects [4], resection cavities, tumor recurrence and tissue relaxation in the follow-up scans. While recent deep learning-based deformable registration (DLDR) methods [2,6,9,10,13] have achieved remarkable registration performance in many medical applications, these registration approaches often ignored the absent correspondence problem in the pre-operative and post-recurrence images. To address this issue, we extend our deep learning-based method described in [17] by introducing affine pre-alignment and non-linear instance optimization as post-processing to our method. DIRAC leverages conditional Laplacian Pyramid Image Registration Networks (cLapIRN) [16] as the backbone network, jointly estimates the bidirectional deformation fields and explicitly locates regions with absent correspondence. By excluding the regions with absent correspondence in the similarity measure during training, DIRAC improves the target registration error of landmarks in pre-operative and follow-up images, especially for those near the tumour regions.

3   Methods

We propose a 3-step registration pipeline for pre-operative and follow-up brain MRI scans which consists of 1) a gradient descent-based affine registration method, 2) a deformable image registration method with absent correspondence (DIRAC), and 3) a non-linear instance optimization method. Let B and F be the pre-operative (baseline) scan B and post-recurrence (follow-up) scan defined over a n-D mutual spatial domain $\Omega \subseteq \mathbb{R}^n$. Our goal is to establish a dense non-linear correspondence between the pre-operative scan and the post-recurrence scan of the same subject. In this paper, we focus on 3D registration, i.e., $n = 3$ and $\Omega \subseteq \mathbb{R}^3$.

3.1   Affine Registration

Although all MRI scans provided by the challenge are rigidly registered to the same anatomical template [1], we found that there are large linear misalignments between the pre-operative and follow-up images in cases suffering from serious tumor mass effect. To factor out the possible linear misalignment between MRI scans B and F, we register T1-weighted B and F scans using the iterative affine registration method.

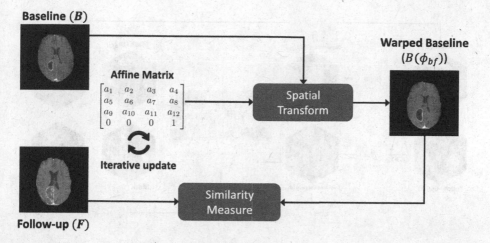

Fig. 1. Overview of the affine registration (Step 1). Our method optimizes the affine matrix using instance optimization. Only the baseline scan registered to the follow-up scan is shown for brevity.

Figure 1 depicts the overview of the affine registration. The affine registration method starts by initializing two identity matrices as initial affine transformation and creating image pyramids with N_{level} levels using trilinear interpolation for B and F. Then, we iteratively optimize the solutions by minimizing a suitable distance measure that quantifies alignment quality using the Adam optimizer [11] and a coarse-to-fine multi-resolution iteratively registration scheme. In this step, we use the Normalized Gradient Fields (NGF) distance measure [8]. Formally, the NGF is defined as:

$$\text{NGF}(B,F) = \int_{\Omega} 1 - \frac{\langle \nabla B, \nabla F \rangle^2}{||\nabla B||_{\epsilon}^2 ||\nabla F||_{\epsilon}^2} \tag{1}$$

where $\langle x, y \rangle := x^{\top} y$, $||x||_{\epsilon} = \sqrt{x^{\top} x + \epsilon}$ and ϵ is an edge parameter controlling the level of influence of image gradients. The value of NGF is minimized when the gradients of B and F are aligned. The result with the minimal distance measure is selected as intermediate result.

3.2 Unsupervised Deformable Registration with Absent Correspondences Estimation

Assume that baseline scan B and follow-up scan F are affinely aligned in step 1 such that the main source of misalignment between B and F is non-linear, we then apply DIRAC [17] to further align B and F in an bidirectional manner. Since multi-parametric MRI sequences of each time-point, including T1 contrast-enhanced (T1ce), T2, T2 Fluid Attenuated (Flair) and T1-weighted (T1), are provided for each case in the BraTS-Reg challenge, we utilize all MRI modalities of the brain MRI scans in this step, i.e., B and F are 4-channel pre-operative and

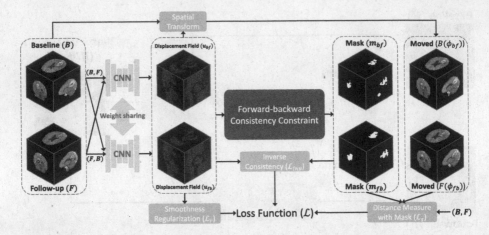

Fig. 2. Overview of the proposed deformable image registration method with absent correspondence. Our method jointly estimates the bidirectional deformation fields and locates regions with absent correspondence (denoted as mask). The regions with absent correspondence are excluded in the similarity measure during training. For brevity, the magnitude loss of the masks is omitted in the figure.

post-recurrence scans, respectively. Specifically, we parameterize the problem with a function $f_\theta(F, B) = (\boldsymbol{u}_{fb}, \boldsymbol{u}_{bf})$ cLapIRN [16], where θ is a set of learning parameters and $\boldsymbol{u}_{bf}$ represents the displacement field that transform B to align with F, i.e., $B(x + \boldsymbol{u}_{bf}(x))$ and $F(x)$ define similar anatomical locations for each voxel $x \in \Omega$ (except voxels with absent correspondence). Figure 2 illustrates the overview of DIRAC. DIRAC leverages the bidirectional displacement fields and a forward-backward consistency locate regions with absent correspondence and excludes them in the similarity measure during training phase.

Forward-Backward Consistency. Given the deformation fields $\phi_{bf} = Id + \boldsymbol{u}_{bf}$ and $\phi_{fb} = Id + \boldsymbol{u}_{fb}$, where Id is the identity transform and $\boldsymbol{u}$ is the corresponding displacement vector field, we calculate the forward-backward error δ_{bf} for B to F as:

$$\delta_{bf}(x) = |\boldsymbol{u}_{bf}(x) + \boldsymbol{u}_{fb}(x + \boldsymbol{u}_{bf}(x))|_2. \tag{2}$$

Based on the observation that regions without true correspondences would have higher forward-backward error in solutions, we create a mask m_{bf} and mark $m_{bf}(x) = 1$ whenever the forward-backward error $\delta_{bf}(x)$ is larger than the pre-defined threshold $\tau_{bf}(x)$. The pre-defined threshold is defined as:

$$\tau_{bf} = \sum_{x \in \{x \,|\, F(x) > 0\}} \frac{1}{N_f} \left(|\boldsymbol{u}_{bf}(x) + \boldsymbol{u}_{fb}(x + \boldsymbol{u}_{bf}(x))|_2 \right) + \alpha, \tag{3}$$

Table 1. Parameters used in the registration pipeline. NCC-SP: Negative Local Cross-correlation with Similarity Pyramid.

Parameters	Methods		
	Affine	**DIRAC**	**Inst. Opt.**
Input MRI sequences	T1ce	T1, T1ce, T2, Flair	T1ce, T2
Number of levels N_{level}	3	3	5
Max. image dimension N_{max}	(64, 64, 40)	(160, 160, 80)	(240, 240, 155)
Min. image dimension N_{min}	(16, 16, 16)	(40, 40, 20)	(80, 80, 80)
Learning rate per level	[1e−2, 5e−3, 2e−3]	[1e−4, 1e−4, 1e−4]	[1e−2, 5e−3, 5e−3, 3e−3, 3e−3]
Max. iteration per level N_{iter}	[90, 90, 90]	–	[150, 100, 100, 100, 50]
Distance measure	NGF($\epsilon = 0.01$)	NCC-SP($w = 7$)	NCC($w = 3$)
Max. number of grid points	–	$160 \times 160 \times 80$	$64 \times 64 \times 64$
Min. number of grid points	–	$40 \times 40 \times 20$	$32 \times 32 \times 32$
Weight of Inverse consistency λ_{inv}	–	[0.5, 0.5, 0.5]	[1.0, 2.0, 4.0, 8.0, 10.0]

where α is set to 0.015. Then, we create a binary mask m_{bf} to mark voxels with absent correspondence as follows:

$$m_{bf}(x) = \begin{cases} 1, & \text{if } (A \star \delta_{bf})(x) \geq \tau_{bf} \\ 0, & \text{otherwise} \end{cases} \tag{4}$$

where A denotes an averaging filter of size $(2p+1)^3$ and $\star$ denotes a convolution operator with zero-padding p.

Objective Function. The objective function $\mathcal{L}$ of DIRAC is defined as follows:

$$\mathcal{L} = (1 - \lambda_{reg})\mathcal{L}_s + \lambda_{reg}\mathcal{L}_r + \lambda_{inv}\mathcal{L}_{inv} + \lambda_m(|m_{bf}| + |m_{fb}|) \tag{5}$$

where the masked dissimilarity measure $\mathcal{L}_s$ and the masked inverse consistency loss $\mathcal{L}_{inv}$ are defined as:

$$\mathcal{L}_s = \mathcal{L}_{sim}(B, F(\phi_{fb}), (1 - m_{fb})) + \mathcal{L}_{sim}(F, B(\phi_{bf}), (1 - m_{bf})) \tag{6}$$

and

$$\mathcal{L}_{inv} = \sum_{x \in \Omega} (\delta_{bf}(x)(1 - m_{bf}(x)) + \delta_{fb}(x)(1 - m_{fb}(x))). \tag{7}$$

In this step, we use masked negative local cross-correlation (NCC) with similarity pyramid [18] as the dissimilarity function. To encourage smooth solutions and penalize implausible solutions, we adopt a diffusion regularizer $\mathcal{L}_r = ||\nabla u_{bf}||_2^2 + ||\nabla u_{fb}||_2^2$ during training. We set λ_{reg} and λ_m to 0.4 and 0.01, respectively. For more details, we recommend interested reader also refer to [17].

3.3   Non-rigid Instance Optimization

Due to insufficient amount of training data and discrepancy in distributions between training and test set, the learning-based method in step 2 may produce

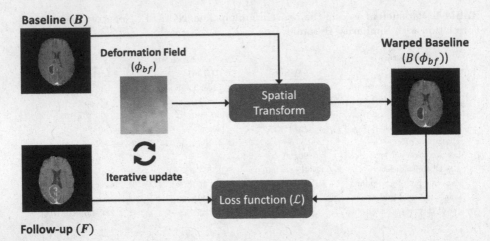

Fig. 3. Overview of the non-rigid instance optimization (Step 3). Initially, the deformation field is initialized with the solution estimated from Step 2. The bidirectional deformation fields are jointly updated using Adam optimizer. For brevity, only baseline scan register to the follow-up scan is shown in the figure.

Table 2. Results on the training set in the BraTS-Reg challenge. MAE_{median} and MAE_{mean} denote the average of median absolute error and mean absolute error of the transformed coordinates and the manually defined coordinates (in millimetre), respectively. Initial: Results before registration.

Methods	MAE_{median}	MAE_{mean}	Robustness
Initial	8.20 ± 7.62	8.65 ± 7.31	–
Ours	2.98 ± 6.25	4.64 ± 11.06	0.78 ± 0.23

biased solutions, especially in cases with small initial misalignment. As such, we introduce a non-rigid instance optimization step to further improve the robustness and registration accuracy of solutions from the previous step. Figure 3 shows the overview of the non-rigid instance optimization. In the final step, the non-parametric deformation is controlled by the same objective function in Eq. 5, except we use NCC as the distance measure. The smoothness regularization coefficients λ_{reg} for each level are set to $[0.25, 0.3, 0.3, 0.35, 0.35]$, respectively. The displacement fields are discretized with trilinear interpolation defined on a uniform control point grid with a fixed number of points. We use an Adam optimizer together with multi-level continuation to avoid local minima.

3.4 Hyperparameters

The hyperparameters of our 3-step approach are summarized in Table 1.

Table 3. Results on the validation set in the BraTS-Reg challenge. MAE and Robustness denote the average of median absolute error and mean absolute error of the transformed coordinates and the manually defined coordinates (in millimetre), respectively. Robustness measures the successful-rate of the registered landmarks. Affine, A-DIRAC and A-DIRAC-IO denote affine registration, DIRAC with affine pre-alignment and our proposed 3-step method, respectively. Initial: Results before registration.

Case	Initial	Affine		A-DIRAC		A-DIRAC-IO	
	MAE	MAE	Robustness	MAE	Robustness	MAE	Robustness
Case 141	13.50	4.26	1.00	1.94	1.00	1.62	1.00
Case 142	14.00	6.12	0.88	3.07	1.00	1.88	1.00
Case 143	16.00	8.98	1.00	2.63	1.00	1.14	1.00
Case 144	15.00	9.52	0.88	3.10	1.00	2.56	1.00
Case 145	17.00	5.14	1.00	2.09	1.00	1.13	1.00
Case 146	17.00	5.74	1.00	1.84	1.00	1.94	1.00
Case 147	1.50	2.03	0.45	2.17	0.60	1.64	0.55
Case 148	3.50	2.90	0.75	1.71	0.90	1.43	0.90
Case 149	9.00	2.22	1.00	1.94	1.00	1.56	1.00
Case 150	4.00	3.65	0.53	2.87	0.63	1.27	0.74
Case 151	3.00	2.13	0.5	1.39	0.75	1.18	0.85
Case 152	5.00	2.11	0.95	1.45	0.84	1.42	0.95
Case 153	2.00	2.04	0.33	1.44	0.67	1.80	0.67
Case 154	2.00	2.61	0.25	2.02	0.4	1.98	0.55
Case 155	2.00	3.09	0.21	2.43	0.37	1.70	0.53
Case 156	7.00	2.84	1.00	2.29	1.00	1.45	1.00
Case 157	10.00	4.90	0.90	2.67	1.00	1.66	1.00
Case 158	4.50	3.48	0.40	1.39	0.80	1.13	1.00
Case 159	6.00	7.28	0.36	2.25	1.00	2.28	1.00
Case 160	4.00	2.55	0.7	2.29	0.80	1.94	0.90
Mean	7.80	4.18	0.70	2.15	0.84	1.64	0.88
Std	5.62	2.30	0.29	0.54	0.21	0.39	0.17
Median	5.50	3.28	0.81	2.13	0.95	1.63	1.00

4   Experiments

Implementation. Our proposed method is implemented with PyTorch 1.8 [19] and trained with an Nvidia Titan RTX GPU and an Intel Core (i7-4790) CPU. We build DIRAC on top of the official implementation of cLapIRN available in [12]. We adopt Adam optimizer [11] with a fixed learning rate 1e−4 and train it from scratch with the training data from the BraTS-Reg challenge.

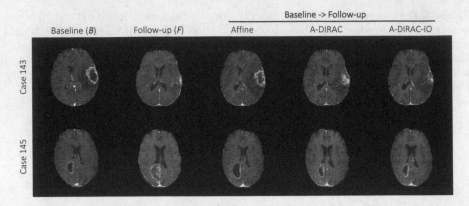

Fig. 4. Example axial T1ce MR slices of resulting warped images (B to F) from affine, A-DIRAC and A-DIRAC-IO registration methods.

Measurements. We quantitatively evaluate our method based on the average of the median absolute error (MAE) and robustness of anatomical landmarks. Specifically, the MAE is defined as:

$$\text{MAE} = \text{Median}_{l \in L}(|x_l^B - \hat{x}_l^B|), \tag{8}$$

where x_l^B is the l-th estimated anatomical landmark in the baseline scan and $\hat{x}_l^B$ is the l-th groundtruth landmark in the baseline scan. The robustness is defined as the ratio of landmarks with improved MAE after registration to all landmarks, following the definition in [1].

Results. For each case in the training and validation set of the BraTS-Reg challenge, we register the pre-operative image scan to the follow-up image scan and use the resulting deformation field to transform the manually defined landmarks in the follow-up scan. In total, there are 140 and 20 pairs of pre-operative and follow-up image scans in the training and validation set, respectively. We follow the evaluation pipeline of the BraTS-Reg challenge and report the average median absolute error MAE and robustness of the training and validation set in Tables 2 and 3.

An example qualitative result is shown in Fig. 4. The reduction of the registration error in the validation set in the pipeline is shown in Table 3. While the MRI scans are pre-registered to a common template, the average median error is reduced from 7.8 mm to 4.18 mm, indicating there exists a large linear misalignment between each case. Furthermore, the median error and robustness are consistently improved after each step, reaching to 1.64 mm average median error. Notably, our MAE is the lowest on the challenge's validation leaderboard.

5   Conclusion

We proposed a 3-step registration method for pre-operative and follow-up brain tumor registration. The method was evaluated with the dataset provided by the BraTS-Reg challenge and ranked 1st place in the 2022 MICCAI BraTS-Reg challenge. By combining the pathological-aware deep learning-based method and instance optimization, we demonstrated the follow-up scan could be accurately registered to the pre-operative scan with an average median absolute error of 1.64 mm. Compared to conventional methods, our method inherits the runtime advantage from deep learning-based approaches and does not require any manual interaction or supervision, demonstrating immense potential in the fully-automated patient-specific registration. We left the further analysis of our method and the comparison to existing methods for future work.

References

1. Baheti, B., et al.: The brain tumor sequence registration challenge: establishing correspondence between pre-operative and follow-up MRI scans of diffuse glioma patients. arXiv preprint arXiv:2112.06979 (2021)
2. Balakrishnan, G., Zhao, A., Sabuncu, M.R., Guttag, J., Dalca, A.V.: An unsupervised learning model for deformable medical image registration. In: Proceedings of the IEEE Conference on Computer Vision and Pattern Recognition, pp. 9252–9260 (2018)
3. Dalca, A.V., Balakrishnan, G., Guttag, J., Sabuncu, M.R.: Unsupervised learning for fast probabilistic diffeomorphic registration. In: Frangi, A.F., Schnabel, J.A., Davatzikos, C., Alberola-López, C., Fichtinger, G. (eds.) MICCAI 2018. LNCS, vol. 11070, pp. 729–738. Springer, Cham (2018). https://doi.org/10.1007/978-3-030-00928-1_82
4. Dean, B.L., et al.: Gliomas: classification with MR imaging. Radiology **174**(2), 411–415 (1990)
5. Han, X., et al.: A deep network for joint registration and reconstruction of images with pathologies. In: Liu, M., Yan, P., Lian, C., Cao, X. (eds.) MLMI 2020. LNCS, vol. 12436, pp. 342–352. Springer, Cham (2020). https://doi.org/10.1007/978-3-030-59861-7_35
6. Heinrich, M.P.: Closing the gap between deep and conventional image registration using probabilistic dense displacement networks. In: Shen, D., et al. (eds.) MICCAI 2019. LNCS, vol. 11769, pp. 50–58. Springer, Cham (2019). https://doi.org/10.1007/978-3-030-32226-7_6
7. Heiss, W.D., Raab, P., Lanfermann, H.: Multimodality assessment of brain tumors and tumor recurrence. J. Nucl. Med. **52**(10), 1585–1600 (2011)
8. Hodneland, E., Lundervold, A., Rørvik, J., Munthe-Kaas, A.Z.: Normalized gradient fields and mutual information for motion correction of DCE-MRI images. In: 2013 8th International Symposium on Image and Signal Processing and Analysis (ISPA), pp. 516–521. IEEE (2013)
9. Hu, X., Kang, M., Huang, W., Scott, M.R., Wiest, R., Reyes, M.: Dual-stream pyramid registration network. In: Shen, D., et al. (eds.) MICCAI 2019. LNCS, vol. 11765, pp. 382–390. Springer, Cham (2019). https://doi.org/10.1007/978-3-030-32245-8_43

10. Kim, B., Kim, J., Lee, J.-G., Kim, D.H., Park, S.H., Ye, J.C.: Unsupervised deformable image registration using cycle-consistent CNN. In: Shen, D., et al. (eds.) MICCAI 2019. LNCS, vol. 11769, pp. 166–174. Springer, Cham (2019). https://doi.org/10.1007/978-3-030-32226-7_19

11. Kingma, D.P., Ba, J.: Adam: a method for stochastic optimization. arXiv preprint arXiv:1412.6980 (2014)

12. Mok, T.C., Chung, A.: Official implementation of conditional deep Laplacian pyramid image registration network. https://github.com/cwmok/Conditional_LapIRN. Accessed 01 Mar 2021

13. Mok, T.C., Chung, A.: Fast symmetric diffeomorphic image registration with convolutional neural networks. In: Proceedings of the IEEE/CVF Conference on Computer Vision and Pattern Recognition, pp. 4644–4653 (2020)

14. Mok, T.C.W., Chung, A.C.S.: Large deformation image registration with anatomy-aware Laplacian pyramid networks. In: Shusharina, N., Heinrich, M.P., Huang, R. (eds.) MICCAI 2020. LNCS, vol. 12587, pp. 61–67. Springer, Cham (2021). https://doi.org/10.1007/978-3-030-71827-5_7

15. Mok, T.C.W., Chung, A.C.S.: Conditional deep Laplacian pyramid image registration network in Learn2Reg challenge. In: Aubreville, M., Zimmerer, D., Heinrich, M. (eds.) MICCAI 2021. LNCS, vol. 13166, pp. 161–167. Springer, Cham (2022). https://doi.org/10.1007/978-3-030-97281-3_23

16. Mok, T.C.W., Chung, A.C.S.: Conditional deformable image registration with convolutional neural network. In: de Bruijne, M., et al. (eds.) MICCAI 2021. LNCS, vol. 12904, pp. 35–45. Springer, Cham (2021). https://doi.org/10.1007/978-3-030-87202-1_4

17. Mok, T.C.W., Chung, A.C.S.: Unsupervised deformable image registration with absent correspondences in pre-operative and post-recurrence brain tumor MRI scans. In: Wang, L., Dou, Q., Fletcher, P.T., Speidel, S., Li, S. (eds.) MICCAI 2022. LNCS, vol. 13436, pp. 25–35. Springer, Cham (2022). https://doi.org/10.1007/978-3-031-16446-0_3

18. Mok, T.C.W., Chung, A.C.S.: Large deformation diffeomorphic image registration with Laplacian pyramid networks. In: Martel, A.L., et al. (eds.) MICCAI 2020. LNCS, vol. 12263, pp. 211–221. Springer, Cham (2020). https://doi.org/10.1007/978-3-030-59716-0_21

19. Paszke, A., Gross, S., Chintala, S., et al.: Automatic differentiation in PyTorch. In: NIPS-W (2017)

20. Price, S.J., Jena, R., Burnet, N.G., Carpenter, T.A., Pickard, J.D., Gillard, J.H.: Predicting patterns of glioma recurrence using diffusion tensor imaging. Eur. Radiol. 17(7), 1675–1684 (2007). https://doi.org/10.1007/s00330-006-0561-2

21. de Vos, B.D., Berendsen, F.F., Viergever, M.A., Staring, M., Išgum, I.: End-to-end unsupervised deformable image registration with a convolutional neural network. In: Cardoso, M.J., et al. (eds.) DLMIA/ML-CDS -2017. LNCS, vol. 10553, pp. 204–212. Springer, Cham (2017). https://doi.org/10.1007/978-3-319-67558-9_24

Unsupervised Method for Intra-patient Registration of Brain Magnetic Resonance Images Based on Objective Function Weighting by Inverse Consistency: Contribution to the BraTS-Reg Challenge

Marek Wodzinski[1,2](✉) ⓘ, Artur Jurgas[1,2] ⓘ, Niccolò Marini[1,3] ⓘ,
Manfredo Atzori[1,4] ⓘ, and Henning Müller[1,5] ⓘ

[1] University of Applied Sciences Western Switzerland Information Systems Institute,
Sierre, Switzerland
wodzinski@agh.edu.pl, marek.wodzinski@hevs.ch
[2] Department of Measurement and Electronics, AGH University of Krakow,
Krakow, Poland
[3] Department of Computer Science, University of Geneva, Geneva, Switzerland
[4] Department of Neuroscience, University of Padova, Padova, Italy
[5] Medical Faculty, University of Geneva, Geneva, Switzerland

Abstract. Registration of brain scans with pathologies is difficult,
yet important research area. The importance of this task motivated
researchers to organize the BraTS-Reg challenge, jointly with IEEE
ISBI 2022 and MICCAI 2022 conferences. The organizers introduced the
task of aligning pre-operative to follow-up magnetic resonance images
of glioma. The main difficulties are connected with the missing data
leading to large, nonrigid, and noninvertible deformations. In this work,
we describe our contributions to both the editions of the BraTS-Reg
challenge. The proposed method is based on combined deep learning
and instance optimization approaches. First, the instance optimization
enriches the state-of-the-art LapIRN method to improve the generalizability and fine-details preservation. Second, an additional objective
function weighting is introduced, based on the inverse consistency. The
proposed method is fully unsupervised and exhibits high registration
quality and robustness. The quantitative results on the external validation set are: (i) IEEE ISBI 2022 edition: 1.85, and 0.86, (ii) MICCAI 2022
edition: 1.71, and 0.86, in terms of the mean of median absolute error
and robustness respectively. The method scored the 1st place during the
IEEE ISBI 2022 version of the challenge and the 3rd place during the
MICCAI 2022. Future work could transfer the inverse consistency-based
weighting directly into the deep network training.

Keywords: Deep Learning · Image Registration · BraTS ·
BraTS-Reg · Brain Tumor · Glioma · Inverse Consistency · Missing
Data

© The Author(s), under exclusive license to Springer Nature Switzerland AG 2023
S. Bakas et al. (Eds.): BrainLes 2022, LNCS 13769, pp. 241–251, 2023.
https://doi.org/10.1007/978-3-031-33842-7_21

1   Introduction

Registration of brain scans acquired using magnetic resonance imaging (MRI) is an active research area. Numerous works addressed the challenge by enforcing diffeomorphic deformations, using both classical [1], as well as deep learning-based (DL) approaches [3,4,7,8]. However, it is still unclear what is the best approach for registering scans containing pathologies.

To answer this question, a Brain Tumor Sequence Registration (BraTS-Reg) challenge was organized in conjunction with IEEE ISBI 2022 and MICCAI 2022 conferences [2]. The challenge organizers proposed a task dedicated to registration of pre-operative MRI scans of patients diagnosed with a brain glioma, to follow-up scans of the same patient acquired after the treatment.

The surgical resection introduces the problem of missing data where the structure of interest is absent in one of the registered images. The problem of missing data in the registration of brain scans induces two main challenges: (i) large, nonrigid deformations caused by the tumor resection (depending on its size), and (ii) non-invertibility of the displacement field in the tumor area (the displacement field is unable to create new structures).

Contribution: In this work, we present our contribution to both the editions of the BraTS-Reg challenge [2]. We propose an unsupervised, hybrid approach, based on a deep neural network followed by an instance optimization (IO) attempting to address the challenge connected with large, nonrigid deformations. We introduce an additional, unsupervised inverse consistency-based weighting of the objective function. We present our motivations behind the method design and show the high quality of the registration in terms of the median absolute error (MAE) and robustness.

2   Methods

2.1   Overview and Preprocessing

The proposed method consists of the following steps: (i) an initial, instance optimization-based affine registration, (ii) calculating the initial displacement field using a modified version of the LapIRN [9], (iii) tuning the displacement field by the instance optimization (IO) based, nonrigid registration method [11], and (iv - MICCAI edition only) an objective function weighting based on the inverse consistency. The ISBI 2022 pipeline is shown in Fig. 1 and the MICCAI 2022 pipeline is shown in Fig. 2.

The basic preprocessing was performed offline by challenge organizers and consisted of resampling the images to the same resolution. The processing pipeline starts with creating the source and target tensors. The tensors are created by concatenating all available modalities in the channel dimension, for both the source and target images. This results in two $4 \times 240 \times 240 \times 155$ volumes. The volumes are normalized channel-wise to [0–1] intensity values. We use the pre-operative scan as the source volume and the follow-up scan as the target volume. The challenge design requires to warp the landmarks annotated in follow-up scans and we decided to not attempt to invert the noninvertible displacement fields, neither to voxelize the landmarks.

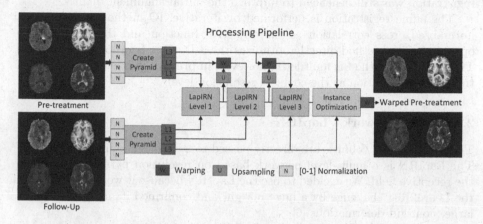

Fig. 1. The IEEE ISBI 2022 registration pipeline. Please note that some connections between LapIRN are omitted for the presentation clarity.

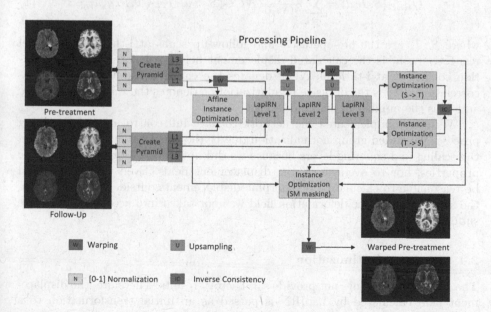

Fig. 2. The MICCAI 2022 registration pipeline. Please note that some connections between LapIRN are omitted for the presentation clarity. Note that during the 2nd edition of the challenge the pipeline starts with an initial affine registration.

2.2 Affine Registration

The process starts with an initial instance optimization-based (IO), iterative affine registration. Even though the volumes were group-wise aligned to the same space by the challenge organizers during preprocessing, the pair-wise affine registration was still beneficial to improve the initial alignment quality.

The affine registration is performed by iterative, IO method with the local normalized cross correlation as the objective function and the Adam as the optimizer. The method directly optimizes the 3-D affine transformation matrix. The proposed method is multilevel, however, in practice it is enough to perform the affine registration at the coarsest resolution level.

2.3 Deep Network - LapIRN

The preprocessed volumes are directly passed to a slightly modified LapIRN [9]. The LapIRN is a multi-level network based on resolution pyramids to enlarge the receptive field. We decided to use the LapIRN because it won two editions of the Learn2Reg challenge by a huge margin and confirmed its ability to recover large, nonrigid deformations [6].

We use the LapIRN to optimize the following objective function:

$$O_{REG}(S, T, u) = \sum_{i=1}^{N} \frac{1}{2^{(N-i)}} (NCC(S_i \circ u_i, T_i) + \theta_i Reg(u_i)), \qquad (1)$$

where S_i, T_i are the pre-operative and follow-up scans at i-th resolution level respectively, u_i is the calculated displacement field, θ_i denotes the regularization coefficient at i-th level, NCC denotes the channel-wise normalized cross-correlation, Reg is the diffusive regularization, $\circ$ denotes the warping operation, and N is the number of pyramid levels.

We have reimplemented the network to have full control over the training process. We added group normalization due to the small batch size and deleted the scaling and squaring layers because we did not want to force diffeomorphic properties, nor to oversmooth the displacement fields. Even though it would be reasonable to calculate diffeomorphic displacements outside the tumor area, the smoothness of the deformation field was not taken into account to rank the submissions.

2.4 Instance Optimization

The LapIRN alone does not provide satisfactory results. Therefore, the displacement field calculated by LapIRN is passed as an initial transformation to a multi-level nonrigid instance optimization (IO) module. The module fine-tunes the displacement field by an iterative optimization implemented using PyTorch autograd. In the original formulation, the method optimizes the same cost function as the LapIRN.

We decided to use the IO because: (i) it improves the ability to register fine details since the displacement fields are optimized for each case separately, (ii) only the unsupervised objective function is used during LapIRN training, and (iii) the registration time is not scored during the challenge. The IO increases the registration time by several seconds which is usually acceptable in applications not requiring real-time alignment.

2.5 Inverse Consistency-Based Weighting

To keep into account the missing data, we introduce an objective function weighting based on the inverse consistency. After the initial registration pipeline, the source and target images are bidirectionally registered again. The registration is performed by several iterations of the IO. Then, the displacement fields are composed and the inverse consistency is calculated. The inverse consistency error is defined as:

$$IC_{err}(u_{st}, u_{ts}) = u_{st}(i) \circ u_{ts}(i), \tag{2}$$

where u_{st}, u_{ts} are the displacement fields from source to target and from target to source respectively, and the $\circ$ denotes the displacement field composition.

The inverse consistency is normalized to $[0\text{--}1]$ range, raised to a given power, negated and smoothed using Gaussian filter with a predefined sigma. Both the sigma and the power are hyperparameters of the method. An exemplary visualization of the exemplary weighting mask is shown in Fig. 3. Importantly, the weighting mask is applied both to the similarity measure and the regularization term. We decided to weight the regularization term because the displacement field is supposed to model tumor resection by the volume contraction which is prohibited by large values of the regularization coefficient.

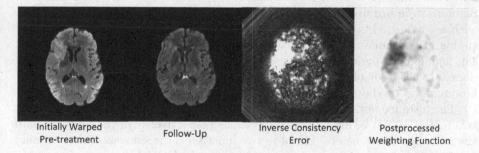

Initially Warped
Pre-treatment   Follow-Up   Inverse Consistency
Error   Postprocessed
Weighting Function

Fig. 3. Visualization of the objective function weighting. Note that small values of the weighting function are close to the tumor.

The intuition behind this approach is connected with the fact that regions without direct correspondences should have large values of the inverse consistency error. Thus, the information can be used to unsupervisedly detect non-corresponding regions and utilize this information in the objective function weighting.

2.6   Dataset and Experimental Setup

The multi-institutional dataset was curated and pre-processed retrospectively by the challenge organizers [2]. The dataset consists of pre-operative and follow-up pairs (of the same patient) diagnosed and treated for glioma. There are four MRI sequences for each pair: (i) T1-weighted (T1), (ii) contrast-enhanced T1-weighted (T1-CE), (iii) T2-weighted (T2), and (iv) fluid-attenuated inversion recovery (FLAIR).

The training set consists of 140 pairs annotated with landmarks varying from 6 to 50 per pair. The landmarks are defined using anatomical markers e.g. midline of the brain, blood vessel bifurcations, and anatomical shape of the cortex. We separated 5% of the training set as an internal validation set not used during the network training.

The external validation set consists of 20 pairs, following the structure of the training set, however, without releasing the landmarks for the pre-operative scans. The evaluation on the external validation set is possible using the challenge infrastructure only. There is also an external test set, however, unavailable for the challenge participants. The test set results will be published in the follow-up challenge summary publication based on container submissions. Therefore, in this paper, we report results for the external validation set only.

All experiments are implemented in PyTorch, extended by PyTorch Lightning [5]. The LapIRN is trained using three pyramid levels. First, the first level is trained until convergence (with frozen weights of the remaining levels), followed by unfreezing the second level, and then finally the third level. We pre-train the network by registering the pairs in a cross-case manner, resulting in almost 18,000 training pairs. The network is then fine-tuned using the pairs representing scans of the same patient. Each iteration consists of registering 100 pairs with a batch size equal to 1. The weighted sum of local channel-wise NCC and diffusive regularization are used as the objective function. The pretraining is performed with a window size equal to 7 pixels, then changed to 3 pixels during the fine-tuning. The regularization coefficients are equal to 1000, 2000, and 4000 in the 1st, 2nd and 3rd pyramid level respectively. The initial learning rate is 0.003 and decays by a factor of 0.99 per iteration. No information about the anatomical landmarks is used during training.

The instance optimization, following the DL-based registration, is run using two resolution levels, for 40 and 20 iterations respectively. All the IO runs share the same hyperparameters. The objective function is the same as during training LapIRN and the hyperparameters are as follows: (i) NCC window size is equal to 3 pixels, (ii) the regularization coefficients are equal to 12500 and 25000 respectively, (iii) the initial learning rate is equal to 0.003. During the last instance optimization call, the inverse consistency is used to perform the similarity measure weighting. The sigma and the power of the inverse consistency map post-processing are both equal to 2. The source code is openly available at [10].

3   Results

The registration is evaluated quantitatively in terms of robustness and median absolute error (MAE) between the anatomical landmarks. The robustness is defined as the ratio of landmarks with improved alignment after registration to all landmarks. The challenge organizers decided to not score the registration time and the deformation field smoothness is used only in case of tie [2].

We show the MAE and robustness statistics on the external validation set in Table 1 and Table 2 for the IEEE ISBI and MICCAI editions respectively. We present the results before the registration, after the affine registration, for the IO and DL-based registration applied separately, for the proposed hybrid approach, and for the hybrid approach extended by unsupervised cost function weighting. These results come from the challenge evaluation platform. An exemplary visualization of the registration results are shown in Fig. 4.

The proposed method scored the first and the third place during the IEEE ISBI 2022 and MICCAI 2022 editions, respectively (however, without statistically significant differences compared to the remaining methods on the podium).

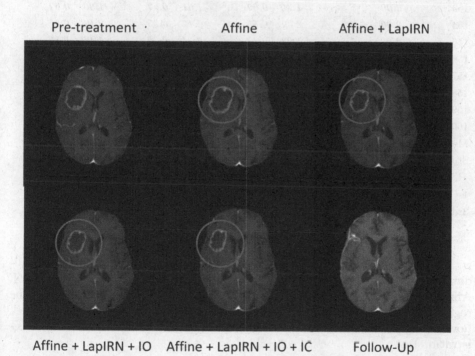

Fig. 4. Exemplary visualization of the registration results. Please note that the inverse consistency-based weighting improves the qualitative results close to the tumor volume. The tumor volume decreases and the quality of registration of fine-details around the tumor is improved. This improvement is not captured by the quantitative results based on the target registration error.

Table 1. Quantitative results on the external validation set during the IEEE ISBI 2022 edition (MAE - Median Absolute Error).

Case	Initial		IO		LapIRN		LapIRN + IO	
ID	MAE	Robustness	MAE	Robustness	MAE	Robustness	MAE	Robustness
141	13.50	–	2.06	1.00	2.78	1.00	**1.94**	1.00
142	14.00	–	4.13	0.86	3.14	0.86	**2.82**	1.00
143	16.00	–	2.00	1.00	4.51	1.00	**1.76**	1.00
144	15.00	–	**3.54**	1.00	5.20	1.00	4.12	1.00
145	17.00	–	1.54	1.00	2.96	1.00	**1.19**	1.00
146	17.00	–	2.26	1.00	3.56	1.00	**2.24**	1.00
147	1.50	–	2.08	0.40	2.41	0.50	**1.79**	0.45
148	3.50	–	**1.30**	0.90	1.99	0.85	1.63	0.80
149	9.00	–	1.66	1.00	1.91	1.00	**1.62**	1.00
150	4.00	–	1.66	0.63	2.34	0.68	**1.32**	0.63
151	3.00	–	1.40	0.80	1.39	0.70	**1.17**	0.80
152	5.00	–	**1.43**	0.95	1.68	0.95	1.46	0.95
153	2.00	–	**1.47**	0.67	1.61	0.67	1.96	0.67
154	2.00	–	2.09	0.55	2.12	0.45	**2.03**	0.55
155	2.00	–	1.93	0.47	2.34	0.42	**1.92**	0.53
156	7.00	–	**1.74**	1.00	2.14	1.00	1.80	1.00
157	10.00	–	2.20	1.00	2.17	1.00	**1.22**	1.00
158	4.50	–	1.43	0.90	1.81	0.90	**1.19**	1.00
159	6.00	–	2.46	1.00	2.57	1.00	**2.18**	1.00
160	4.00	–	**1.59**	0.90	2.39	0.90	1.75	0.90
Mean	7.80	–	2.00	0.85	2.55	0.84	**1.85**	0.86
StdDev	5.62	–	0.72	0.20	0.95	0.20	**0.67**	0.19
Median	5.50	–	1.83	0.92	2.34	0.92	**1.77**	1.0
1st quartile	3.38	–	1.52	0.77	1.96	0.70	**1.42**	0.77
3rd quartile	13.63	–	2.12	1.00	2.82	1.00	**1.98**	1.00

The average registration time (RTX GeForce 3090 Ti) on the external validation set is: 1.3, 1.4, 21.8, 57.9 s respectively for the Affine, Affine + LapIRN, Affine + LapIRN + IO, Affine + LapIRN + IO + IC version respectively. The registration time is increased by the IO modules that could be further optimized, however, in practice the real-time alignment is not crucial for the discussed registration task.

Table 2. Quantitative results on the external validation set during the MICCAI 2022 edition (MAE - Median Absolute Error). The initial errors are reported in Table 1.

Case ID	Affine		LapIRN		LapIRN + IO		LapIRN + IO + IC	
	MAE	Robustness	MAE	Robustness	MAE	Robustness	MAE	Robustness
141	4.39	1.00	2.62	1.00	1.82	1.00	**1.82**	1.00
142	6.13	0.88	3.12	1.00	2.79	1.00	**1.92**	1.00
143	8.50	0.88	3.07	1.00	2.56	1.00	**1.88**	1.00
144	9.46	0.88	2.99	1.00	**2.31**	1.00	2.62	1.00
145	4.99	1.00	2.15	1.00	1.10	1.00	**1.08**	1.00
146	6.40	1.00	2.33	1.00	1.73	1.00	**1.66**	1.00
147	2.17	0.15	2.34	0.35	2.11	0.45	**1.64**	0.45
148	2.86	0.80	2.00	0.85	**1.57**	0.80	1.67	0.90
149	2.34	1.00	2.10	1.00	1.65	1.00	**1.61**	1.00
150	3.99	0.37	2.78	0.47	1.34	0.63	**1.28**	0.63
151	2.10	0.60	1.71	0.60	**1.30**	0.85	1.31	0.85
152	2.14	0.95	1.65	0.84	**1.43**	0.89	1.51	0.89
153	1.90	0.50	2.00	0.42	1.74	0.67	**1.66**	0.75
154	2.45	0.30	1.99	0.45	2.03	0.40	**1.98**	0.45
155	2.88	0.22	2.91	0.42	**2.01**	0.42	2.03	0.42
156	3.29	1.00	2.79	1.00	**1.48**	1.00	1.53	1.00
157	5.86	0.90	2.99	1.00	**1.52**	1.00	1.58	1.00
158	3.75	0.40	2.56	0.80	1.16	1.00	**1.16**	1.00
159	7.78	0.36	2.75	1.00	**2.30**	1.00	2.37	1.00
160	2.72	0.80	2.66	0.70	**1.79**	0.90	1.80	0.90
Mean	4.31	0.70	2.48	0.70	1.79	0.85	**1.71**	0.86
StdDev	2.32	0.30	0.46	0.25	0.46	0.22	**0.38**	0.21
Median	3.52	0.84	2.59	0.93	1.74	1.00	**1.66**	1.00
1st quartile	2.42	0.39	2.08	0.57	**1.47**	0.77	1.53	0.83
3rd quartile	5.93	0.96	2.82	1.00	2.05	1.00	**1.89**	1.00

4 Discussion and Conclusion

The results confirm that the proposed hybrid approach, based on both deep learning and instance optimization (IO), improves the quantitative results compared to the methods used separately. Interestingly, the IO alone (extended by the IO-based affine registration) provides slightly better results than the LapIRN without any further tuning. This is expected because the IO optimizes each case separately and we do not use any supervision other than the unsupervised objective function to guide the training process. Interestingly, the worst robustness is reported for cases with a low initial error, suggesting that the unsupervised registration cannot improve the results more.

The objective function weighting further improves the results. From the quantitative perspective the difference is not significant, however, it is connected with the characteristic of target registration error (TRE). The TRE is not dedicated to the evaluation of the image registration with missing data because the corresponding points cannot be annotated directly in the missing volume. Therefore, the correlation between the TRE and the qualitative results nearby the tumor is limited.

Our method has several limitations. First, we do not use information about sparse landmarks during training. We think that it would be possible to use the landmarks as a weak-supervision, however, with MAE at the level of 1.71 pixel, there is not much space for further improvements, and such a method would probably learn only the annotators' preferences. Second, we did not extensively explored the use of different modalities. Probably the use of modality used for the annotation would slightly improve the quantitative results. What is more, tuning the hyperparameters to just a subset of the available modalities could possibly further improve the results. Moreover, the inverse consistency weighting significantly increases the registration time (from several seconds to almost one minute). However, we think that future work could introduce the objective function weighting directly into the deep network training and significantly decrease the registration time.

In our opinion, several decisions regarding the challenge setup should be rethought. First, the MAE and the related robustness should not be used as the only evaluation criteria for image registration with missing data. The evaluation landmarks cannot be chosen directly within the tumor volume because it is missing in the target scan. Additional metrics, based e.g. on the relative tumor volume [11] could be used to evaluate the registration quality. Second, it could be considered to score the submissions using the displacement field smoothness outside the tumor volume (and the recurrences), as well as the registration time. Moreover, uploading the displacement fields directly instead of the transformed landmarks would enable the organizers to calculate all the statistics automatically using the challenge evaluation platform.

To conclude, we proposed a hybrid approach based on the DL and IO as a contribution to the BraTS-Reg challenge. We have shown that the proposed method improves the alignment for majority of the external validation cases with high robustness. The proposed objective function weighting based on the inverse consistency further improved the results. The method could be further extended by directly incorporating the unsupervised objective function weighting during the deep network training.

Acknowledgements and Compliance With Ethical Standards. This research study was conducted retrospectively using human subject data made available in open access by BraTS-Reg Challenge organizers [2]. Ethical approval was not required as confirmed by the license attached with the open access data. The authors declare no conflict of interest. The authors would like to thank the organizers for their help with the submission of the Singularity container. This research was supported in part by PLGrid Infrastructure.

References

1. Avants, B., et al.: Symmetric diffeomorphic image registration with cross-correlation: evaluating automated labeling of elderly and neurodegenerative brain. Med. Image Anal. **12**, 26–41 (2008)
2. Baheti, B., Waldmannstetter, D., Chakrabarty, S., et al.: The brain tumor sequence registration challenge: establishing correspondence between pre-operative and follow-up MRI scans of diffuse glioma patients (2021). arXiv:2112.0697
3. Balakrishnan, G., et al.: VoxelMorph: a learning framework for deformable medical image registration. IEEE Trans. Med. Imaging **38**(8), 1788–1800 (2019)
4. Dalca, A., et al.: Unsupervised learning of probabilistic diffeomorphic registration for images and surfaces. Med. Image Anal. **57**, 226–236 (2019)
5. Falcon, W., Cho, K.: A framework for contrastive self-supervised learning and designing a new approach. arXiv preprint: arXiv:2009.00104 (2020)
6. Hering, A., et al.: Learn2Reg: comprehensive multi-task medical image registration challenge, dataset and evaluation in the era of deep learning. arXiv preprint: arXiv:2112.04489 (2021)
7. Hoffmann, M., et al.: SynthMorph: learning contrast-invariant registration without acquired images. IEEE Trans. Med. Imaging. Early Access (2021)
8. Mok, T., Chung, A.: Fast symmetric diffeomorphic image registration with convolutional neural networks. In: IEEE CVPR, pp. 4644–4653 (2020)
9. Mok, T.C.W., Chung, A.C.S.: Large deformation diffeomorphic image registration with Laplacian pyramid networks. In: Martel, A.L., et al. (eds.) MICCAI 2020. LNCS, vol. 12263, pp. 211–221. Springer, Cham (2020). https://doi.org/10.1007/978-3-030-59716-0_21
10. Wodzinski, M., Jurgas, A.: Source code (2022). https://github.com/MWod/BraTS_Reg
11. Wodzinski, M., et al.: Semi-Supervised deep learning-based image registration method with volume penalty for real-time breast tumor bed localization. Sensors **21**(12), 1–14 (2021)

Employing ConvexAdam for BraTS-Reg

Christoph Großbröhmer$^{(\boxtimes)}$, Hanna Siebert , Lasse Hansen ,
and Mattias P. Heinrich

Institute of Medical Informatics, Universität zu Lübeck, Lübeck, Germany
{c.grossbroehmer,h.siebert,l.hansen,mattias.heinrich}@uni-luebeck.de

Abstract. Multiparametric MRI registration between pre- and postoperative brain scans, which is the subject of the BraTS-Reg Challenge, poses a complex problem to solve due to large deformations and missing correspondences. We make use of hand-crafted geometric features, coupled convex optimisation, and an Adam-based instance optimisation. Our method only requires few trainable parameters and is able to perform accurate image alignment while using smooth and plausible deformation fields. For our challenge submission, we achieved a mean median target registration error of 1.77 mm on the validation dataset. ConvexAdam ranks 2nd both in the ISBI-2022 and MICCAI-2022 BraTS-Reg Challenge.

Keywords: BraTS-Reg · Medical Image Registration · Convex Optimisation

1 Introduction

The problem of image registration between pre-operative and follow-up brain tumour multiparametric MRI scans is, next to its clinical relevance, characterised by its difficulty. Strong deformations induced by tumour volume change as well as possible tissue relaxation following treatment poses a challenge, limiting the use of off-the-shelf registration algorithms. Furthermore, the registration process is error-prone due to missing correspondences caused by treatment and tumour reoccurrences, as well as image intensity distribution shifts following pathophysiological processes.

The Brain Tumor Sequence Registration (BraTS-Reg) challenge [2] aims to find registration techniques suited for this specific task and stands in the tradition of multiple BraTS segmentation challenges using similar data, prompting the incorporation of segmentation knowledge acquired through those challenges. With regard to this specific setting, our proposed method consists of

- hand-crafted modality and contrast invariant features to overcome intensity shifts,
- a coupled convex optimisation with respect to discretised displacements to capture large motions induced by mass effect and
- an instance optimisation for final fine-grained displacement prediction.

Furthermore, we investigate the incorporation of semantic segmentations from nnU-Nets.

S. Bakas et al. (Eds.): BrainLes 2022, LNCS 13769, pp. 252–261, 2023.
https://doi.org/10.1007/978-3-031-33842-7_22

2   Methods

The main idea of this challenge submission consists of three parts: Meaningful image features Sect. (2.1) are used to compute a discrete correlation-based cost tensor which is subject to a coupled convex optimisation scheme regarding feature similarity and spatial smoothness Sect. (2.2). To refine this intermediate displacement field, we employ an additional Adam-based instance optimisation Sect. (2.3). An overview of the whole registration pipeline is presented in Fig. 1.

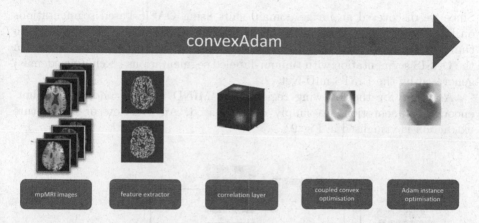

Fig. 1. Pipeline of our registration method: Input features are extracted from mpMRI images and given to a correlation layer, which computes a discrete cost tensor with respect to possible displacements within a predefined range. The displacement field is calculated by performing coupled convex optimisation and finalised by Adam-based instance optimisation.

2.1   Feature Extraction

One of the findings of Learn2Reg [8], a similar challenge with multiple registration tasks, has been the demonstration of the distinct benefit of using additional semantic information, such as high-quality segmentations, in image registration. Therefore, to improve registration, we tried to leverage a combination of hand-crafted and automatically generated features.

We use MIND-SSC [7] to extract locally discriminative image features robust to varying intensity profiles on all four image domains (T1, T1ce, T2, FLAIR), resulting in a 48-dimensional descriptor per voxel.

To obtain additional segmentations we employ two trained versions of the nnU-Net [9], a powerful self-configuring version of the U-Net:

1. BraTS nnU-Net: A model that has been trained for Task 1 of the *Medical Decathlon Challenge* [1] on a subset of data used for the 2016 and 2017 Brain

Tumor Segmentation (BraTS) challenges and therefore using multiparametric MRI of the same modalities (T1, T1ce, T2, FLAIR) as BraTS-Reg [3,11]. Target structures were limited to three tumour sub-regions, namely edema, enhancing and non-enhancing tumour. The model is publicly available[1].

2. OASIS nnU-Net: A model that has been trained for Task 3 of the *Learn2Reg Challenge 2021* [8] on T1-weighted, skull stripped MRIs for inter-patient brain registration. Target ROIs include a total of 35 different anatomical structures. The model has been used as a feature extractor for the Convex-Adam submission of this task [12].

Since we discovered an image domain shift using OASIS-based segmentations on BraTS-Reg image data due to large anatomical distortions originating from tumours, we simply merge both models by overwriting corresponding voxels in the OASIS segmentation with tumour-labeled segmentations (excluding edemas) generated by the BraTS nnU-Net.

As input for the following registration, MIND features and the one-hot-encoded segmentation are simply concatenated. An overview of our feature extraction is visualised in Fig. 2.

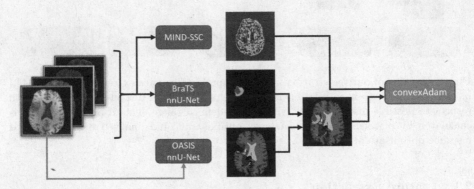

Fig. 2. Feature extraction: All MRI domains (T1, T1ce, T2, FLAIR) are used to create locally descriptive MIND features (top) and segmentations of tumorous structures (middle). An additional OASIS nnU-Net produces a detailed brain segmentation (bottom).

2.2 Convex Optimisation

One formulation of the image registration problem is that one has to find the optimal local matching of corresponding image elements while maintaining the plausibility of the deformation. Analogous to [6], our method splits this coupled problem into two convex optimisable problems: To estimate the optimal local

---

[1] https://github.com/MIC-DKFZ/nnUNet.

displacements, we first create a cost tensor mapping the similarities of corresponding patches. A correlation layer computes the sum-of-squared-differences
for possible displacements within a fixed search range using an efficient box filter.
A coupled convex optimisation performed on this cost tensor leads to an efficient global regularisation: First, a locally smooth displacement field is derived
from the positions of the lowest costs (i.e. argmin) in the cost tensor to ensure
feature similarity. Second, global smoothness is promoted by adding costs penal-
ising spatial discrepancies of displacements. Both steps are performed alternately
converging to a global smooth optimum. In this specific setting, with the possibility of large mass-effect induced deformations we employ a search range from
$24 \times 24 \times 24$ mm to $30 \times 30 \times 30$ mm. To account for missing correspondences
derived from medical treatment and long duration between scans, we enforce
additional inverse consistency by performing the same procedure with swapped
inputs and minimising the inverse consistency error between the forward and
backward displacement fields.

2.3 Adam Instance Optimisation

The intermediate displacement field serves as in initialisation for an instance
optimisation scheme with respect to deformation smoothness, enforced through
a weighted diffusion regularisation and B-Spline-Interpolation, and feature similarity. Utilising Adam [10] for gradient descent, the refined displacement field is
used to warp the input follow-up scan.

3   Multiparametric Registration

We submitted our method both to the BraTS-Reg-ISBI and BraTS-Reg-
MICCAI Challenge with minor adaptations. An overview of the submissions
is shown in Table 1.

Table 1. Challenge Submissions & Results

Challenge	MRI modalities	Feature Extraction	Convex Optimisation	Adam Instance Optimisation	Final Rank
ISBI	T1 T1ce T2 FLAIR	MIND Radius: 2 Dilation: 2	Spacing: 6 Capture range: 5	Spacing: 2 Iterations: 150 λ_{Reg}: 1	**2**
MICCAI	T1ce	MIND Radius: 2 Dilation: 2	Spacing: 6 Capture range: 4	Spacing: 2 Iterations: 80 λ_{Reg}: 0.75	**2**

3.1   BraTS-Reg-ISBI

We investigate different strategies of combining image features for registration. *MIND* denotes registration with concatenated MIND-SSC features computed on all 4 modalities, while *SEG* describes the registration using solely one-hot-encoded merged nnU-Net segmentations. Furthermore, we explore leveraging the high-quality tumour segmentations produced by the BRATS nnU-Net to combat the problem of missing correspondences. We pursue two strategies by masking out voxels with either tumour labels (*mask_T*) or tumour and edema labels (*mask_TE*) both for convex and Adam instance optimisation.

The easy-to-use registration framework *deedsBCV* [5], which also utilises MIND-SSC features and discrete optimisation, is employed on FLAIR-MRI-Scans and serves as a baseline. Analogous to prior challenge entries [4], we create spheres at keypoint locations and treat them as labels to be warped in order to translate the keypoints along with image registration. To obtain the coordinates of the warped keypoints, we simply calculate the centre of mass of each keypoint's label.

To assess the quality of our registrations consistent with the BraTS-Reg challenge, we calculate the median absolute error between landmark coordinates of each pair of pre-operative and follow-up images. For each experiment, we report the mean median (meanTRE) and median median target registration error (medianTRE) across all images, as well as the mean robustness score (mRS), which denotes the mean fraction of improved landmark coordinates. Results on the BraTS-Reg's training data are presented in Table 2.

The challenge organisers provided an automatic evaluation of registrations on validation data on their hardware. Results are reported in Table 3. Qualitative registration results are shown in Fig. 3.

Table 2. Results on BraTS-Reg-ISBI training dataset. All registration errors are denoted in *mm*. Experiments

	meanTRE	medianTRE	mRS
intial	8.2000	5.5000	/
deeds	3.2587	2.6928	0.7199
MIND	2.5622	2.2624	0.7639
SEG	11.3274	6.2815	0.2778
mask_T	2.5619	2.2569	0.7620
mask_TE	2.5618	2.2630	0.7620
MIND_T1ce*	2.4139	2.1428	0.7788

With MIND features, our method was able to outperform deeds in accuracy by about 0.7 mm (meanTRE), 0.4 mm (medianTRE) and about 4% in robustness (mRS) on the training set. However, the desired boost derived from including

Table 3. Results on BraTS-Reg-ISBI validation dataset. All registration errors are denoted in *mm*.

	meanTRE	medianTRE	mRS
intial	7.8000	5.5000	/
deeds	2.6321	2.1429	0.8071
MIND	1.8562	1.8645	0.8537
MIND_T1ce*	1.8163	1.7443	0.8756

semantic information could not be shown. Instead, the registration fails when relying solely on the merged nnU-Net segmentations. Consequently, all experiments combining MIND features and segmentations led to worse results compared to using only MIND features, and are therefore not listed. Our hypothesis is that the domain gap between OASIS and BraTS was wider than anticipated, and could not be overcome by our strategy of merging with the high-quality tumour segmentations. Upon visual inspection, the quality of generated labels differed greatly between patients.

Restricting the registration to non-tumorous structures did neither benefit nor harm the methods' performance. We suspect the geometric features in the masked tumour segmentation to lack correspondences, already limiting their influence on the deformation field. In both cases, this area would mainly be subject to regularisation.

On the validation dataset, the results of *MIND* could be reproduced by archiving a mean median TRE of 1.86 mm. Therefore, it was chosen as our starting point for hyperparameter optimisation.

Table 4. Results of our BraTS-Reg-MICCAI challenge submission for training and validation datasets. All registration errors are denoted in *mm*.

		meanTRE	medianTRE	mRS
Training Dataset	initial	8.1750	5.5000	/
	submission	2.3267	2.1331	0.8750
Validation Dataset	initial	7.8000	5.5000	/
	submission	2.2897	1.7654	0.8705

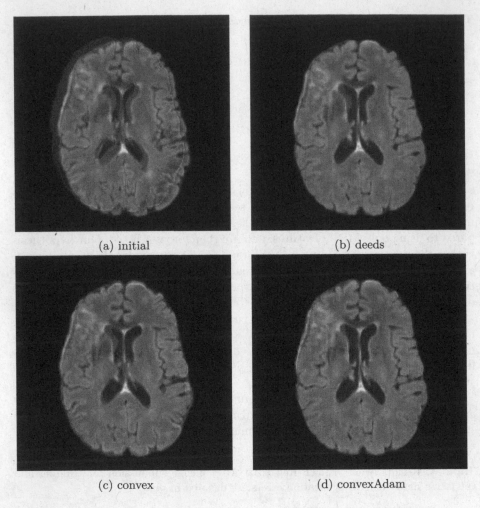

(a) initial

(b) deeds

(c) convex

(d) convexAdam

Fig. 3. Qualitative registration results on FLAIR MRI Scans. Colourmap overlay (a) before registration, (b) after baseline registration with deeds, (c) after coupled convex optimisation, and (d) after coupled convex optimisation and subsequent Adam instance optimisation.

3.2   BraTS-Reg-MICCAI

Building on the method submitted for ISBI, we could improve registration accuracy by limiting the feature extraction to contrast-enhanced MRI images (denoted *MIND_T1ce** in Tables 2 and 3) only. Neglecting the other modalities led to an overall boost in performance by 0.15 mm and 0.04 mm for the ISBI training and validation dataset respectively. Furthermore, we performed a hyperparameter grid search on the capture range and density of MIND, Inverse Consistency, and the number of iterations for Adam instance optimisation, resulting in the set of hyperparameters shown in Table 1. Our final results on BraTS-Reg-MICCAI training and validation data are denoted in Table 4.

4 Additional Experiments

We additionally investigated the quality of geometric features in conjunction with our method by evaluating intermodal registration as well as registration inference speed.

4.1 Intermodal Registration

In order to assess the modality-dependent feature quality, we employed convexAdam with MIND features crafted for every MRI modality independently and evaluated registration performance on the training dataset, resulting in meanTREs presented in Table 5.

Table 5. Mean median TRE of intermodal registration using MIND features in mm on deprecated training data. Columns and rows denote source and target domain respectively.

	T1	T1ce	FLAIR	T2
T1	3.1865	3.0206	3.6013	3.2879
T1ce	3.3590	2.4411	3.6121	3.2865
FLAIR	3.5450	3.2045	3.2061	3.4509
T2	3.3043	2.9128	3.5744	3.0159

As expected, intermodal registration is always outperformed by intramodal registration. However, even the worst constellation archives a median mean TRE of 3.61 mm, trailing only 0.36 mm behind deeds performance. The best result is archived by omitting all modalities but T1ce, which even exceeded our method with MIND Features derived from all available scans.

4.2 Registration Speed

To evaluate the inference speed of our registration approach we measured the computational time for each component of our submitted methods for both challenges. Table 6 depicts the mean runtime evaluated over the BraTS-Reg-MICCAI validation dataset using an NVIDIA GeForce RTX 2080 Ti.

As expected, both limiting the feature extraction to one modality and reducing the instance optimisation iterations lead to a faster inference throughout all components.

Table 6. Mean computational speed in seconds

Submission	Feature Extraction	Convex Optimisation	Adam Instance Optimisation	Full Registration
ISBI	1.65	0.21	2.98	5.47
MICCAI	0.50	0.13	0.74	1.64

5   Conclusion

Our contribution to BraTS-Reg'22 consists of the adaption of the convexAdam method for multiparametric MRI images. Since our experiments of including semantic segmentations in the registration process did not yield any improvement, the method of our submission is limited to multimodal geometric image features. Our method ranks second in both the BraTS-Reg-ISBI and the BraTS-Reg-MICCAI challenges, validating ConvexAdam as a lightweight, fast and comprehensible tool for the registration of pathologic multiparametric brain MRIs. Although our contribution to the BraTS-Reg challenge is limited to multimodal image features without leveraging any additional segmentations, we still believe in strong benefits from including semantic information and will further investigate the combination of geometric and semantic information for image registration.

References

1. Antonelli, M., Reinke, A., Bakas, S., Farahani, K., Kopp-Schneider, A., Landman, B.A., et al.: The medical segmentation decathlon. Nat. Commun. **13**(4128), 1–13 (2022). https://doi.org/10.1038/s41467-022-30695-9
2. Baheti, B., et al.: The brain tumor sequence registration challenge: establishing correspondence between pre-operative and follow-up MRI scans of diffuse glioma patients. arXiv, December 2021. https://doi.org/10.48550/arXiv.2112.06979
3. Bakas, S., Reyes, M., Jakab, A., Bauer, S., Rempfler, M., Crimi, A., Shinohara, R., et al.: Identifying the Best Machine Learning Algorithms for Brain Tumor Segmentation, Progression Assessment, and Overall Survival Prediction in the BRATS Challenge. arXiv, November 2018. https://doi.org/10.48550/arXiv.1811.02629
4. Heinrich, M.P.: Intra-operative ultrasound to MRI fusion with a public multimodal discrete registration tool. In: Stoyanov, D., Taylor, Z., Aylward, S., Tavares, J.M.R.S., Xiao, Y., Simpson, A., Martel, A., Maier-Hein, L., Li, S., Rivaz, H., Reinertsen, I., Chabanas, M., Farahani, K. (eds.) POCUS/BIVPCS/CuRIOUS/CPM -2018. LNCS, vol. 11042, pp. 159–164. Springer, Cham (2018). https://doi.org/10.1007/978-3-030-01045-4_19
5. Heinrich, M.P., Jenkinson, M., Brady, M., Schnabel, J.A.: MRF-based deformable registration and ventilation estimation of lung CT. IEEE Trans. Med. Imaging **32**(7), 1239–1248 (2013). https://doi.org/10.1109/TMI.2013.2246577
6. Heinrich, M.P., Papież, B.W., Schnabel, J.A., Handels, H.: Non-parametric discrete registration with convex optimisation. In: Ourselin, S., Modat, M. (eds.) WBIR 2014. LNCS, vol. 8545, pp. 51–61. Springer, Cham (2014). https://doi.org/10.1007/978-3-319-08554-8_6

7. Heinrich, M.P., Jenkinson, M., Papież, B.W., Brady, S.M., Schnabel, J.A.: Towards realtime multimodal fusion for image-guided interventions using self-similarities. In: Mori, K., Sakuma, I., Sato, Y., Barillot, C., Navab, N. (eds.) MICCAI 2013. LNCS, vol. 8149, pp. 187–194. Springer, Heidelberg (2013). https://doi.org/10.1007/978-3-642-40811-3_24

8. Hering, A., Hansen, L., Mok, T.C.W., Chung, A.C.S., Siebert, H., Häger, S., et al.: Learn2Reg: comprehensive multi-task medical image registration challenge, dataset and evaluation in the era of deep learning. IEEE Trans. Med. Imaging **42**, 697–712 (2022). https://doi.org/10.1109/TMI.2022.3213983

9. Isensee, F., Jaeger, P.F., Kohl, S.A.A., Petersen, J., Maier-Hein, K.H.: nnU-Net: a self-configuring method for deep learning-based biomedical image segmentation. Nat. Methods **18**, 203–211 (2021). https://doi.org/10.1038/s41592-020-01008-z

10. Kingma, D.P., Ba, J.: Adam: a method for stochastic optimization, December 2014. arXiv:arxiv.org/abs/1412.6980v9

11. Menze, B.H., et al.: The multimodal brain tumor image segmentation benchmark (BRATS). IEEE Trans. Med. Imaging **34**(10), 1993–2024 (2014). https://doi.org/10.1109/TMI.2014.2377694

12. Siebert, H., Hansen, L., Heinrich, M.P.: Fast 3D registration with accurate optimisation and little learning for Learn2Reg 2021, December 2021. arXiv:arxiv.org/abs/2112.03053v1

Iterative Method to Register Longitudinal MRI Acquisitions in Neurosurgical Context

Luca Canalini[1,2(✉)], Jan Klein[1], Annika Gerken[1], Stefan Heldmann[3], Alessa Hering[3,4], and Horst K. Hahn[1,2]

[1] Fraunhofer MEVIS, Institute for Digital Medicine, Bremen, Germany
luca.canalini@mevis.fraunhofer.de
[2] University of Bremen, Bremen, Germany
[3] Fraunhofer MEVIS, Institute for Digital Medicine, Lübeck, Germany
[4] Diagnostic Image Analysis Group, Radboud University Medical Center, Nijmegen, The Netherlands

Abstract. The visual comparison of MRI images obtained before and after neurosurgical procedures is useful to identify tumor recurrences in postoperative images. Image registration algorithms are utilized to establish precise correspondences between subsequent acquisitions. The changes observable in subsequent MRI acquisitions can be tackled by methods combining rigid and non-rigid registration. A rigid step is useful to accommodate global transformations, due, for example, to the different positions and orientations of the patient's head within the scanning device. Furthermore, brain shift caused by tumor resection can only be tackled by non-rigid approaches. In this work, we propose an automatic iterative method to register pre- and postoperative MRI acquisitions. First, the solution rigidly registers two subsequent images. Then, a deformable registration is computed. The T1-CE and T2 MRI sequences are used to guide the registration process. The method is proposed as a solution to the BraTS-Reg challenge. The method improves the average median absolute error from 7.8 mm to 1.98 mm in the validation set.

1 Introduction

In neurosurgery for tumor resection, preoperative magnetic resonance imaging (MRI) data is acquired to plan the further removal. Thus, MRI images are obtained at successive postoperative stages to follow the development of the resection cavity and to spot any tumor recurrence. Figure 1 shows two subsequent MRI acquisitions obtained before and after neurosurgical resection. The visual analysis of post-operative data can be difficult. In fact, signs of enhancing tumor regrowth can be confused with the effects of adjuvant postsurgical treatments applied on the brain tissues. A comparison with pre-operative data can be helpful to improve the understanding of follow-up acquisitions. Registration algorithms are utilized to establish precise correspondences between MRI

S. Bakas et al. (Eds.): BrainLes 2022, LNCS 13769, pp. 262–272, 2023.
https://doi.org/10.1007/978-3-031-33842-7_23

images acquired at different stages. The first step of a registration solution usually consists of the computation of a rigid or an affine transformation. This step is useful to register to the same reference system subsequent images, in which the patient's head might assume different orientations and locations within the scanning device. More complex deformations visible in follow-up stages are caused by the tumor resection. In particular, brain shift phenomenon mostly affects the areas surrounding pathological area, which usually gets more deformed than the rest of intracranial locations. Thus, a deformable solution, which can locally register the brain tissues, is necessary.

Several solutions to register subsequent MRI acquisitions have been already proposed. A method to register corresponding healthy tissues of two longitudinal images is developed by [1]. The same authors propose a method to register pre-operative MRI data with subsequent images acquired after tumor resection [2]. Another solution is investigated by [3], in which pathological tissues are excluded from the computation of the distance measure. Furthermore, the authors in [5] propose a semi-automatic method to register pre-operative, post-operative, and follow-up images of individual patients. Besides, in [4] the authors propose a method to register pre-operative and post recurrence brain tumor images. The acquisitions are registered by excluding the pathological tissues from the image-correspondence term.

In this work, we propose an iterative solution that first performs a rigid alignment of two successive scans, and second computes a deformation field to non-rigidly register the brain tissues.

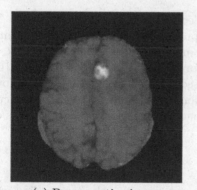
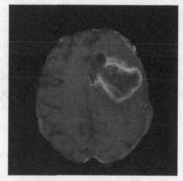

(a) Pre-operative image   (b) Post-operative image

Fig. 1. Example of subsequent MRI T1-CE acquisitions of the validation set of the BraTS-Reg dataset. In subfigure a, the hyperintense area is represented by the pathological tissues, which has to be removed. In subfigure b, the hypointense resection cavity is visible, together with post-operatively induced edema.

2   BraTS-Reg Challenge

In the BraTS-Reg challenge, organized at the ISBI 2022 conference, participants are asked to develop automatic registration solutions to improve the registration of pre- and post-operative MRI volumes [6]. The dataset released with the challenge includes 200 pairs of MRI volumes obtained before and after neurosurgical resection. Each pair includes two images, one acquired before surgery, the second one after the resection. Each case is described by four different MRI sequences: native T1, contrast enhanced T1-weighted (T1-CE), T2-weighted (T2) and T2 Fluid Attenuated Inversion Recovery (FLAIR). The data is divided into training, validation, and test set. The training set includes 140 pairs of volumes, with corresponding landmarks in each pair of volumes. These landmarks are obtained on anatomical locations such as blood vessel bifurcations, the anatomical shape of the cortex, and anatomical landmarks of the midline of the brain. The total number of landmarks varies from case to case and across all cases in the range of 6–50 per scan. The validation set consists of 20 pairs of volume, and only includes the MRI volumes and the landmarks of the post-operative cases. Finally, the test set of 40 pairs is not provided to the challenge participants.

The volumes of each pair have previously preregistered to a common reference [6]. However, several cases in the training and validation sets have a poor alignment. An example is shown in Fig. 2. Thus, before applying any deformable solution, an improvement of the initial alignment is advisable.

3   Method

The fixed and moving images can be modeled as functions $\mathcal{F}, \mathcal{M} : \mathbb{R}^3 \to \mathbb{R}$. The goal of the proposed image registration approaches is to generate a deformation $y : \Omega \to \mathbb{R}^3$ that aligns the two images $\mathcal{F}$ and $\mathcal{M}$ on the field of view $\Omega \subset \mathbb{R}^3$ such that $\mathcal{F}(x)$ and $\mathcal{M}(y(x))$ are similar for $x \in \Omega$. The proposed method is a variational image registration approach based on [7], in which the registration of two volumes corresponds to the minimization of a discretized objective function $\mathcal{J}(\mathcal{F}, \mathcal{M}, y)$. In particular, the proposed image registration method consists of a parametric and a non-parametric steps.

3.1   Parametric Registration

The first step consists of a parametric approach, in which the registration problem is based on the estimation of limited number of transformation parameters. In particular, a rigid registration technique, restricted to the search of rotations and translations parameters, is used. Thus, the deformation can modelled as follows:

$$y(x) = Qx + b \tag{1}$$

where $Q \in \mathbb{R}^{3x3}, \det(Q) = 1, b \in \mathbb{R}^3$. In the parametric approach, the minimization of the objective function corresponds to the minimization of a similarity measure $\mathcal{D}$

$$\mathcal{J}(\mathcal{F}, \mathcal{M}, y) = \mathcal{D}(\mathcal{F}, \mathcal{M}(y)) \tag{2}$$

measuring the similarity between the fixed and warped moving image. Hence, the registration parameters are modified in order to generate a transformation which can reduce the distance between the reference and warped moving images. In the proposed solution, we use the normalized gradient field (NGF) as distance measure:

$$\text{NGF}(R, T) = \frac{1}{2} \int_{\Omega} 1 - \left(\frac{\langle \nabla R(x), \nabla T(x) \rangle_{\varepsilon_R \varepsilon_T}}{\|\nabla T(x)\|_{\varepsilon_T} \|\nabla R(x)\|_{\varepsilon_R}} \right)^2 dx \tag{3}$$

where $\langle x, y \rangle_{\varepsilon} := x^\top y + \varepsilon$, $\|x\|_{\varepsilon} := \sqrt{\langle x, x \rangle_{\varepsilon^2}}$ and $\varepsilon_R, \varepsilon_T > 0$ are the so-called edge-parameters controlling influence of noise in the images. The transformation obtained in the parametric registration is utilized to initialize the following non-parametric registration.

3.2 Non-parametric Registration

The non-parametric approach aims to predict a deformation vector field y that provides a different transformation for each voxel position. To limit the number possible solutions, the registration problem introduces additional regularization terms. Thus, the objective function is written as

$$\mathcal{J}(\mathcal{F}, \mathcal{M}, y) = \mathcal{D}(\mathcal{F}, \mathcal{M}(y)) + \alpha \mathcal{R}(y) + \gamma \mathcal{V}(y) \tag{4}$$

This function is composed of the NGF distance measure and two regularization terms, limiting the range of possible transformations and making the deformation more plausible. The first one is the curvature regularizer

$$\mathcal{R}(y) = \int_{\Omega} \sum_{k=1}^{3} \|\Delta y(x)\|^2 dx \tag{5}$$

which penalizes deformation fields having too large second derivatives. To limit even further the available solutions, another regularization term

$$\mathcal{V}(y) = \int_{\Omega} \psi(\det \nabla y(x)) dx \tag{6}$$

is added to the objective function, where $\psi(t) = (t-1)^2/t$ for $t > 0$ and $\psi(t) := \infty$ for $t \leq 0$. The volume change control is used to reduce foldings in the deformation field y that may be generated during the minimization of the cost function. Folding in the deformation field represents an unrealistic transformation that the minimization process may lead to. The two hyperparameters γ and α control the influence of the regularization terms on the loss function. The choice of the optimal transformation parameters is conducted by using the quasi-Newton l-BGFS [8], due to its speed and memory efficiency.

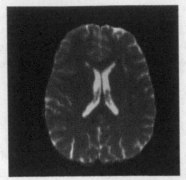

(a) Pre-operative image

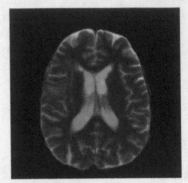

(b) Post-operative image

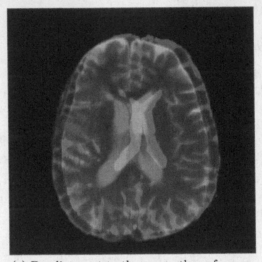

(c) Prealignment to the same atlas reference.

Fig. 2. Example of overlap between pre- and post-operative acquisitions based on the affine prealignement to the same atlas reference. The initial registration is performed for all the volumes available in the BraTS-Reg dataset. As can be observed, the two subsequent acquisitions are poorly prealigned. Before the deformable registration, the proposed method improves the initial alignment by rigidly registering the acquisitions of each MRI pair.

3.3 Multi-level Variational Registration Method

Multi-level approaches register images at different scales (L). Multi-level registration demonstrated to be useful to avoid local minima in the optimization of the objective function, and to speed up computational runtimes [10–13]. The deformation field is initially computed on the coarsest level and the images are downsampled by a factor equal to 2^{L-1}. On a finer level, the previously computed deformation fields are utilized as an initial guess by warping the moving image. At each level, the moving and fixed images are downsampled.

Registration Parameters. Our solution proposes a registration performed on three levels ($L = 3$). The values of the stopping criteria for the optimization process are empirically set: the minimal progress, the minimal gradient, the relative one, the minimum step length are set to 0.001, and the maximum number of iterations is set to 100. The loss weighting parameters are empirically set to $\alpha = 0.1$ and $\gamma = 1$.

3.4 Choice of the MRI Sequence

The two steps in the proposed registration method can use only an MRI sequence at a time. Thus, we first verified on the training set of the BraTS-Reg challenge dataset which sequence is the best to guide the registration in both the rigid and non-rigid steps. More details about the process of choosing the best MRI sequence to guide the deformable registration step is available in [9]. Our final solution uses the T2 and T1-CE sequences to guide respectively the rigid and deformable registration steps.

4 Evaluation

The proposed method is first designed by computing the registration results on 140 pairs of the training set of the BraTS-Reg dataset [6], whose which initial median absolute error (MAE) computed on the corresponding landmarks is 8.2 mm. Second, it is validated on 20 pairs of volumes of the validation set of the BraTS-Reg dataset [6]. The initial median absolute error (MAE) computed on the corresponding landmarks is 7.8 mm. The first column *ID* in Table 1 identifies the pairs of volumes of the validation set to be registered, and the initial MAEs for each pair of volumes are also reported, together with the mean absolute error (in the second and third columns of Table 1. The deformation field output by the proposed method is used to warp the landmarks of the post-operative acquisitions. The goal of the registration algorithm is to reduce the MAE. The numerical results presented in this manuscript are computed by utilizing the challenge evaluation online platform.

5 Results

In the training set, the initial MAE is reduced to 2.69 mm. Moreover, on the validation set, the average MAE gets reduced to 1.98 mm. In particular, the forth and fifth columns in Table 1 report the values obtained after registering the

Table 1. Initial and final registration errors. The first column shows the IDs of the validation set, and the second and third ones contain the initial registration errors. The results obtained by our method are available in the last three columns.

ID	Initial registration errors		Registration results		
	Median Absolute Error	Mean Absolute Error	Median absolute Error	Mean Absolute Error	Robustness
141	13.50	14.13	1.91	3.00	1.00
142	14.00	16.38	3.43	4.83	1.00
143	16.00	15.38	3.24	3.92	1.00
144	15.00	15.75	4.07	6.04	1.00
145	17.00	17.88	2.32	4.05	1.00
146	17.00	16.50	1.83	2.47	1.00
147	1.50	4.80	1.82	2.28	0.50
148	3.50	5.15	1.27	1.50	0.85
149	9.00	9.42	1.64	2.09	1.00
150	4.00	3.32	1.13	1.52	0.68
151	3.00	2.95	1.39	1.55	0.80
152	5.00	4.84	1.35	1.70	0.95
153	2.00	2.83	1.82	2.61	0.67
154	2.00	1.95	2.09	2.13	0.55
155	2.00	3.26	1.86	1.99	0.53
156	7.00	8.80	1.71	4.86	0.90
157	10.00	9.60	1.46	2.21	0.90
158	4.50	4.70	1.25	2.05	0.90
159	6.00	6.45	2.08	2.40	1.00
160	4.00	4.20	1.95	1.93	0.80
Mean	7.80	8.41	1.98	2.76	0.85
StdDev	5.62	5.54	0.77	1.29	0.17
Median	5.50	5.80	1.82	2.25	0.90
25quantile	3.38	3.98	1.44	1.97	0.77
75quantile	13.63	14.44	2.08	3.23	1.00

volumes of validation set and applying the computed deformation fields on the landmarks. Furthermore, the robustness results are reported in the last column of the same table. Examples of qualitative results can be observed in Figs. 3, 4, for T1-CE and T2 images. In particular, Fig. 4 compares the results obtained in the rigid step, and the outcome achieved by applying also the deformable registration.

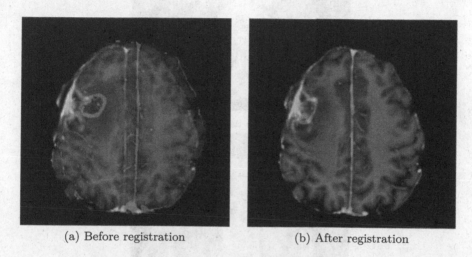

(a) Before registration   (b) After registration

Fig. 3. Example of registration results visualized on MRI T1-CE acqusitions.

6   Discussion

The method leads to a significant improvement of the MAE, which from 7.9 mm gets reduced to 1.98mm. Moreover, for all the cases, the method improves the baseline values. The mean robustness is 0.87, and only for two cases it is lower than 0.6. Figure 4 shows how the rigid registration helps to improve the initial overlap between two subsequent acquisitions. However, only a rigid transformation is not sufficient to locally compensate the brain shift due to the resection, as it can be noticed by observing the lateral ventricles. Instead, the deformable step, starting the minimization process from the prealignment set in the first step, can accommodate the local displacements due to tumor resection.

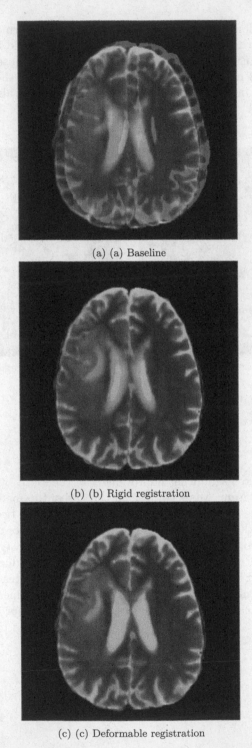

(a) (a) Baseline

(b) (b) Rigid registration

(c) (c) Deformable registration

Fig. 4. Example of two-step registration method proposed for the challenge.

7   Conclusion

Our method improves the registration results for all the cases of the validation set of BraTs-Reg dataset. As future work, we believe it would be beneficial to exclude the contribution of the pathological tissues from the distance measure. In fact, these structures do not show correspondences in both pre- and post-surgical stages. Thus, the registration could further be improved by only corresponding (healthy) tissues in the registration process.

Funding Information. This work was funded by the H2020 Marie-Curie ITN TRA-BIT (765148) project. LC is supported by the Translational Brain Imaging Training Network (TRABIT) under the European Union's 'Horizon 2020' Research and Innovation Program (Grant agreement ID: 765148).

References

1. Chitphakdithai, N., Duncan, J.S.: Pairwise registration of images with missing correspondences due to resection. In: Proceedings IEEE International Symposium on Biomedical Imaging: from Nano to Macro. IEEE International Symposium on Biomedical Imaging, p. 1025 (2010). https://doi.org/10.1109/ISBI.2010.5490164
2. Chitphakdithai, N., Chiang, V.L., Duncan, J.S.: Non-rigid registration of longitudinal brain tumor treatment MRI. In: Conference proceedings : Annual International Conference of the IEEE Engineering in Medicine and Biology Society. IEEE Engineering in Medicine and Biology Society. Conference, p. 4893 (2011). https://doi.org/10.1109/IEMBS.2011.6091212
3. Han, X., et al.: Patient-specific registration of pre-operative and post-recurrence brain tumor MRI scans. In: Crimi, A., Bakas, S., Kuijf, H., Keyvan, F., Reyes, M., van Walsum, T. (eds.) BrainLes 2018. LNCS, vol. 11383, pp. 105–114. Springer, Cham (2019). https://doi.org/10.1007/978-3-030-11723-8_10
4. Kwon, D., Niethammer, M., Akbari, H., Bilello, M., Davatzikos, C., Pohl, K.M.: PORTR: pre-operative and post-recurrence brain tumor registration. IEEE Trans. Med. Imaging **33**(3), 651 (2014). https://doi.org/10.1109/TMI.2013.2293478
5. van der Hoorn, A., Yan, J.-L., Larkin, T.J., Boonzaier, N.R., Matys, T., Price, S.J.: Validation of a semi-automatic co-registration of MRI scans in patients with brain tumors during treatment follow-up. NMR Biomed. **29**(7), 882–889 (2016). https://doi.org/10.1002/nbm.3538
6. Baheti, B., et al.: The brain tumor sequence registration challenge: establishing correspondence between pre-operative and follow-up MRI scans of diffuse glioma patients (2021). arXiv:2112.06979. https://doi.org/10.48550/arXiv.2112.06979
7. Modersitzki, J.: Fair: Flexible Algorithms for Image Registration. Society for Industrial and Applied Mathematics (2009). https://archive.siam.org/books/fa06
8. Liu, D.C., Nocedal, J.: On the limited memory BFGS method for large scale optimization. Math. Program. **45**(1), 503–528 (1989). https://doi.org/10.1007/BF01589116
9. Canalini, L., et al.: Quantitative evaluation of the influence of multiple MRI sequences and of pathological tissues on the registration of longitudinal data acquired during brain tumor treatment. Front. Neuroimaging **1**, 977491 (2022). https://doi.org/10.3389/fnimg.2022.977491

10. Hering, A., van Ginneken, B., Heldmann, S.: mlVIRNET: multilevel variational image registration network. In: Shen, D., et al. (eds.) MICCAI 2019. LNCS, vol. 11769, pp. 257–265. Springer, Cham (2019). https://doi.org/10.1007/978-3-030-32226-7_29

11. Hering, A., Häger, S., Moltz, J., Lessmann, N., Heldmann, S., van Ginneken, B.: CNN-based lung CT registration with multiple anatomical constraints. Med. Image Anal. **72**, 102139 (2021). https://doi.org/10.1016/j.media.2021.102139

12. Mok, T.C.W., Chung, A.C.S.: Large deformation diffeomorphic image registration with Laplacian pyramid networks. In: Martel, A.L., et al. (eds.) MICCAI 2020. LNCS, vol. 12263, pp. 211–221. Springer, Cham (2020). https://doi.org/10.1007/978-3-030-59716-0_21

13. Meng, M., Bi, L., Feng, D., Kim, J.: Non-iterative coarse-to-fine registration based on single-pass deep cumulative learning. In: Wang, L., Dou, Q., Fletcher, P.T., Speidel, S., Li, S. (eds.) Medical Image Computing and Computer Assisted Intervention - MICCAI 2022. MICCAI 2022. Lecture Notes in Computer Science, vol. 13436, pp. 88–97. Springer, Cham. https://doi.org/10.1007/978-3-031-16446-0_9

Brain Tumor Sequence Registration
with Non-iterative Coarse-To-Fine Networks
and Dual Deep Supervision

Mingyuan Meng[1] , Lei Bi[1]([⊠]) , Dagan Feng[1,2] , and Jinman Kim[1]

[1] School of Computer Science, The University of Sydney, Sydney, Australia
lei.bi@sydney.edu.au
[2] Med-X Research Institute, Shanghai Jiao Tong University, Shanghai, China

Abstract. In this study, we focus on brain tumor sequence registration between pre-operative and follow-up Magnetic Resonance Imaging (MRI) scans of brain glioma patients, in the context of Brain Tumor Sequence Registration challenge (BraTS-Reg 2022). Brain tumor registration is a fundamental requirement in brain image analysis for quantifying tumor changes. This is a challenging task due to large deformations and missing correspondences between pre-operative and follow-up scans. For this task, we adopt our recently proposed Non-Iterative Coarse-to-finE registration Networks (NICE-Net) – a deep learning-based method for coarse-to-fine registering images with large deformations. To overcome missing correspondences, we extend the NICE-Net by introducing dual deep supervision, where a deep self-supervised loss based on image similarity and a deep weakly-supervised loss based on manually annotated landmarks are deeply embedded into the NICE-Net. At the BraTS-Reg 2022, our method achieved a competitive result on the validation set (mean absolute error: 3.387) and placed 4th in the final testing phase (Score: 0.3544).

Keywords: Image Registration · Coarse-to-fine Networks · Deep Supervision

1 Introduction

Deformable image registration aims to establish a dense, non-linear correspondence between a pair of images, which is a crucial step in a variety of clinical tasks such as organ atlas creation and tumor monitoring [1]. Due to pathological changes (e.g., tumor growth) or inter-patient anatomy variations, medical images usually carry many non-linear local deformations. Therefore, unlike the commonly used natural image registration tasks such as photo stitching [2], medical image analysis heavily relies on deformable image registration. However, deformable image registration is still an intractable problem due to image shape and appearance variations [3], especially for image pairs containing pathology-affected tissue changes.

To establish a fair benchmark environment for deformable registration methods, Baheti et al. [4] organized a Brain Tumor Sequence Registration challenge (BraTS-Reg

S. Bakas et al. (Eds.): BrainLes 2022, LNCS 13769, pp. 273–282, 2023.
https://doi.org/10.1007/978-3-031-33842-7_24

2022), focusing on brain tumor sequence registration between pre-operative and follow-up Magnetic Resonance Imaging (MRI) scans of brain glioma patients. Brain tumor registration is clinically important as it can advance the understanding of gliomas and aids in analyzing the tissue resulting in tumor relapse [5]. However, this is a challenging task because: (i) brain tumors usually cause large deformations in brain anatomy, and (ii) there are missing correspondences between the tumor in the pre-operative scan and the resection cavity in the follow-up scan [4].

Traditional methods attempt to solve deformable registration as an iterative optimization problem [6], which is usually time-consuming and has inspired a tendency toward faster deep registration methods based on deep learning [7]. To register image pairs with large deformations, coarse-to-fine deep registration methods were widely used and are regarded as the state-of-the-art [8–13]. Typically, coarse-to-fine registration was implemented by iteratively warping an image with multiple cascaded networks [8, 9] or with multiple network iterations [10]. Recently, non-iterative coarse-to-fine registration methods were proposed to perform coarse-to-fine registration with a single network in a single iteration [11–13], which have demonstrated state-of-the-art registration accuracy even when compared with methods using multiple cascaded networks or multiple network iterations.

In this study, we adopt our recently proposed deep registration method – Non-Iterative Coarse-to-finE registration Networks (NICE-Net) [13]. The NICE-Net performs multiple steps of coarse-to-fine registration in a single network iteration, which is optimized for image pairs with large deformations and has shown state-of-the-art performance on inter-patient brain MRI registration [13]. However, the NICE-Net was not optimized for brain tumor registration with missing correspondences. We extend the NICE-Net by introducing dual deep supervision, where a deep self-supervised loss based on image similarity and a deep weakly-supervised loss based on manually annotated landmarks (ground truth) are deeply embedded into each coarse-to-fine registration step of the NICE-Net. The deep self-supervised loss can leverage the information within image appearance (e.g., texture and intensity pattern), while the deep weakly-supervised loss can leverage ground truth information to overcome the missing correspondences between pre-operative and follow-up scans.

2   Materials and Methods

2.1   Dataset and Data Preprocessing

The BraTS-Reg 2022 dataset was curated from multiple institutions, containing pairs of pre-operative and follow-up brain MRI scans of the same patient diagnosed and treated for gliomas. The training set contains 140 pairs of multi-parametric MRI scans along with landmark annotations. The multi-parametric MRI sequences include native T1-weighted (T1), contrast-enhanced T1-weighted (T1CE), T2-weighted (T2), and T2 Fluid Attenuated Inversion Recovery (FLAIR) images. The landmark annotations include the landmark coordinates in the baseline scan and their corresponding coordinates in the follow-up scan, which were manually annotated by clinical experts and are regarded as ground truth (refer to [4] for more details about landmark annotations). The validation set contains 20 pairs of MRI scans and was provided to validate the developed registration methods. Finally, the registration methods are submitted in a containerized form to be evaluated on a hidden testing set.

We preprocessed the provided images with the following steps: (i) we cropped and padded each MRI image from $240 \times 240 \times 155$ to $144 \times 192 \times 160$ with the coordinates of $(48:192, 32:224, -5:155)$, and (ii) we normalized each MRI image within the range of 0 and 1 through min-max normalization.

2.2 Non-iterative Coarse-To-Fine Registration Networks

Image registration aims to find a spatial transformation ϕ that warps a moving image I_m to a fixed image I_f, so that the warped image $I_m \circ \phi$ is spatially aligned with the fixed image I_f. In this study, the I_m and I_f are two volumes defined in a 3D spatial domain $\Omega \subset \mathbb{R}^3$, and the ϕ is parameterized as a displacement field [14]. Our method is based on our recently proposed NICE-Net (Non-Iterative Coarse-to-finE registration Networks) [13]. The architecture of the NICE-Net is shown in Fig. 1, which consists of a feature learning encoder and a coarse-to-fine registration decoder. We employed the NICE-Net to perform four steps of coarse-to-fine registration. At the ith step for $i \in \{1, 2, 3, 4\}$, a transformation ϕ_i is produced, with the ϕ_1 as the coarsest transformation and the ϕ_4 as the finest transformation. We created two image pyramids as the input, downsampling the I_f and I_m with trilinear interpolation by a factor of $0.5^{(4-i)}$ to obtain I_f^i and I_m^i for $i \in \{1, 2, 3, 4\}$ with $I_f^4 = I_f$ and $I_m^4 = I_m$. In addition, the coordinates of the landmark in the I_f and I_m are denoted as L_f and L_m. Along with the downsampling of I_f and I_m, the L_f and L_m were also downsampled as L_f^i and L_m^i for $i \in \{1, 2, 3, 4\}$ with $L_f^4 = L_f$ and $L_m^4 = L_m$.

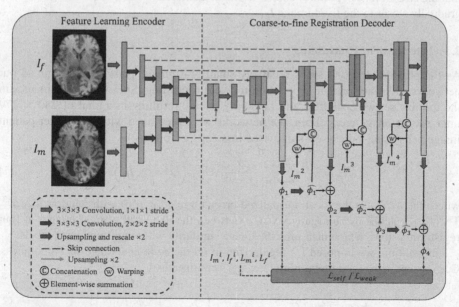

Fig. 1. Architecture of the NICE-Net that performs four steps of coarse-to-fine registration.

The feature learning encoder has two paths to separately extract features from the I_f and I_m, which is different from the deep registration methods that learn coupled features from the concatenated I_f and I_m [8, 9, 14, 15]. Specifically, the encoder has two identical, weight-shared paths that take I_f and I_m as input. Each path consists of five successive $3 \times 3 \times 3$ convolutional layers, followed by LeakyReLU activation with parameter 0.2. Except for the first convolutional layer, each convolutional layer has a stride of 2 to reduce the resolution of feature maps.

The coarse-to-fine registration decoder performs four steps of registration in a coarse-to-fine manner. Specifically, the decoder has five successive $3 \times 3 \times 3$ convolutional layers to cumulate features from different sources, followed by LeakyReLU activation with parameter 0.2. Except for the last convolutional layer, an upsampling layer is used after each convolutional layer to increase the resolution of feature maps by a factor of 2. The first convolutional layer is used to cumulate features from the encoder, while the first (coarsest) registration step is performed at the second convolutional layer and produces the ϕ_1. The ϕ_1 is upsampled by a factor of 2 (as $\widehat{\phi_1}$) and then warps the $I_m{}^2$. The warped image $I_m{}^2 \circ \widehat{\phi_1}$ and the $\widehat{\phi_1}$ are fed into a convolutional layer to extract features and then are leveraged at the second registration step. The second registration step produces a displacement field based on the cumulated features at the third convolution layer, and voxel-wisely add the displacement field to $\widehat{\phi_1}$ to obtain ϕ_2. We repeat this process until ϕ_4 is obtained.

During training, all the output ϕ_1, ϕ_2, ϕ_3, and ϕ_4 are supervised by a deep self-supervised loss $\mathcal{L}_{self}$ and/or a deep weakly-supervised loss $\mathcal{L}_{weak}$ (detailed in Sect. 2.3 and Sect. 2.4). During inference, only ϕ_4 is used to warp the I_m to align with the I_f. We present exemplified registration results of the NICE-Net in Fig. 2, which shows that the NICE-Net can perform coarse-to-fine registration to make the moving image I_m gradually closer to the fixed image I_f.

2.3   Inter-patient Pretraining

As the provided training set is relatively small (140 image pairs), we pretrained our networks with inter-patient registration to avoid overfitting. Specifically, all images in the training set were shuffled and randomly paired, resulting in a total of 280×279 inter-patient image pairs. Then, the networks were pretrained with these inter-patient image pairs using a deep self-supervised loss $\mathcal{L}_{self}$ as follows:

$$\mathcal{L}_{self} = -\sum\nolimits_{i=1}^{4} \frac{1}{2^{(4-i)}} NCC_w\left(I_m{}^{i} \circ \phi_i, I_f{}^{i}\right), \tag{1}$$

where the NCC_w is the local normalized cross-correlation [16] with window size w^3. The $\mathcal{L}_{self}$ calculates the negative NCC_w between the fixed and warped images at four registration steps, which measures the image similarity without ground truth labels.

In addition, we imposed L2 regularization on the ϕ_i to encourage its smoothness. Consequently, the total pretraining loss $\mathcal{L}_{pre}$ is defined as:

$$\mathcal{L}_{Pre} = \mathcal{L}_{self} + \sum\nolimits_{i=1}^{4} \frac{1}{2^{(4-i)}}\left(\sum\nolimits_{p \in \Omega} ||\nabla\phi_i(\boldsymbol{p})||^2\right). \tag{2}$$

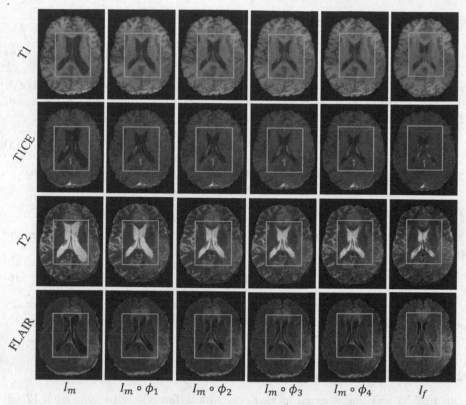

Fig. 2. Exemplified registration results with NICE-Net. Red boxes highlight the regions with major changes, gradually being closer to the fixed image I_f after each registration step. The same red bounding box has been placed at the same location for better visual comparison.

2.4 Intra-patient Training with Dual Deep Supervision

After the inter-patient pretraining, our networks were further trained for intra-patient registration with the 140 intra-patient image pairs in the training set. In addition to the deep self-supervised loss $\mathcal{L}_{self}$ used during pretraining, we also introduced a deep weakly-supervised loss $\mathcal{L}_{weak}$ as follows:

$$\mathcal{L}_{weak} = \sum_{i=1}^{4} 2^{(4-i)} MSE\left(L_m^{\ i} \circ \phi_i, L_f^{\ i}\right), \tag{3}$$

where the *MSE* is the mean square error between the coordinates of two sets of landmarks. The $\mathcal{L}_{weak}$ penalizes the distance between the fixed and warped landmarks at four registration steps, which leverages the information within the landmark labels to overcome the missing correspondences between pre-operative and follow-up scans.

In addition, as the landmark labels are sparse, the displacement fields should be smooth so that the landmark labels can impose more influence on the displacement fields. Therefore, in addition to the L2 regularization used during pretraining, we adopted an additional regularization loss that explicitly penalizes the negative Jacobian determinants

[17], making the total regularization loss $\mathcal{L}_{reg}$ as:

$$\mathcal{L}_{reg} = \sum\nolimits_{i=1}^{4} \frac{1}{2^{(4-i)}} \left[\lambda \cdot JD(\phi_i) + \sum\nolimits_{p \in \Omega} ||\nabla \phi_i(\boldsymbol{p})||^2 \right], \tag{4}$$

where the JD is regularization loss penalizing the negative Jacobian determinants of ϕ_i (refer to [17]) and the λ is a regularization parameter that adjusts the smoothness of displacement fields. Finally, the total training loss $\mathcal{L}_{train}$ is defined as:

$$\mathcal{L}_{Train} = \mathcal{L}_{self} + \mu \mathcal{L}_{weak} + \sigma \mathcal{L}_{reg}, \tag{5}$$

where the μ and σ are two parameters that adjust the magnitude of each loss term.

2.5 Pair-Specific Fine-Tuning

We fine-tuned the trained networks for each inferred image pair and then used the fine-tuned networks for inference. The loss used for pair-specific fine-tuning is:

$$\mathcal{L}_{Fine} = \mathcal{L}_{self} + \sigma \mathcal{L}_{reg}. \tag{6}$$

As ground truth labels are not required, pair-specific fine-tuning can be used for any unseen image pairs and this has been demonstrated to improve the registration accuracy of deep registration methods [14, 18].

2.6 Implementation Details

Our method was implemented using Keras with a Tensorflow backend on a 12 GB Titan V GPU. We used an Adam optimizer with a batch size of 1. Our networks were (inter-patient) pretrained for 50,000 iterations with a learning rate of 10^{-4} and then were (intra-patient) trained for another 14,000 iterations (100 epochs) with a learning rate of 10^{-5}. We trained four networks for four MRI sequences (T1, T1CE, T2, and FLAIR) and combined them by averaging their outputs. During inference, for each inferred image pair, we fine-tuned the trained networks for 20 iterations with a learning rate of 10^{-5}. The σ and μ were set as 1.0 and 0.01 to ensure that the $\mathcal{L}_{self}$, $\sigma \mathcal{L}_{reg}$, and $\mu \mathcal{L}_{weak}$ had close values, while the λ and w were optimized based on validation results. Our method achieved the best validation results when $\lambda = 10^{-4}$ and $w = 3.0$.

2.7 Evaluation Metrics

The registration accuracy was evaluated based on manually annotated landmarks in terms of Mean Absolute Error (MAE) and Robustness. MAE is calculated between the landmark coordinates in the pre-operative scan and in the warped follow-up scan, where a lower MAE generally indicates more accurate registration. Robustness is a successful-rate metric in the range of [0, 1], describing the percentage of landmarks improving their MAE after registration. In addition, the smoothness of the displacement field was evaluated by the number of negative Jacobian determinants (NJD). As the ϕ is smooth and invertible at the voxel p where the Jacobian determinant is positive ($|J\phi(p)| > 0$) [19], a lower NJD indicates a smoother displacement field.

Brain Tumor Sequence Registration with Non-iterative Coarse 279

3 Results and Discussion

Our validation results are summarized in Table 1. We trained four networks with four MRI sequences (T1, T1CE, T2, and FLAIR) and report their validation results respectively. Among the four networks, the network using T1CE achieved the best validation results (MAE: 3.486; Robustness: 0.818), followed by the networks using T1 (MAE: 3.917; Robustness: 0.785), FLAIR (MAE: 4.127; Robustness: 0.787), and T2 (MAE: 4.156; Robustness: 0.748). We combined these networks by averaging their outputs, in which we first combined all four networks and then removed the networks with relatively lower validation results one by one, resulting in three network ensembles (T1/T1CE/T2/FLAIR, T1/T1CE/FLAIR, and T1/T1CE). We found that all three ensembles achieved better validation results and produced smoother displacement fields, which suggests that combining different MRI sequences improves brain tumor registration. Combining more MRI sequences consistently improved NJDs as averaging more displacement fields together naturally resulted in a smoother displacement field. However, combining more MRI sequences cannot guarantee better registration accuracy. Among different ensembles, the T1/T1CE ensemble achieved the best validation results (MAE: 3.392; Robustness: 0.827), while further combining T2 and FLAIR networks resulted in lower validation results. In addition, combining the T1/T1CE networks by 0.3/0.7-weighted averaging further improved the performance and achieved our best validation results (MAE: 3.387; Robustness: 0.831). Therefore, we submitted this ensemble to be evaluated on the testing set, which made us place 4th in the final testing phase (Score: 0.3544) [4]. We also attempted to train a single network with multi-channel image pairs (concatenating MRI sequences into multiple channels), but this approach resulted in worse validation results.

Table 1. Validation results of our method using different MRI sequences.

MRI sequence	MAE	Robustness	NJD
T1	3.917	0.785	94.70
T1CE	3.486	0.818	68.65
T2	4.156	0.748	69.70
FLAIR	4.127	0.787	100.00
T1/T1CE/T2/FLAIR	3.445	0.826	**0.30**
T1/T1CE/FLAIR	3.432	0.826	0.65
T1/T1CE	3.392	0.827	2.65
T1/T1CE (weighted by 0.3/0.7)	**3.387**	**0.831**	3.60

Bold: the lowest MAE, the highest Robustness, and the lowest NJD are in bold.

In addition, we performed an ablation study to explore the contributions of dual deep supervision and pair-specific fine-tuning. In the ablation study, all four MRI sequences were used, and the deep weakly-supervised loss $\mathcal{L}_{weak}$ and/or the pair-specific fine-tuning process were excluded. The MAE results of the ablation study are shown in Table 2.

Since pair-specific fine-tuning was not performed on the training set, the corresponding results are missing in Table 2. We found that using both $\mathcal{L}_{self}$ and $\mathcal{L}_{weak}$ (i.e. dual deep supervision) resulted in lower MAE than merely using $\mathcal{L}_{self}$. This is because ground truth information (landmark labels) was leveraged through the $\mathcal{L}_{weak}$, which helped to find the existing correspondences between images and thus relieved the challenges introduced by missing correspondences. However, when $\mathcal{L}_{weak}$ was used, the training MAE (=1.026) became much lower than the validation MAE (=3.521), indicating heavy overfitting. This is attributed to the fact that the provided training set is small (140 pairs) and the landmark labels are sparse (6–20 landmarks per pair). We suggest that a larger, well-labeled (more landmarks) training set will contribute to better registration performance. Also, we found that pair-specific fine-tuning can consistently contribute to lower MAE. This is consistent with existing studies [14, 18] where pair-specific fine-tuning (also named test-specific refinement or instance-specific optimization) was demonstrated to improve the registration accuracy. Pair-specific fine-tuning can improve the network's adaptability to image shape/appearance variations because the network can have chances to adjust the learned weights for each unseen image pair during inference.

Our method has some limitations and we suggest better performance potentially could be obtained by addressing them. Firstly, we omitted affine registration as all MRI scans provided by the challenge organizers have been rigidly registered to the same anatomical template [4]. However, we found that the first-place team adopted additional affine registration and this dramatically improved their registration performance [20]. This suggests that there still exist large linear misalignments between the provided MRI scans, and therefore additional affine registration is required. Secondly, as manually annotated landmarks are expensive to acquire, the provided landmark labels are sparse and thus led to heavy overfitting. For this limitation, automatic landmark detection methods could be considered to produce additional landmark labels. Finally, we adopted NICE-Net to perform four steps of coarse-to-fine registration. However, this step number (four steps) was empirically chosen without full exploration. We suggest that performing more steps of coarse-to-fine registration might result in better registration performance.

Table 2. MAE results of the ablation study on the training and validation sets.

$\mathcal{L}_{self}$	$\mathcal{L}_{weak}$	PSFT	Training set	Validation set
√	×	×	4.375	3.716
√	×	√	/	3.598
√	√	×	**1.026**	3.521
√	√	√	/	**3.445**

Bold: the lowest MAE on each set is in bold. PSFT: pair-specific fine-tuning.

4   Conclusion

We outline a deep learning-based deformable registration method for brain tumor sequence registration in the context of BraTS-Reg 2022. Our method adopts our recently proposed NICE-Net as the backbone to handle the large deformations between pre-operative and follow-up MRI scans. Dual deep supervision, including a deep self-supervised loss based on image similarity and a deep weakly-supervised loss based on manually annotated landmarks, is deeply embedded into the NICE-Net, so as to overcome the missing correspondences between the tumor in the pre-operative scan and the resection cavity in the follow-up scan. In addition, pair-specific fine-tuning is adopted during inference to improve the network's adaptability to testing variations. Our method achieved a competitive result on the BraTS-Reg validation set (MAE: 3.387; Robustness: 0.831) and placed 4th in the final testing phase (Score: 0.3544).

References

1. Haskins, G., Kruger, U., Yan, P.: Deep learning in medical image registration: a survey. Mach. Vis. Appl. **31**(1–2), 1–18 (2020)
2. Meng, M., Liu, S.: High-quality panorama stitching based on asymmetric bidirectional optical flow. In: International Conference on Computational Intelligence and Applications, pp. 118–122 (2020)
3. Meng, M., Bi, L., Fulham, M., Feng, D.D., Kim, J.: Enhancing medical image registration via appearance adjustment networks. Neuroimage **259**, 119444 (2022)
4. Baheti, B., Waldmannstetter, D., Chakrabarty, S., Akbari, H., et al.: The brain tumor sequence registration challenge: Establishing correspondence between pre-operative and follow-up mri scans of diffuse glioma patients. arXiv preprint, arXiv:2112.06979 (2021)
5. Kwon, D., Niethammer, M., Akbari, H., Bilello, M., Davatzikos, C., Pohl, K.M.: PORTR: pre-operative and post-recurrence brain tumor registration. IEEE Trans. Med. Imaging **33**(3), 651–667 (2013)
6. Sotiras, A., Davatzikos, C., Paragios, N.: Deformable medical image registration: a survey. IEEE Trans. Med. Imaging **32**(7), 1153–1190 (2013)
7. Xiao, H., et al.: A review of deep learning-based three-dimensional medical image registration methods. Quant. Imaging Med. Surg. **11**(12), 4895–4916 (2021)
8. Zhao, S., Dong, Y., Chang, E.I., Xu, Y., et al.: Recursive cascaded networks for unsupervised medical image registration. In: IEEE International Conference on Computer Vision, pp. 10600–10610 (2019)
9. Mok, T.C., Chung, A.C.: Large deformation diffeomorphic image registration with laplacian pyramid networks. In: International Conference on Medical Image Computing and Computer-Assisted Intervention, pp. 211–221. Springer, Cham (2020). https://doi.org/10.1007/978-3-030-59716-0_21
10. Shu, Y., Wang, H., Xiao, B., Bi, X., Li, W.: Medical image registration based on uncoupled learning and accumulative enhancement. In: International Conference on Medical Image Computing and Computer-Assisted Intervention, pp. 3–13. Springer, Cham (2021). https://doi.org/10.1007/978-3-030-87202-1_1
11. Kang, M., Hu, X., Huang, W., Scott, M.R., Reyes, M.: Dual-stream pyramid registration network. Med. Image Anal. **78**, 102374 (2022)
12. Lv, J., et al.: Joint progressive and coarse-to-fine registration of brain MRI via deformation field integration and non-rigid feature fusion. IEEE Trans. Med. Imaging **41**(10), 2788–2802 (2022)

13. Meng, M., Bi, L., Feng, D., Kim, J.: Non-iterative coarse-to-fine registration based on single-pass deep cumulative learning. In: International Conference on Medical Image Computing and Computer-Assisted Intervention, pp. 88–97. Springer, Cham (2022). https://doi.org/10.1007/978-3-031-16446-0_9

14. Balakrishnan, G., Zhao, A., Sabuncu, M.R., Guttag, J., Dalca, A.V.: Voxelmorph: a learning framework for deformable medical image registration. IEEE Trans. Med. Imaging **38**(8), 1788–1800 (2019)

15. Dalca, A.V., Balakrishnan, G., Guttag, J., Sabuncu, M.R.: Unsupervised learning of probabilistic diffeomorphic registration for images and surfaces. Med. Image Anal. **57**, 226–236 (2019)

16. Avants, B.B., Epstein, C.L., Grossman, M., Gee, J.C.: Symmetric diffeomorphic image registration with cross-correlation: evaluating automated labeling of elderly and neurodegenerative brain. Med. Image Anal. **12**(1), 26–41 (2008)

17. Kuang, D., Schmah, T.: Faim–a convnet method for unsupervised 3d medical image registration. In: International Workshop on Machine Learning in Medical Imaging, pp. 646–654. Springer, Cham (2019). https://doi.org/10.1007/978-3-030-32692-0_74

18. Lee, M.C., Oktay, O., Schuh, A., Schaap, M., Glocker, B.: Image-and-spatial transformer networks for structure-guided image registration. In: International Conference on Medical Image Computing and Computer-Assisted Intervention, pp. 337–345. Springer, Cham (2019). https://doi.org/10.1007/978-3-030-32245-8_38

19. Ashburner, J.: A fast diffeomorphic image registration algorithm. Neuroimage **38**(1), 95–113 (2007)

20. Mok, T.C., Chung, A.C.: Robust Image Registration with Absent Correspondences in Preoperative and Follow-up Brain MRI Scans of Diffuse Glioma Patients. arXiv preprint, arXiv:2210.11045 (2022)

Author Index

S. Bakas et al. (Eds.): BrainLes 2022, LNCS 13769, pp. 283–285, 2023.
https://doi.org/10.1007/978-3-031-33842-7

Printed in the United States
by Baker & Taylor Publisher Services